SICK MONEY

SICK MONEY

THE TRUTH ABOUT THE GLOBAL PHARMACEUTICAL INDUSTRY

BILLY KENBER

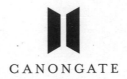

CANONGATE

First published in Great Britain in 2021
by Canongate Books Ltd, 14 High Street, Edinburgh EH1 1TE

canongate.co.uk

1

British Library Cataloguing-in-Publication Data
A catalogue record for this book is available on
request from the British Library

ISBN 978183885 025 8
Export ISBN 978 1 83885 026 5

Typeset in Garamond MT Std by
Palimpsest Book Production Limited, Falkirk, Stirlingshire

Printed and bound in Great Britain by Clays Ltd, Elcograf S.p.A.

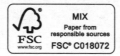

For Sam

Contents

A note to readers   ix

Introduction   1
Prologue – A house near Lake Ontario   7
1. Apothecaries, pills and guns   29
2. AZT – the first AIDS drug   50
3. The hunt for blockbusters   83
4. How to price a drug   103
5. Dirty pharma   127
6. The trick   148
7. The acquisition game   188
8. A one-sided tug of war   211
9. The drugs we get   241
10. Hard science   271
11. Fighting back   293
12. A reckoning   315
Epilogue – Concordia's fall   346

Acknowledgements   358
Notes and references   361
Index   407

A note to readers

When it comes to drug prices, what you see is rarely what you get. Just like a used car lot, the price on display is unlikely to be the price many people pay and some customers can expect much better deals than others.

Drug companies publish list prices for brand-name drugs but beneath this often lies a host of secret trade prices; prices that differ depending on who is buying. Governments mandate certain discounts, health insurers and other players negotiate confidential price reductions and wholesalers and pharmacists all take their cut. These price concessions all affect exactly how much a drug manufacturer actually receives. The system in the US is particularly complex. Here, powerful middlemen known as pharmacy benefit managers (PBMs) have inserted themselves between insurance companies and drugmakers, negotiating an opaque web of rebates that may or may not be passed on to the benefit of consumers. PBMs are supposed to use their bargaining power to drive down prices but the system incentivises companies to charge higher prices in order to offer larger rebates and secure preferred status on the list of drugs covered by a health plan. Rebates received from drugmakers are bundled up across different medicines, ensuring that even the health insurance companies who work with PBMs are often left in the dark about exactly how much they have paid for a specific drug.

If this all sounds a mystifying system, it's not a coincidence – the market has deliberately been forced into this shape. Amid the opacity, huge sums of money grease the selling of medicines around the world.

Because the prices actually received by manufacturers for a drug can vary significantly from contract to contract and are often closely guarded commercial secrets, prices for individual drugs described in this book are generally list prices, and so do not include confidential discounts and rebates negotiated with different parties. Figures for overall spending on pharmaceuticals, however, are for the sums manufacturers actually receive after rebates and discounts are removed at an aggregate level.

For first-in-class treatments, particularly those launched several decades ago, there was generally little pressure for companies to offer significant discounts to published prices. More recently, as we shall see, there can be significant gaps between list and net prices, particularly in the United States in therapeutic areas saturated with similar drugs. Even when health providers have secured sizeable discounts, the list price of a drug is still critically important for many patients. Most US healthcare plans require policyholders to make a contribution based on a percentage of a medication's published price, or to pay the full price of a medicine until they have met a high spending limit known as a deductible. Uninsured patients pay list prices unless a company has made arrangements to offer cheap medicines to those in poverty.

The prices for products sold in the US by Concordia Healthcare, a drug company we will follow in several chapters, are list prices drawn from Elsevier's Gold Standard Drug Database. Concordia did not disclose sufficiently detailed sales information to appear in a dataset maintained by SSR Health, which collects estimated net price data. However, in some cases, court hearings, financial filings and management statements in earnings calls confirm in percentage terms the scale of price rises imposed by the company. More information on the pricing of individual drugs can be found in the reference notes, which should be read in conjunction with the main text.

Finally, currencies are given in British pounds, US and Canadian dollars and Euros as appropriate. For those countries which use other currencies, conversions have been made to reflect currency rates at the time of the transaction or price change described.

Introduction

The first reports to reach the Western public were buried towards the back of newspapers. Terse accounts told of a mysterious pneumonia outbreak afflicting a couple of dozen people in the industrial city of Wuhan, China. It was a New Year curiosity but no real cause for alarm. Then the mysterious virus started to escalate. Hundreds of people coming down with respiratory problems and a fever. Hospital beds filling fast. The death toll rising. Wuhan was closed to outsiders as government officials oversaw the rushed construction of new medical facilities.

The novel coronavirus – named SARS-CoV-2 – was believed to have originated in bats before making the jump to humans. By mid-January 2020 scientists had decoded the virus's genome sequence and published it but they could do little to stop its spread. Soon it was in Europe, fast infecting thousands in the chalets and après-ski bars of the Italian Alps. By late March the world had shut down.

With economies paralysed and healthcare systems at risk of being overwhelmed by the influx of previously healthy patients struck down with the new virus, all eyes turned to science and the hope that treatments could be identified and developed. Above all, over the months that followed, the world held its breath for a vaccine: the only clear route to returning life to its normal axis.

Instrumental to this effort would be the vast $1 trillion global industry dedicated to the discovery, production and sale of medicines. The pandemic vividly illustrated the importance of these companies – from large drugmakers producing billions of vaccine doses to the smaller biotechs who helped develop groundbreaking new vaccine technologies. It was an indication of the debt society owes to the grit and ingenuity of scientists and the machinery that helps translate their efforts into medicines. But it also exposed the industry's flaws and served as a reminder of some of its worst impulses.

The pharmaceutical industry's success in helping to deliver vaccines was largely the result of governments in the US and Europe committing billions in public funding to make up for drug companies' reluctance to invest in areas long considered insufficiently profitable. Meanwhile, the public-spirited actions of some drugmakers, coaxed by university scientists into selling vaccines at cost, served only to highlight the contrast with the rest of the industry's avaricious business-as-usual approach. Even those large drug companies who promised to eschew profits from a vaccine made it clear this would only be while the pandemic raged, reserving the right to make a fortune in future if, as expected, it were to become a seasonal virus.

For others, a global health emergency was as good a time as any to make a killing. The head of one large pharmaceutical company boasted to investors that a coronavirus vaccine generating monthly sales of more than $1 billion would see price rises once the initial crisis was averted. Another drugmaker charged up to $3,000 per patient for an existing drug repurposed as a five-day treatment for Covid-19 that shortened hospital stays but had no impact on mortality rates. Rich countries were allowed to buy up the vast majority of early vaccine stocks while drug companies declined to share manufacturing know-how and intellectual property rights with less well-off nations.

The sense of duty to the common good displayed by a handful of drug companies marked only a brief suspension of the slavish adherence to the best interests of shareholders and the ideology which normally governs decision-making: maximise profits, no matter the cost.

Since the Second World War a succession of pharmacological revolutions have transformed healthcare, dramatically improving life expectancy and saving countless lives. For much of that time, large pharmaceutical companies and the scientists who led them were revered; viewed as both vital engines of economic growth and as corporations with a sense of moral purpose. Underlying this was a simple premise: a social contract where society traded a period of exclusivity guaranteed by patent law as the reward for expensive but worthy research into discovering novel drug therapies, followed by medicines becoming cheap commodities readily prescribed by doctors around the globe. The deal guaranteed healthy compensation for those companies which navigated the long odds of drug development – where nine out of ten drugs fail in clinical trials – and expected, in return, that this would not be exploited by profiteering.

But in recent years, the delicate equilibrium between private profit and public benefit which was once central to the drug industry has shifted. The social contract has broken and the giants of Big Pharma have fallen from their perch as some of the most respected companies in the world to become the comic-book villains of Hollywood films and hit television series.

While the industry hopes that its role in developing Covid-19 vaccines will help to restore its standing, the reputational collapse it suffered happened for good reason. On the other side of the ledger to the innovative products the pharmaceutical industry brings to market sits a lengthy charge sheet: the drugs with minimal clinical benefits; the lawsuits and lobbying; the marketing abuses and bribes paid to doctors; the tricks and tactics used to artificially extend patent lengths and, above all, the often sky-high prices charged for medicines.

In many countries, drug prices have never been higher and have never risen faster. During the 2010s, inflation-adjusted drug prices in the United States rose at a faster rate than in any other decade. Across Europe, patients are being denied drugs that could save their lives because the health systems of some of the richest countries on earth can't afford to meet the prices demanded. In Africa and vast swathes of the subcontinent, billions have become accustomed to having no access to many modern medications.

This drug-pricing crisis is not limited to the newest drugs protected by patents. It afflicts old medicines too, as was conspicuously demonstrated by pyrimethamine, a small white pill the same size and shape as the aspirin or paracetamol tablets found in every bathroom cabinet. The drug, developed by scientists in the 1950s as an antimalarial, is used to treat a parasitic infection which can cause serious health issues for pregnant women and those with compromised immune systems, including patients with AIDS. In 2015, Martin Shkreli, a former hedge-fund manager, drew front-page headlines when he hiked the price of the drug from $17.50 to $750 per pill.[1] Far from shrinking from the sudden scrutiny, Shkreli revelled in the notoriety it brought. Did he regret raising the price? No, he said. If anything, he wished he'd raised it more.

The established players of Big Pharma were quick to distance themselves and denounce Shkreli's behaviour. But whilst his actions – and those of other price-hiking businessmen – were extreme, the reality is they were symptoms of the industry's wider transformation over the preceding decades. These research-free, profiteering companies were the legacy of how detached many drugmakers had become from the science-led forebears who had focused on developing useful treatments and selling them at a reasonable price.

You don't need to discover drugs to get rich from them any more. Access to medicine is a fundamental human right but for many executives pharmaceuticals have become little more than financial assets, to be flipped, dealt, exploited and manipulated in a myriad of creative and profitable ways. For some, this is an opportunistic response to flawed markets and a lack of resistance from health systems and insurers. For others, particularly the large research-driven companies of Big Pharma, it is driven by shifting attitudes in boardrooms, new ideas about how to run a company and price medicines and by the legitimate challenges of translating scientific knowledge into clinically useful products.

The result is a financialised industry where companies appear to have few limits on the lengths to which they will go to wring as much money as possible from life-saving medicines. We live in a world where the previously unthinkable has become a reality. A world where new drugs cost millions for a single patient and old drugs rocket in price by thousands of per cent at the whim of speculators.

A world where a South African drug company is prepared to destroy stocks of a medication for children with cancer rather than continue to sell it at a price it considers too low. A world where a twice-monthly lottery is held by a Swiss pharmaceutical giant with a unique prize: the winners will see their child cured of a genetic disorder and the losers will likely see theirs die tragically young. A world where a young Canadian woman dies without access to a breakthrough therapy because the American manufacturer doesn't want to jeopardise future sales. A world where patients have become pawns in the efforts of drug companies to gouge ever-higher prices from insurers and health systems.

This transformation is not simply a tale of greed and naked capitalism. It is a tale, too, of unintended consequences. Of efforts in the key US market to help a few gravely ill children who had been all but abandoned by medical science and of revolutions in drug discovery which failed to deliver on their promise. Of hesitant drug executives persuaded to follow their rivals in setting ever-higher prices and of billion-dollar acquisitions to fill the vacuum left by emptying laboratories. Of, as one industry observer puts it, the 'ugly situation where health systems are horrified by the price of new drugs, where industry profit margins are really high, but where R&D is so expensive that many investors think it is losing them money'.[2]

We stand at the beginning of an era in which new approaches to treating and curing sickness, from using the body's own immune system to fight diseases, to gene editing and lab-made antibodies, hold untold promise. And yet, without radical change, health systems will struggle to afford these therapies and offer them to all who need them.

To understand what has happened we first need to look backwards: to trace how, unnoticed, the original social contract was chipped away by the MBA-wielding lawyers and hedge-fund bosses who took over from scientists as the kings of pharma. We will meet the people who, sometimes unwittingly, prompted huge changes in the way the pharmaceutical industry approaches the sale of medicines. And we will encounter those small but dedicated groups of activists, doctors, patients and businessmen and women leading the fight back. Among them, the middle-class American housewives smuggling insulin across the border to post life-saving vials to strangers and the communities of hepatitis C patients brought together by the internet to secure cut-price versions of $1,000 pills from the generic drug factories of India.

But before that it's time to meet an entrepreneur whose story illustrates just how far the pharmaceutical industry has moved from its founding principles over the past four decades or so. We join him in early 2013 as he sets out to get rich.

PROLOGUE

A house near Lake Ontario

The gold rush was in full swing and Mark Thompson wanted a piece of the action.

It was early in 2013, the middle of a brutally cold winter in the affluent Canadian city of Oakville, and ice was forming on the edges of Lake Ontario. In the front room of a low-slung townhouse close by, Thompson, a stocky forty-five-year-old former lawyer, was busy making plans. He had spent long enough watching others make their fortunes in the pharmaceutical industry; it was time to make his.

Thompson believed he had spotted an opportunity that others had missed. The industry is broadly split into two types of company. On one side are the research-led businesses who spend billions trying to develop new treatments. On the other are the generic manufacturers making cheap copies of the drugs discovered by research-led firms once they are no longer protected by a patent. Generic medicines manufacturing is often a numbers game, with fierce competition meaning margins are low and profits come from selling pills costing a few pennies or cents in huge numbers.

Thompson wasn't interested in paying researchers to hunch over microscopes and Petri dishes, hoping that, somehow, at some point years down the line, they would make a discovery that might prove clinically useful and commercially viable. Nor did he have much appetite for the costly business of building a factory and trying to squeeze out a profit within the cut-throat market for common generic drugs. He saw a third way: a new kind of drug company which could enjoy the windfalls of Big Pharma without the high research costs and overheads. 'The two biggest risks in the pharma business are R [for research] in R&D – trying to find new molecules – and launching new products, trying to change doctors' minds,' he would later say.[1] 'We don't do either of those things.'

It was old drugs that interested him or, as he preferred to call them, 'mature, cash-producing assets'.[2] These were not the common generic pills used by hundreds of millions of people but drugs which had fallen from favour, still taken by a small number of patients but largely forgotten by the wider world. For Thompson, these ageing products could, with a bit of care and attention, allow him to fulfil the dreams of so many entrepreneurs, paving the way to a life of fast cars, luxury homes and Caribbean jaunts.

But by the time spring began to thaw the ice on the lake, Thompson was still struggling to get the business started. He spent hours poring through a list of pharmaceutical assets produced by Torreya Partners, a Manhattan investment bank specialising in healthcare. It listed hundreds of different drugs which had been put up for sale – from opportunities to invest in the development of experimental new treatments to licences for long-established products. Companies were typically open to selling off these older assets because the revenue streams – though still amounting to millions of dollars a year for each medicine – were tiny compared with their bestselling drugs. Thompson had hired a young executive at Torreya to help him. However, with little more than a phone number and a company name, Concordia Healthcare, Thompson was struggling to persuade an established drugmaker to sell him the right product at the right price.

He was after drugs with some very specific characteristics. It didn't matter to him what kind of ailment or disease they treated – unlike other specialist drug companies, he didn't plan to limit himself to one or two therapeutic areas. But it was important doctors were already familiar with the medicines so there was no need to invest in a large sales team, and that there was reason to believe others wouldn't enter the market any time soon. Newly discovered drugs are protected from competition by patents but the drugs he was after would likely be too old to have much patent life, if any, left. Instead, they needed to have other characteristics which kept competition at bay. Above all, the drugs had to have a loyal group of patients who had taken the product for years and would continue to do so, ensuring they would provide a steady cash stream. His plan was to use a tax-efficient structure similar to one used by his previous employer, Biovail, and buy the assets through a Barbados-based subsidiary, thereby paying far lower taxes than would be due in the US or Canada. The low Caribbean tax rate, and low-cost financing later available to fund the acquisitions, would allow him to outbid others for the rights to drugs and still generate strong cash flow. Perhaps he could also find ways to increase revenues from the drugs too. A former colleague summed it up as: 'Buy drugs, use cheap financing and throw off a ton of cash. That was Mark's idea.'

Finally, he thought he had found the assets he was after. Shionogi, the US subsidiary of a long-established Japanese pharmaceutical company, was selling the rights to three drugs: a head-lice treatment with the brand name Ulesfia, an anti-inflammatory called Orapred, and Kapvay, which was used as a treatment for children with ADHD. Kapvay was the most valuable, bringing in revenues of $4 million a month, but its patent was due to expire in the autumn, meaning generic manufacturers would soon be free to sell cheaper versions. Orapred was also likely to face competition the following year. Ulesfia, on the other hand, was patent-protected for more than a decade and, as a topical lotion, was much harder for generic companies to secure regulatory approval for than orally-administered pills. Thompson expected it to kick out $2 or $3 million a month for years to come.[3]

Benj Garrett, the young Torreya executive hired by Thompson, was on hand to help him land the deal. All that was left was for Thompson to get the funds together to meet Shionogi's asking price. In early May 2013 he had been able to raise $6 million from business associates buying shares in the company. Investment banks and private equity firms offered another $24 million in loans with interest rates of up to 18 per cent, reflecting the high-risk nature of a fledgling start-up. He would need rapid growth if he was to pay off the debt, but he'd got enough together to buy the three drugs. The deal was done for $27.9 million, with a maximum of $6 million more due if sales of Kapvay hit certain targets.

The deal was tiny, of no significance to the wider pharmaceutical industry or to those taking or paying for the medicines involved. So it is little surprise that no one took much notice of what happened next. Several weeks after acquiring the drugs, Thompson increased the price of all three medicines. By the start of 2014, Kapvay's price had risen by more than 50 per cent, while Ulesfia was up by 43 per cent and Orapred had undergone a more modest 10 per cent price rise. The market didn't care, the company would say in subsequent filings, with no 'adverse prescription volume effect' reported.[4]

Concordia Healthcare, the business Thompson would later boast of having 'started from scratch in my living room', was up and running.[5]

Thompson had never expected to end up in the pharmaceutical industry. He spent his twenties at university, studying for under-graduate and master's degrees in political science at York University in Toronto, before becoming a law student at the University of Ottawa. He qualified as a lawyer in 1998 and spent two years ploughing through paperwork as an associate at a Canadian law firm, working on commercial transactions, real estate and corporate finance, before taking a job in business development at IMAX Corporation, the giant cinema screen company. It was while at IMAX in early 2001 that he was approached by a headhunter recruiting for a fast-growing pharmaceutical company called Biovail. 'I knew nothing about the industry at this point. I didn't know anything about Biovail either,' Thompson later said. But he had young children and wasn't enjoying the heavy travel required by his IMAX role so he decided to take the plunge.[6]

Biovail was in the midst of an expansion. It had been founded by Eugene Melnyk, a college dropout turned self-made billionaire who was born in Canada but had moved to Barbados. Melnyk, whose father died when he was a teenager, grew up at the racetracks around Toronto and made his first fortune from a medical publishing company he started in his twenties. He sold off that interest in 1989 to focus on manufacturing pharmaceuticals. The company, which took on the name Biovail in 1994, specialised in finding ways to tweak existing off-patent drugs into a 'sustained release' version that need only be taken once or twice a day, instead of three or four times. Sometimes the improved version would be licensed back to the company which originally discovered it and sold under a brand name. On other occasions, the tweak gave Melnyk's company a head-start of a few years over rival generic manufacturers who would have to find their own way to match the more patient-friendly format. At the time Thompson was approached, Biovail was broadening its operations into buying the rights to branded drugs and selling them through a newly hired sales team in the United States.

Thompson started work as a junior in-house lawyer in May 2001 and began learning the ropes, working initially on corporate financing and contracts for new acquisitions. After a few years, by now well-acquainted with the products Biovail was buying, his boss asked him to move out of the legal division and into a new business acquisitions role, tasked with finding assets – individual drugs or whole companies – for Biovail to purchase. The company was growing fast, although there were rumblings of problems in the works when the company missed its earning estimates in 2003 and blamed an accident involving a truck shipping its anti-depressant – an excuse which didn't hold up to scrutiny.

By late 2004, having only worked in business development for a matter of months, Thompson decided it was time to leave. He wanted to do his own thing, 'to start my own business and work for myself,' he later said.[7] The former lawyer left in early 2005, joining three former Biovail colleagues in a new venture called Legacy Pharma. Like Concordia a decade later, Legacy focused on buying the rights to well-established, off-patent medications used by a group of loyal patients who would likely need the drugs for the rest of their lives – generating a reliable income stream for investors in the process.

The company lined up four-decades-old drugs and attempted to raise money to pay for them by selling shares in an initial public offering (IPO) in the summer of 2005, seeking CAD$150 million. It intended to boost revenues by increasing the price of the drugs soon after acquiring them, but the figures mooted were relatively modest: between 10 and 20 per cent.[8]

However, Legacy Pharma would quickly prove an embarrassing failure. The planned IPO was abandoned in September 2005 amid scepticism that investors would put funds into 'a drug manufacturer that didn't yet own the rights to produce any drugs'.[9] The firm had agreed to buy the brand names for several drugs from a Croatian company but the deal was pulled, costing Legacy $5 million.[10] Undaunted, Thompson and his former colleagues tried again, renaming the company Tribute Pharmaceuticals. This time, they were able to partner with a New York private equity firm, Fortress Investments, which provided a war chest. But persuading companies to sell or license the rights to existing drugs proved a slow grind and when Thompson left the company two years later, it still hadn't managed to acquire any drugs.[11]

While Thompson was trying, and ultimately failing, to get his own company off the ground, the disquiet at Biovail continued. Regulators in the United States and in Canada were investigating possible accounting fraud and Melnyk, whose profile had risen dramatically after he bought the Ottawa Senators, an NHL ice hockey team, in 2003, was locked in an increasingly bitter fight for control of the business. Thompson went back to work with the Biovail founder who, after a corporate dispute, broke with his old company and spent CAD$100 million setting up a new one: Trimel Pharmaceuticals. The business was established by Melnyk, a long-time Biovail executive called Bruce Brydon, and Thompson, whose role was to find the technologies the company hoped to use to improve existing drugs with expired patents, in much the same way Biovail had once used 'sustained release' technology.

Trimel went on to sign deals for several inventions including a special bioadhesive gel which stuck to the inside of the nose and allowed a drug to be delivered over a longer period of time. The company put it to use as a testosterone treatment for men and also funded trials which explored whether a testosterone patch would give women better orgasms. Trimel talked up the results it claimed to be seeing in clinical trials and in 2011 performed a reverse takeover – a method of going public in which a company takes over an existing but inactive 'shell company' and secures a stock market listing far faster than can be achieved through an IPO. However, it was still yet to bring anything to market and Thompson, who saw himself as 'basically the guy who did everything and went and sourced the products', had had enough.[12] He left the company and took a job at a small Canadian investment bank, but soon decided the work wasn't for him.

In December 2012, Thompson filed papers with the Ontario Business Corporation setting up a new corporate entity. At the same time he opened a subsidiary in Barbados: Concordia Pharmaceuticals Inc. International companies based in Barbados pay taxes of around 1 or 2 per cent depending on the size of their profits, and a treaty with Canada then allows the money to be passed on to the parent company with no further tax charges.

He was aided soon after the launch by several former Biovail colleagues, among them Wayne Kreppner, who would become president and chief operating officer, and an accountant called John McCleery. The Shionogi drugs, boosted by price increases, brought in steady profits of $2 million a month.[13] Ulesfia, the head-lice treatment, was promoted on social media and patients were offered a coupon which limited the out-of-pocket cost for those with insurance to $10. Kapvay only had a short window of exclusivity but the company was making the most of it, with price rises taken by Shionogi and Concordia increasing the cost per pill of the medicine from around $2 to more than $4 in the space of two years.[14] The drugs earned back the price Concordia paid for them within twelve months of the acquisition.[15]

More deals followed. Kapvay was due to see its patent expire in

October 2013 and Torreya learnt that a generic manufacturer, Par Pharmaceuticals, was poised to launch a cheaper version. With Torreya's help, Concordia agreed a deal with Par to supply the drug and receive half of the rival company's profits. In exchange, Concordia agreed not to launch its own generic version for at least five years, thereby avoiding competition which could drive the price down.[16]

There were opportunities everywhere. In October, Concordia bought a mail order company which made cold calls to try and sell supplies for diabetic patients including medicines, specially designed shoes and back braces. It was up for sale on the orders of the US government over allegations the previous owners had illegally paid kickbacks for customer referrals and had submitted false claims to federal healthcare programmes.[17] A month after that $15 million deal came the $58 million purchase of a small biotech company which sold a laser-activated drug used to treat two rare cancers.

By late 2013, Concordia was ready to go public, using a reverse takeover in the same way Trimel Pharmaceuticals had floated a couple of years earlier. The subsequent share offering was a success, raising nearly CAD$35 million, and Concordia was tipped in the financial press as a stock to watch in the year ahead.

In filings accompanying the public offering, Concordia's strategy was laid out in more detail. The company explained that its business model focused 'on acquiring legacy pharmaceutical products that either enjoy market exclusivity through technical, manufacturing or economic barriers to competition, or otherwise maintain . . . predictable prescription demand'.[18]

Concordia boasted of a 'post-acquisition value enhancement program . . . [to] improve the financial performance of acquired drugs'. In short, it would improve earnings by imposing price increases and integrating acquisitions into the company's 'tax-efficient structure'. The report highlighted the benefits of these products having 'minimal competitive threats' from generics or other products and, crucially, their 'financial stability with upside potential' because of the 'pricing inelasticity'. Translated from corporate speak, this meant the products had a reliable patient base which would keep taking the drugs regardless of price changes. They also planned to cut deals for 'authorised generics' to preserve revenue when patent-protected drugs lost that protection.

Public companies must also disclose known risks to investors, a wide-ranging list of everything that might go wrong from competitive threats to personnel issues and macroeconomic changes. Among those listed in Concordia's annual report in 2013 were several relating to the price of drugs. Whilst it expected to retain its status as the sole supplier of several drugs because of 'economic barriers to competition', increased sales revenue might drive interest from generic companies looking to launch competing versions.

The report also noted its reliance on governments and private health insurers being willing to pay for its products in an environment in which 'third-party payers increasingly challenge the pricing of pharmaceutical products'.[19] In other words, every time the company pushed a price higher, it risked drawing unwanted attention from insurers, pharmacy benefit managers and government-run healthcare programmes. But for now, Concordia was unstoppable and Thompson and his board's thirst for more deals to grow the size of the company showed no signs of abating.

Donnatal had first been sold by A.H. Robins Company, Inc. in the 1930s. Originally made from a combination of extracts from deadly nightshade plants and the sedative anticonvulsant drug phenobarbital and used to treat irritable bowel syndrome (IBS), during the 1970s and 1980s it was one of America's bestselling medicines. Over the ensuing years, sales fell as it was overtaken by more modern alternatives and by 2002 the marketing rights ended up in the hands of Paul Manning, the multi-millionaire founder of a baby-formula company in Virginia. The existing manufacturer, Wyeth, had planned to stop making the drug because of low sales, but Manning bought the rights, outsourced manufacturing and hired two employees to look after it, creating a steady income for his company, PBM Pharmaceuticals, of a little more than $1 million a year.[20]

The drug, sold in both liquid and tablet form, was so old it pre-
dated a requirement for drugmakers to demonstrate that new
medicines were not simply safe for patients but were actually effective treatments. As a result, there was a risk that the Food and Drug
Administration (FDA), the US agency responsible for regulating
medicines, could intervene any day. A clinical trial demonstrating the
drug's efficacy had been completed decades earlier but the FDA had
never reviewed the evidence.

Despite its age, thousands of patients a year still took the drug.
Among them was Lori Kessell, who, like several members of her
family, suffered from stomach problems. A hysterectomy when she
was thirty-eight left her with scar tissue which worsened over time
and an operation to remove her gallbladder a couple of years later
also contributed to her abdominal pain. 'It got progressively worse
as I got older,' she says.[21] By her late forties over-the-counter
medicines were no longer cutting it and she sought help from a
doctor.

The former tile-fitter, who lives in the small town of North
Brunswick, just off the New Jersey turnpike, spent years trying several
different medicines before finding Donnatal. 'It's been a really good
pill for me, an incredibly good pill for me,' she says. Without treatment, she would be doubled over with severe abdominal pain caused
by spasms in her colon.

'It could last for hours like that,' she says. 'I know if I take that
pill [Donnatal] within five minutes that pill will work, it's amazing.
That pill was a godsend. It's something I really feel I can't live
without.'[22]

In 2011, a year after Manning sold his baby-formula business for
$800 million, he hired Kevin Combs, a drug industry veteran, to
oversee Donnatal and search for other assets to build the business
up. Combs was just a few months into the job when, out of the
blue, the FDA said they were taking another look at Donnatal. He
duly dusted off clinical trial data dating back to the early 1980s and
paid a consultancy firm to run a fresh analysis of the results, expecting
that the FDA would finally be asking the manufacturer to prove that

the drug actually worked. The FDA's communications led to several rival companies withdrawing from the market but the anticipated hearing to assess Donnatal's efficacy never happened. Instead, the clear-out left PBM as the drug's sole manufacturer.

The study Combs had commissioned revealed evidence of how effective Donnatal was compared with other IBS treatments, creating an opportunity, he believed, to increase the drug's low price. He hired pricing consultants who spent months studying the market before recommending a range of possible prices. After much deliberation, Combs priced it at just over half the cost of newer patent-protected IBS drugs.

In 2011, a bottle of Donnatal pills had a list price of around $43, but by May 2014 this had risen to $393.[23] With a new marketing campaign and a sales force hired to promote the drug, revenues rose from $2 million a year before the FDA's intervention to nearly $50 million in 2013.[24] PBM Pharmaceuticals was rebranded as Revive Pharmaceuticals in a nod to the drug's rejuvenation.

In January 2014 Combs went to the J.P. Morgan Healthcare Conference, a huge annual gathering of pharmaceutical industry executives held at the St Francis Hotel in San Francisco. With a $200 million line of credit, he was on the hunt for drugs to add to the company's portfolio. But after spending the five-day event exchanging company information sheets, he returned to Virginia to discover that five companies wanted to buy Donnatal. When the bids came back, there was a clear winner. Concordia had blown away the competition with a bid more than double the value of the second-highest. For $200 million in cash and shares in Concordia worth $65 million, Donnatal was theirs.

Combs was due to work with Concordia for four months as the product was transferred and so a few weeks after completing the deal, Thompson and three colleagues, including Kreppner, the chief operations officer, and Dan Peisert, a business development executive, flew down to Virginia. During a meeting at Revive's office in Charlottesville, Combs said Peisert told him that Concordia planned to raise the price to two or three times its current level. '[He] basically told me I'm stupid, I could have made so much more money off of this,' Combs says.

Combs was incredulous. 'You've just bought a Ferrari and you're gonna just drive the thing right off a cliff in your first week,' he told the visiting executives.[25] Peisert strongly denies Combs's account of the conversation. Despite the significant price increase under PBM, Concordia doubled the price – taking the list price of a bottle to nearly $800. Another price rise followed the next year.[26] The company didn't appear to be too worried about ruffling feathers in the pursuit of maximising profits; what they were doing was perfectly legal and any ethical concerns didn't seem to matter in the face of the millions that could be made.

'What Concordia did after they acquired it was ridiculous,' Combs says. 'It took me a while to understand that they didn't care about building a company. They thought, "You might get to $200 million in three years [by better promoting the drug], we're gonna get the $200 million in six months".

'The whole model for them was to acquire assets, raise the price and flip the company for as much money as they could,' he says.[27] He wasn't the only one who would regret his boss's decision to sell Donnatal to Concordia. One spring morning, Kessell discovered that her local pharmacist wouldn't fulfil her latest prescription because the dramatic price rise meant they would lose money in doing so. Her health insurer hadn't increased how much it would reimburse the pharmacy and the difference amounted to hundreds of dollars. They wanted her to accept a different medication instead. 'I kind of lost my mind,' Kessell recalls. 'You can't imagine being doubled over in pain because of your health problems when a simple little pill could just take care of that problem.' The issue got ironed out and she was able to collect her bottle of Donnatal pills, but from then on she was worried her insurer could decide to stop covering it at any moment. Kessell began to hoard the pills, taking them only when the pain became unbearable.

Several years later, in October 2019, her fears would come to pass when she dropped off a prescription and was told it had been denied by her insurer. Donnatal was no longer covered – it was simply too expensive.

Back in Canada, Thompson was in no mood to slow down. In an earnings call with analysts in late March 2014, he was ebullient. He'd just announced the Donnatal deal and the Shionogi assets had, he said, 'performed extremely well for us,' leaving him 'really, really happy with the way that worked out.' He promised that more deals were on the way.

'We have some good-sized transactions we're looking at, and we're going to steer away from the smaller guys from now on,' Thompson said.[28]

By now, the company had a clear playbook and it soon found another asset that would fit the bill – a niche product with a stable and loyal patient base which produced a steady cash flow and allowed them to increase the price. In September, Concordia was ready to announce the deal, again brokered by Torreya Partners.

Zonegran, the brand name for an anti-epileptic drug called zonisamide, had been discovered by scientists in the 1970s and initially used to treat psychiatric diseases. It was first commercialised as a treatment to help prevent seizures in adults by Dainippon Pharmaceutical in Japan in 1989. By the time it came on Concordia's radar in 2014, the rights to sell the drug in the US had been passed around. Dainippon initially struck a deal to license Zonegran to the Irish drugmaker Elan Pharmaceuticals at the time of its US launch in 2000. In 2004, the rights were sold to an American subsidiary of the Japanese firm Eisai. Both companies had subsequently been rapped for promoting the drug on an 'off-label' basis – for indications such as migraines, eating disorders and weight loss for which it didn't have regulatory approval. Elan entered a guilty plea and paid more than $200 million in a settlement reached in 2010, while Eisai agreed to pay $11 million to settle charges that it had continued the illicit behaviour.[29]

The drug's patent had expired in 2005 and, as a result, there were at least nine cheaper competing generic versions available for

American patients. However, it was still attractive to Concordia because doctors are often reluctant to move patients with epilepsy to a version of the drug from a different manufacturer once their seizures are under control. As a result, Zonegran had been able to maintain a small but profitable share of the market.

With Torreya advising, Concordia used a new loan to pay Eisai $90 million to buy the rights to sell the drug in the US and Puerto Rico. Eisai would continue to manufacture the drug on Concordia's behalf, but the Canadian company was now in charge of pricing and marketing the medication. Sales of the drug had been sliding for several years but it still generated around $30 million a year in revenue. After Concordia acquired it the list price increased by nearly half, from $650 per bottle of pills to $935, with comments from Thompson to analysts suggesting the company pocketed around half of this price rise after paying rebates to ensure the drug was covered by insurers.[30]

By September, the company's share price had increased by 350 per cent and early investors were jubilant. Hedge fund managers particularly loved the tax structure, which meant Concordia could overpay for assets when competing with companies paying full US tax and still make a killing. James Hodgins, chief investment officer at the Toronto fund Curvature Hedge Strategies, predicted a lustrous future. 'There's a lot of value to be split between the buyer and the seller,' he told a Canadian newspaper. 'It's effectively an arbitrage. Repeat until rich.'[31]

The low tax rate also meant the business might make a tempting target for acquisition by a large American drugmaker looking to cut their own tax bills through a tax inversion. By merging with the smaller firm, the larger business could relocate its headquarters from the United States to a country with a much lower rate of corporate tax. In November 2015, the pharmaceutical giant Pfizer announced plans to merge with an Irish drug company, Allergan, in a $160 billion deal which would have dramatically reduced its exposure to US taxes.[32]

Concordia's growth was extraordinary for a company which had been founded less than eighteen months earlier. It had taken advantage of a strong market and cheap debt to make ever-bigger acquisitions at a rapid pace. But it also benefited from the slipstream created by a much larger rival: Valeant.

The drug company Thompson had previously worked at, Biovail, had merged with an American firm, Valeant, in 2010. The deal allowed Valeant to become a Canadian company and enjoy the tax-efficient structure set up under Melnyk's ownership. With Mike Pearson, a hard-drinking, no-nonsense former management consultant, at the helm, Valeant embarked on an enormous acquisition spree against which Concordia's own efforts paled in comparison. Valeant bought dozens of drug companies and stripped down overheads to keep costs as low as possible.

Whatever Pearson was doing seemed to be working. Shortly after he took over, Valeant's stock traded for less than eight dollars. By the autumn of 2012 it had topped $120 and was hurtling up the list of Canada's largest companies with little sign of slowing. Bill Ackman's Pershing Square and Jeffrey Ubben's ValueAct Capital, two prominent hedge funds, were among those backing the company.

When investors looked at Concordia, they saw a smaller, earlier version of Valeant. Several dubbed it 'Baby Valeant' or the 'Poor Man's Valeant'. Like Concordia, Valeant had a growth-by-acquisition strategy, a low-tax structure and a willingness to implement significant price rises. Pearson was a bigger, louder, brasher version of Thompson and, while Valeant soared, Concordia's chief executive didn't shy away from comparisons between the two companies. 'We're an M&A [mergers and acquisitions] driven company, very similar to Valeant,' Thompson told the Canadian business news channel BNN Bloomberg in March 2015. 'It's ironic because Valeant when Mike Pearson took over, the company was [in] a very similar position to what we are now. He's done a very good job in terms of acquisitions.'[33]

For the time being, whenever Concordia was seeking fresh financing from banks or investors, there was an easy story to tell about the company's business model and where it might end up. For those who'd arrived too late to get on board Valeant's rocketship, here was a second bite at the cherry. 'Valeant, at one point, was the

most valuable company on the Toronto Stock Exchange, worth more
than the Canadian banks,' said Niall McGee, a reporter at the *Globe
and Mail* who covered Thompson's company. 'Concordia really benefited from that momentum.'[34]

Concordia's shareholders were well on their way to significant
riches, but the company still hadn't landed a deal on the scale needed
to reach the next level. It was becoming an increasingly competitive
landscape for acquiring pharmaceutical assets, with more than $100
billion in deals done in the first quarter of 2015.[35] Thompson was
tired of doing deals in the tens of millions, or at best low hundreds.
In late 2014, the financing had been lined up ready for the next
acquisition and it was waiting to be spent.

Thompson, whose goal for 2015 was to double the size of the
company, looked at dozens of potential transactions.[36] Torreya tried
to interest him in a company called Arbor Pharmaceuticals, but he
felt the asking price was too high. Then, during the annual J.P. Morgan
Healthcare Conference in San Francisco, Dan Peisert, Concordia's
VP of business development, went for a coffee with executives from
Covis. The companies had been in touch the previous year about
the possible sale of a single asset. Now Covis was offering something
much more juicy: a package of the US rights to twelve brand-name
drugs, along with several authorised generics (unbranded generic
versions of the company's own branded drugs).

Covis had been set up in Switzerland in 2011 by the private equity
firm Cerberus Capital Management. The drugs it was selling had been
acquired from Big Pharma companies including GlaxoSmithKline,
Sanofi-Aventis and AstraZeneca, with these firms often continuing to
make the products for Covis to sell. Sensing a potentially game-
changing deal, Peisert called Thompson, who was also in town for the
conference, and urged him to 'sit down with these guys'.[37] Thompson
quickly arranged a meeting. Ten days later, Concordia sent a term sheet
to Covis outlining their offer.

Internally, not everyone at Concordia was convinced by the deal,
dubbed 'Project Phoenix'. Valeant had looked at the Covis assets but
baulked at the asking price. Paperwork subsequently filed by

Concordia revealed that Covis had spent just over $230 million acquiring the twelve branded drugs; now the assets, along with five authorised generic versions and the licence to a small Australian drug, had an asking price of $1.2 billion.

Also concerning was how much more room there might be left to, in the industry lingo, 'take price'. Under Cerberus's ownership, the Covis products had already enjoyed rapid revenue growth driven by price increases. Six drugs had at least trebled in price under Covis's watch and there were already signs that the number of prescriptions were falling.[38]

Thompson, however, had made his mind up and RBC Capital Markets, which stood to make significant fees from a commercial loan which helped to fund the deal, also advised him to go for it. With the board's agreement, the deal was announced in mid-March. To fund the purchase, Concordia issued eight-year bonds with a 7 per cent yield worth $735 million, raised around $275 million from a share offering and secured a $700 million credit facility from a group of Canadian banks.[39]

After acquiring the drugs, Concordia sold on three products with low sales and increased prices on others. One Covis drug, Dutoprol, had a price of $16 for thirty pills when the private-equity-backed fund bought it from AstraZeneca in February 2014. It had reached $82 when Concordia acquired it and Thompson's company promptly doubled that. As a result it topped a list of the industry's 'biggest price gougers' produced later that year, with the invoice price for US pharmacies rising by more than 900 per cent in the space of twelve months.[40] Another newly acquired drug, the blood-pressure medicine Dibenzyline, had seen a ten-fold price increase in the space of a year in the run-up to Concordia's acquisition. Undeterred, under the new ownership two price rises took the drug from $88 a pill to $240.[41] At that price, a year's supply for one patient would cost hundreds of thousands of dollars.

Concordia told analysts that 'they have not experienced payor push back to the company's aggressive price increases.'[42] However, price rises were hitting prescription volumes, as a research firm called

Pacific Square Research (PSR) discovered when it later dug into the data. When Concordia increased the price of the heart drug Lanoxin after buying the asset from Covis revenue quickly rose from around $55,000 a week to more than $200,000. But sales fell back to $140,000 within months as the number of prescriptions dropped in response to the price hike, PSR found.[43]

The Covis deal really put Concordia on the map. That summer, the company listed on the Nasdaq Stock Exchange, with Thompson and other executives travelling to New York to ring the opening bell. Television footage captured him grinning as he and a huddle of drab-suited executives applauded the market opening. The mid-August listing gave them better access to financing from US institutions and some of the bigger players were now on hand to offer funds and advice. Goldman Sachs, the investment bank once memorably described by *Rolling Stone* magazine as a 'giant vampire squid wrapped around the face of humanity, relentlessly jamming its blood funnel into anything that smells like money', had come on board and began to exert some influence.[44] The bank recruited Ed Borkowski, a fifteen-year industry veteran who had previously been chief financial officer at the generics company Mylan. Borkowski, who was brought in to try and add some more experience to the fast-growing operation, joined the board in June 2015.

With a growing market cap came growing attention. In the same month that Concordia became a US listed company it announced it had reached a settlement with the US Federal Trade Commission over the deal it had struck with Par Pharmaceuticals to divide up the spoils of a generic version of Kapvay, the ADHD treatment which was one of the original three drugs acquired in 2013.

Although Concordia had described it as a supply agreement, the FTC claimed it was in reality an illegal deal not to compete in the market for generic versions of Kapvay. The FTC said that Concordia had agreed not to launch its own authorised generic for five years. Instead, it received between one-third and one-half of Par's profits.[45] Concordia didn't launch an authorised generic until December 2014, after learning of the FTC's investigation. In a settlement agreed with the consumer regulator, Concordia was banned from reaching deals with other companies to delay or block the entry of an authorised generic and was not allowed to enforce its agreement with Par, including the profit-sharing deal.

The settlement was little more than an inconvenience as Concordia continued its ascent. Investors noticed that Thompson had begun to change the way he dressed. He grew his hair and swept it back over his head, giving him a well-groomed grey mane to go with his tightly kept goatee. His suits became sharper and he stopped wearing a tie, instead accessorising his open-collar shirts with colourful pocket handkerchiefs.

His new appearance, with, as one acquaintance who noticed the change put it, a 'good watch, good shoes, all those kind of things', raised eyebrows among investors in Canada who were used to working with staid corporate types. But Thompson was out to enjoy the rewards of his success. He'd bought a new family home in August 2014, splashing out $3 million on a huge six-bedroom house with a swimming pool on a quiet, tree-lined street in Oakville. In 2015 his pay package jumped to nearly $9 million, including a $2 million performance bonus and $4 million in shares, as well as additional stock options.[46]

In January 2015, Concordia took out a huge $3,000-a-night suite at a luxury hotel at the top of Nob Hill in San Francisco for the J.P. Morgan Healthcare Conference. David Maris, the analyst who had blown apart Biovail's truck accident excuse for lacklustre earnings in 2003 by obtaining evidence it had been almost empty, was shocked by the extravagance when he was invited for a meeting. 'Here's a company that's trying to be like, "We're going to save the [health] system money,"' he says. 'When you're a mid-sized or small company and you're that lavish it's always a red flag.'[47]

Thompson and other senior executives were rarely at the company's Canadian headquarters as they flew around the world in search of more deals. A month before the Covis deal was announced, the company had treated itself to a new toy. Concordia signed a five-year lease for a $30 million private jet, a French-made Dassault Falcon

2000. The jet was a thing of beauty. Its spacious cabin, with wood panelling and plush leather seats, had room for ten passengers and the aircraft was capable of flying non-stop from London to New York at up to 550 miles per hour.

During the summer of 2015, the Falcon 2000 made regular trips across the Atlantic to Luton airport, north of London. Another major deal was brewing; one which, if they could pull it off, would launch Concordia into a new stratosphere. Having previously spoken of his determination to focus on North America where he felt he knew the market, Thompson was now ready to go global.

The company had alighted on a British pharmaceutical company as its route there. Amdipharm Mercury, or AMCo, had been created only a few years earlier by the London private equity fund Cinven. It had amassed nearly 200 off-patent drugs which were sold in 100 countries, although a significant majority of the sales were in the UK.[48] Private equity houses like to get in, try and improve a business and then, after just a few years, make an exit. Cinven was no different. It had first considered selling AMCo in February 2015, with Reuters reporting that it hoped to get as much as $2.6 billion for the business.

However Concordia, with its rocket-fuelled rise, was under pressure from shareholders hungry for more growth and had to keep making acquisitions. Worse still, there were few other companies available with this sort of portfolio of products in the United Kingdom and other overseas markets.

'There just weren't that many companies like AMCo that either had been available or were perceived to be available any time soon,' one former executive says. 'There were several other bidders in there as well so that kind of pushed the price up.'

An analyst covering the company highlighted the predicament. 'Once you get onto this treadmill of making acquisitions on a regular basis, you can't stop because then people lose interest and they sell your stock,' he says. 'Everyone's looking for where's the next transaction?'

As a result, Concordia, with the urging of bankers from Goldman Sachs, agreed to pay a hefty premium for the business. When the deal was clinched, it was worth an eye-watering $3.5 billion, almost $1 billion more than the sale price floated earlier that year. Cinven had earned several times the sum it had invested in assembling AMCo and also received shares in Concordia. The Cinven partner behind the deal, Supraj Rajagopalan, hailed AMCo as 'one of the most successful deals we've ever done'[49] The price tag meant Concordia would be highly leveraged with debts of over $3 billion – at least six times the enlarged company's expected earnings – but it would more than double the size of the company.

Less than three years after he had first registered the company, Thompson had seemingly struck gold. His stocks in Concordia were worth nearly $200 million.[50] He drove an orange Lamborghini Aventador worth $400,000 and had a Porsche Cayenne in the garage, as well as motorbikes, snowmobiles, off-road vehicles and a pick-up truck.

At the same time, patients like Lori Kessell were rationing their medication, fearful on each trip to fill her prescription that the increased price of Donnatal might mean her insurer no longer covered it, but on Wall Street and Bay Street – the Canadian equivalent – investors loved the company. The drug industry had become a financial playground, and Thompson was playing the game perfectly, turning Concordia into one of the hottest stocks in Canada.

The initial reaction of the market to the news of the AMCo deal was positive, with shares in Concordia rising in early trading to $89.10, a new record which gave the company a valuation of more than $3.9 billion.[51] Anyone investing when it first went public in December 2013 now held shares worth more than fourteen times what they had paid for them.

Soon, however, doubts began to creep in. As well as taking on a lot of debt, Concordia needed to raise at least half a billion dollars from an equity issue to pay for the deal. In a break from the more traditional approach of Canadian companies, it planned to find the money in a sale to US financial institutions, something that would take weeks. But trouble was brewing for the pharmaceutical industry.

The sale launched two weeks later, on September 21, 2015. Concordia could barely have picked a worse time. That morning, hours into the sale, Hillary Clinton posted a Twitter message responding to a story on the front page of that morning's *New York Times* which had revealed the news that Martin Shkreli had increased the price of an old, off-patent drug, Daraprim, by more than 4,000 per cent overnight.[52]

Clinton, at the time the heavy favourite to become the next US president, posted a comment alongside a link to the article: 'Price gouging like this in the specialty drug market is outrageous. Tomorrow I'll lay out a plan to take it on. -H.'[53]

Within seconds, the arrows next to biopharma stocks began to turn red. A sell-off had begun, and suddenly Concordia's future was deeply uncertain.

CHAPTER ONE

Apothecaries, pills and guns

It began with a stroke of fortune. An absent-minded Scottish scientist neglected to close the window in his London laboratory as he left for a month's holiday in his country home. When he returned from Suffolk, Alexander Fleming was greeted with a collection of Petri dishes discarded from a previous experiment and waiting to be disinfected for reuse. That summer in 1928 he had been studying *Staphylococcus aureus*, a common bacteria which, undisturbed for several weeks, had spread across the shallow glass plates. One plate, however, was different. Here a blue-green mould had developed and at its edges the bacteria had disappeared. The substance responsible, which Fleming called 'mould juice', was a rare strain of the mould *penicillium* – he had discovered one of the world's first antibiotics.

Fleming wrote up his findings for publication in a medical journal but he gave up on the substance he'd extracted from the mould, penicillin, after a year, unable to isolate the unstable compound and concluding that it was likely to be too toxic for clinical use anyway.[1] His discovery therefore remained undeveloped for another decade. In the meantime, the research director at German chemical company Bayer, Gerhard Domagk, had identified that a red dye, which was given the name Prontosil, cured infections caused by the bacterium streptococcus. French scientists subsequently identified the reason it was effective: a chemical in the sulphonamide group which became the basis of sulpha drugs made by dozens of pharmaceutical companies. Domagk's breakthrough in 1932 was the most significant discovery since his compatriot Paul Ehrlich's 1909 discovery of Salvarsan, a treatment for syphilis, and it reopened the hunt for what Ehrlich had termed 'magic bullets': chemicals which could target and kill microorganisms without harming the host.

In 1938, the biochemist Ernst Chain, a German Jewish emigré who had been recruited to work at the Sir William Dunn School of Pathology in Oxford, decided to join that search for compounds with antibacterial properties. He read Fleming's earlier paper on penicillin and suggested to his supervisor, the Australian-born Howard Florey, that they try to isolate the active substance from the mould juice Fleming had captured.[2] They were eventually able to extract and semi-purify penicillin as a brown powder. By the spring of 1940, as war raged in Europe, it was ready to be tested on animals. Following the same procedure Domagk had used to test Prontosil, several mice were infected with a virulent bacteria and half were then injected with penicillin. The next morning, the mice that had received penicillin were still alive while the others were dead.[3]

Buoyed by the success of the experiment, the scientists turned their Oxford laboratory into a factory, rigging up a complicated system of baths, toilet cisterns and milk churns to produce enough penicillin for human testing.[4] The first patient treated was Albert Alexander, a forty-three-year-old policeman with a face wound which had become badly infected.[5] After being injected with penicillin he began to improve within hours but Florey and Chain's supply of the drug was very small, so small in fact that they took to extracting penicillin from his urine and re-using it. After several days, they ran out of penicillin and had to stop the treatment. The policeman died a month later.[6]

Their lab couldn't scale up production any further so it was clear that Chain and Florey needed help. The British drug industry was itself relatively small and it was struggling with wartime demands to begin manufacturing medications which had previously been the exclusive domain of German pharmaceutical companies. With little prospect of assistance from domestic firms, Florey and a colleague called Norman Heatley travelled to the United States with hopes of securing the help of American drugmakers. On July 9, 1941, they were in Washington DC visiting the US Department of Agriculture where they expected to meet a senior administrator responsible for four research laboratories. The man they sought was away on a trip, however, and in his place, serving as Acting Assistant Chief of the Bureau of Agricultural and Industrial Chemistry, was Percy Wells. As luck would have it, Wells had spent the last decade specialising in mould fermentation and so when he heard Florey explain his predicament he knew exactly where to turn. That afternoon he sent a telegram to his former colleagues who had just been relocated to the Northern Regional Research Laboratory (NRRL) in Peoria, Illinois.[7] The reply came back the same day: 'Suggest they visit Peoria for discussions. Laboratory in position to cooperate immediately', the missive concluded.[8]

Florey and Heatley visited a few days later and the team in Peoria were soon put to work trying to improve the yield. The NRRL scientists rapidly made some important breakthroughs. One member of the team, Andrew Moyer, who had years of experience in growing moulds, switched out the brewer's yeast used by the British researchers for large quantities of corn steep liquor, a change which resulted in a thirty-fold increase in production. Government scientists also experimented with switching from growing surface cultures to using deep-tank fermentation, which proved far more effective.[9]

These advances helped to persuade American manufacturers to join efforts to make the antibiotic on a mass scale. Alfred Richards, an American pharmacology professor who had been tasked with overseeing medical and scientific projects with the potential to bolster the war effort, initially struggled to convince drug companies to help. They were sceptical of their ability to produce the quantity of penicillin required for medical testing and of the risks investment would represent. Richards' requests were twice rejected. It was only at the third time of asking, at a meeting held less than a fortnight after the Pearl Harbor attacks had brought the United States into the war, that the mood changed. Drug executives were presented with a report showing the impact the corn steep medium had made on increasing the yield. This led George Merck, the president of Merck & Co., to make the decisive move. He pledged his company's support, saying that, 'if these results could be confirmed in their laboratories it was possible to produce the kilo of material for Florey, and industry would do it!'[10]

Merck was joined by three other drug companies – Pfizer, Lederle and E.R. Squibb – in taking up the task. They struck agreements to share information and successes but scaling up production proved tough going. Six months after that December 1941 meeting, Merck had only produced enough to treat eleven patients.[11] Fortunately, government scientists once again came through with a critical discovery. In 1942, the Peoria team launched a search for different strains of penicillium mould in the hope that they might be able to locate one which would prove more productive than that captured by Fleming. With the help of the US military, strains were obtained from soil collected all over the world but it was one drawn from a mouldy cantaloupe melon bought in 1943 at a local market in the Illinois town where the research laboratory was based which proved to be the best.[12] It could produce as much as 100 times more penicillin than Fleming's strain, and X-rays and UV rays were used to increase its productivity further still.[13]

By the spring of 1944, boosted by government funding, tax breaks and Pfizer's experience with deep-tank fermentation, twenty-one factories were at work, among them a converted ice plant in Brooklyn which housed fourteen vast 7,500 gallon tanks.[14] Posters on the walls of fermentation plants declared penicillin 'the new life-saving drug' which 'Saves Soldiers' Lives!' Workers were urged on with the words: 'Men who might have died will live . . . if YOU give this job everything you've got!'[15] When D-Day arrived in June 1944, penicillin was in sufficient supply to save thousands of soldiers' lives during the Normandy landings and subsequent Battle for France. By the end of the war, drug companies were producing millions of sterile packages each month, enough for it to be released for civilian use.[16]

* * *

Penicillin was hailed as the first 'wonder drug' and the successful drive to produce it on a mass scale would help to launch the modern pharmaceutical industry. For much of the preceding century, medicine had been the preserve of apothecaries and quack doctors who hawked nostrums to the unsuspecting public. These were little more than folk remedies, mixtures of herbs, alcohol, opium and cocaine packaged up and sold with evocative names and elaborate promises. Among the most popular were a 'cure-all' brandy-based concoction sold in Britain as Dr Samuel Solomon's Cordial Balm of Gilead and Lydia E. Pinkman's Vegetable Compound available in the United States as a 'women's tonic'.[17] Another American treatment, Kopp's Baby's Friend, was a mixture of sugar, water and the powerful painkiller morphine, which was sold as a means of calming infants into the early part of the twentieth century.[18]

Those selling the ointments and powders were under no obligation to disclose what was inside; in fact this was typically a closely held trade secret, and nor was there any requirement to demonstrate that they were safe to consume or could deliver the promised benefits. By the start of the twentieth century, pressure to regulate the sale of nostrums, which, somewhat misleadingly, were known as patent medicines even though they didn't rely on patents and often had few medicinal qualities, led to legislation on both sides of the Atlantic. In the United States, the 1906 Pure Food and Drugs Act and subsequent amendments banned medicines from being labelled with false claims, although it would take another thirty years before regulators were able to ban dangerous ingredients.

As so-called patent medicines gradually began to fall out of favour, a new type of drug company was on the rise selling 'ethical drugs' with products rooted in science. During the nineteenth century, advances in organic chemistry had enabled the isolation of specific active substances extracted from plants which could be purified and used as medications. These early drugs were typically compounded by pharmacists for patients as they waited in their shop but some began to see the potential of making these products on a larger scale. Among the first was Heinrich Emanuel Merck, the descendant of generations of apothecaries in the German town of Darmstadt. The expanding business he oversaw began selling morphine commercially in 1827 and by the close of the century had expanded to the United States, where pharmacists were also beginning to move into manufacturing on a larger scale.

Pfizer can trace its roots back to 1848 when it was founded by two German immigrants who opened a small chemical plant in Brooklyn. A few years later, Edward Robinson Squibb, a former naval doctor, opened a similar business nearby. Both flourished during the American Civil War from 1861 to 1865 when there was great demand for painkillers and other treatments including morphine, iodine and chloroform. In the years that followed several of the other modern pharmaceutical giants were established. Parke-Davis was founded in Detroit in 1866, a year after the war had finished. Eli Lilly, a chemist who had served as a colonel on the Union side, opened a manufacturing facility in Indianapolis in 1876 and began producing the antimalarial quinine. Abbott Laboratories began making alkaloids near Chicago in 1888, a couple of years after Upjohn had started producing drugs in Kalamazoo, Michigan.

In the same period, dye manufacturers in Germany and Switzerland were experimenting with the possible medicinal benefits of their products. These companies were some of the first to employ chemists, among them Felix Hoffmann, who in 1897, while working for the German dyemaker Bayer, then F. Bayer & Co., managed to synthesise pure acetylsalicylic acid.[19] The new drug removed the stomach irritation which plagued users of salicylic acid, the most commonly available pain reliever sold by rivals. It was given the trade name aspirin and would remain one of the most widely used medications in the world more than a century later. Another of the bestselling medicines of the period was Salvarsan, the syphilis treatment discovered by Ehrlich when experimenting with chemical dyes, but most medicines were simple, purified versions of naturally-occurring substances. The discovery of new drugs remained rare. In part, this was because of the industry's relationship with scientists and the medical establishment's deep-seated mistrust of commercial motives. The idea of these early pharmaceutical companies carrying out scientific research was met with great scepticism if not outright horror. The intrusion of commerce into the world of science was seen as an affront to the unbridled pursuit of truth and knowledge to serve the public good.

The British Medical Research Council, the American Pharmacological Association and the French Académie Impériale de Médecine all opposed cooperation between scientists and the drug industry in the early twentieth century, and this mindset extended to the use of patents.[20] It was believed that scientists should not seek to prevent the flow of information and ideas by patenting something which could have medical uses. Medical researchers would frequently refuse to cooperate with clinical trials 'merely because the products to be tested were patented' and it wasn't until 1950 that the British Medical Association dropped this opposition.[21] German companies, however, took a different view.[22] After developing a stable and pure form of acetylsalicylic acid in 1897, F. Bayer & Co. rushed to patent aspirin wherever possible. The company received a patent in the United States and was initially successful in Britain, too, although it was overturned a few years later after a court ruled it had previously been synthesised.

When the First World War broke out in 1914, German companies were the global leaders in the fledgling pharmaceutical industry, but the conflict forced firms in Britain, France and America to catch up. The American government passed a law which confiscated patent rights from German firms and awarded them to domestic companies. The conflict engulfing Europe meant many of the German-made chemicals needed to make important drugs were in short supply and, with necessity the mother of invention, governments tasked pharmaceutical companies with finding alternative means of creating these medicines. Burroughs Wellcome, the British firm with the most advanced scientific capabilities, came up with a substitute for the German drug Salvarsan within a year and also made versions of aspirin and a treatment for typhoid.[23]

Something similar would happen during the Second World War

two decades later when companies were once again forced to compensate for lost supply routes. That conflict also created demand for
treatments for exotic diseases which had previously been of no
significant concern to Western armed forces. The business historian
Thomas Corley has described how Japanese advances removed British
access to the bark needed to make quinine, forcing drug companies
to develop alternative antimalarials.[24] Later in the war, a vaccine
against mite-borne typhus was developed within six months to aid
soldiers sent to fight campaigns in the Far East.

In the immediate aftermath of the First World War Britain passed
a law prohibiting patents on a chemical substance and restricting
drugmakers to patents on a specific method of manufacturing. This
codified the medical establishment's philosophical opposition to
patenting but it was also a pragmatic move designed to help British
chemical manufacturers who had fallen behind their German counterparts and saw an opportunity to make and sell compounds
discovered by foreign rivals.[25]

In the interwar years, large drug companies invested in substantial
facilities dedicated to carrying out research which might lead to new
products. Parke-Davis, which had led the way by building the first
American pharmaceutical research laboratory in 1902, expanded the
facility, while Merck opened its large New Jersey laboratory in 1933
and Eli Lilly staff began working at the Lilly Research Laboratories
a year later. Others, however, remained unsophisticated manufacturers
with little scientific expertise and forays into developing their own
products could end in disaster amid the fast-and-loose regulatory
regime of the time. In 1937, a Tennessee manufacturer, S.E.
Massengill, decided to make a sulfa drug more palatable for children
by selling it as a syrup, adding a chemical called dietyhlene glycol to
give it a sweet almond flavour. The chosen chemical was in fact a
deadly poison normally used in antifreeze and the concoction killed
more than a hundred people before it was taken off the market.[26]
Legislation passed the following year required American manufacturers to demonstrate that their products were safe, placing a new
emphasis on scientific rigour which extended to how drugs were

marketed. The 1938 Food, Drug and Cosmetic Act handed control over the sale of some powerful drugs to doctors by requiring a prescription, encouraging drugmakers to switch their marketing focus from patients to doctors.

By the end of the Second World War, pharmaceutical companies in Europe and America were well positioned to embrace the tremendous commercial opportunities now opening up. Penicillin had revealed the incredible possibilities of pharmaceutical intervention, raising the possibility of harnessing microbiology to cure diseases. After Selman Waksman, a chemist at Rutgers University in America, laid out a method for discovering new antibiotics, companies implanted large-scale screening programmes and identified more than two dozen new ones during the 1950s.[27] Meanwhile, peace and prosperity would create vast potential markets. In Britain, a rebuilding government established the National Health Service, which would pay for medicines for millions of people, while the Finance Act 1944 had created incentives for investing in research by allowing it to be offset for tax purposes.[28]

It was in the post-war years that the modern drug industry took shape. German manufacturers had been dominant for the first half of the century but the US government's support for penicillin production helped to turn American companies into powerhouses. Penicillin, sold by dozens of companies, became the bestselling drug of the era and the US quickly became the world's pharmacy. By the end of the 1940s, American firms were making half of the world's drugs.[29]

This dominance of German and then American companies had been boosted by their willingness to seek patents for pharmaceutical and manufacturing advances, and by an expansion in what they were able to patent. In Britain, however, the lingering resistance to patenting products with therapeutic uses came to a head during the Oxford team's development of penicillin.

There had been no question of Fleming seeking a patent for penicillin since at that time patents weren't granted for naturally occurring substances. The work of the Oxford team, however, raised the possibility of pursuing legal protection for the processes involved in producing the drug. The headstrong biochemist Ernst Chain was a strong proponent, arguing it would bring in valuable revenue for the laboratory and prevent others seeking one at a later date.[30] But the idea provoked strong opposition from establishment figures including from Sir Edward Mellanby, the secretary of the Medical Research Council, whom Florey had consulted on the dilemma and whose intervention proved decisive. Mellanby did not believe research-minded scientists should seek patents.[31] It was still thought unbecoming, if not unethical, to pursue such a nakedly commercial move, particularly when penicillin came from a naturally occurring substance and was a life-saving medicine.

On the other side of the Atlantic there were no such reservations and the US Department of Agriculture would obtain patent protection for key parts of the process of producing penicillin. Moyer, the microbiologist who had made the crucial intervention of using the corn steep medium was, as a government employee, prohibited from obtaining a US patent for his invention but was later able to obtain the foreign rights. Several American firms obtained patents of their own on different parts of the processes they had come up with for manufacturing penicillin at scale.

In the aftermath of the conflict, British authorities concluded that the failure to patent Florey and Chain's work had been a significant error of judgement. Although the US government patents were licensed out without charge, British firms were now forced to pay royalties to American manufacturers for the rights to use their techniques for growing the mould through deep-vat fermentation. The authorities vowed it would not happen again, setting up the National Research Development Corporation (NRDC) shortly after the war to help academics patent their discoveries.[32] The country's 1919 patent law was revised a year later, allowing patents on drugs themselves rather than only on a manufacturing process.

Thus, the golden age of drug discovery that was beginning would be led by companies propelled, in the wake of two devastating world wars, by a powerful drive to contribute to building a better future for humankind. Pharmaceutical companies were imbued with a strong sense of social purpose which shaped their entire approach to the business of discovering and selling medicines. It was best summed up in a famous speech by George W. Merck, Merck & Co.'s president and chairman and a member of its founding family, delivered at a medical college in Virginia in December 1950. Inventing a transformative new drug, Merck told his audience, was not enough.

'We cannot step aside and say that we have achieved our goal by inventing a new drug or a new way by which to treat presently incurable diseases', he said. It was only when 'the way has been found, with our help, to bring our finest achievement to everyone' that the job had been done. 'We try to remember that medicine is for the people. It is not for the profits', he explained. 'The profits follow, and if we have remembered that, they have never failed to appear.'[33]

Other drug companies were driven by similar sentiments. A few years earlier, Robert Wood Johnson had penned a company credo for Johnson & Johnson, where he was chairman. Like Merck & Co., known outside the US as Merck Sharp & Dohme (MSD), it placed a sense of public duty at the core of its obligations, believing that if they followed that goal the need for profit would look after itself.[34]

'We believe our first responsibility is to the patients, doctors and nurses, to mothers and fathers and all others who use our products and services', the credo read. 'We must constantly strive to provide value, reduce our costs and maintain reasonable prices.' The interests of shareholders were mentioned last, falling behind patients, employees and 'the communities in which we live and work' in the pecking order. 'When we operate according to these principles, the stockholders should receive a fair return', Johnson concluded.[35]

This mantra fed into a hesitation to exploit intellectual property rights, even as companies won important victories on what could be patented. In 1946, MSD began selling streptomycin, which had been discovered in Waksman's laboratory at Rutgers. Streptomycin had been obtained from a naturally occurring microbe found in soil and products of nature were not patentable.[36] However, MSD argued to the US Patent Office that the process of turning the substance extracted from soil into something which could be administered to patients was sufficiently transformative as to mean that streptomycin was not simply something from nature but a new substance in its own right. The argument succeeded and the patent was granted in 1948. MSD, however, was unable to enjoy the spoils of this success. Waksman, concerned at the criticism that might follow if MSD was the only supplier of the drug – particularly if it used this situation to charge high prices – persuaded the company to give up its exclusive rights.[37] Instead MSD's patent was assigned to a public trust set up by Rutgers University and licensed out to eight manufacturers.[38] A few years later, when a pioneering American virologist developed a vaccine for the debilitating and highly contagious disease polio, he decided not to seek a patent. The vaccine belonged to 'the people', Jonas Salk told the American newsman Edward R. Murrow in a 1955 television interview. 'There is no patent,' he said. 'Could you patent the sun?'[39]

Without exclusivity rights, drugmakers were thrown into competition with one another, which required huge investments in advertising and sales efforts as well as having a pronounced effect on prices. With large numbers of companies making penicillin, there was strong price competition and post-war advances in production efficiency were also passed on to consumers. As a result, the cost of penicillin fell dramatically after the war, from $3,955 per pound in 1945 to $282 in 1950.[40] The same thing happened with streptomycin, which dropped from $16 per gram in 1946 to 7 cents per gram a decade later.[41]

The problem for the industry, as the economist Peter Temin has written, was that the size of royalties which had become the norm were very low: MSD, for example, was paid just 2.5 per cent of sales by other manufacturers of the antibiotic it had discovered, streptomycin.[42] Gradually, the commercial rewards that could be reaped if a manufacturer could retain the rights to a drug and enjoy all of the sales revenue for itself became irresistible. Some of the next antibiotics discovered – among them Lederle Laboratories' Aureomycin (chlortetracycline), Parke-Davis's Chloromycetin (chloramphenicol) and Pfizer's Terramycin (oxytetracycline) – were successfully patented and production was more tightly controlled. The patent holders changed tack, either selling the drugs on an exclusive basis or allowing no more than two or three other manufacturers to produce them. This resulted in much higher prices than those for streptomycin or penicillin.[43] By 1956, seventeen antibiotics were sold on an exclusive basis by a single manufacturer, up from just four eight years earlier.[44] The same thing happened with other classes of drugs. While the first generation of steroids had been patented and widely licensed, the next discoveries, launched in the late 1950s, were sold on an exclusive basis.[45]

As drug companies increasingly focused on their own exclusive products, research operations became ever more important. During the 1950s, led by American companies, the amount spent by the pharmaceutical industry globally on research and development doubled as a proportion of sales, from 4 to 8 per cent.[46] British companies raced to catch up, with leading companies Burroughs Wellcome, May & Baker and Imperial Chemical Industries (ICI) all building sizeable new research institutes in the 1950s.[47] Drug companies became fully integrated businesses, bringing in-house each part of the chain from the lab to the factory to the packaging, marketing and eventual sale of the product.

These changes would uncork an extraordinary burst of innovation and the 1950s and 60s were the golden years of drug discovery; but as the industry began to discover its huge profit-making potential, the first problems were also beginning to emerge. By the end of the 1950s, high drug prices and windfall profits were already a subject of public complaint. A report by the Joint Economic Committee in the United States concluded that 'medical care is becoming wonderfully effective and appallingly expensive'.[48] The Federal Trade Commission accused several drug companies of colluding on the prices of some broad-spectrum antibiotics including Pfizer's tetracycline. Apparently tired of the effects of true competition on prices, the small number of companies making each drug had agreed not to compete, meaning prices had remained unchanged for a decade.[49]

The companies' behaviour captured the interest of a powerful Democratic senator, Estes Kefauver, who had held a series of hearings on monopolies and competition in a number of important industries including automobiles and steel. Now he turned his attention to pharmaceuticals. The ensuing hearings focused on four types of drug and centred on the question that would underpin the public's relationship with the pharmaceutical industry: were companies making excessive returns and, in doing so, keeping important medicines out of reach of the less well off? After a year and a half of hearings, Kefauver concluded that they were and produced draft legislation which sought to restrict the size of profits that could be made. Alongside changes to marketing and requirements for the FDA to review a drug's efficacy before approving it, he focused on reducing the period of time in which companies held exclusive rights over a product. The bill proposed that drugmakers might obtain a compulsory licence allowing them to sell a rival's drug after it had been on the market for three years. He also called for a more restrictive approach to granting patents, requiring modified drugs to show they had a 'significantly greater' therapeutic effect compared with the original.[50]

Similar concerns were troubling the authorities in Britain. During the First World War, recognising the critical need for medicines, the British government gave itself legal powers to override patent rights in circumstances where it saw fit to do so. The changes also permitted other companies to apply for a compulsory licence, allowing them to use another company's intellectual property without its permission in exchange for a fee if it could show a monopoly position was being abused. When passing a new Patent Act in 1949, much to the anguish of the pharmaceutical industry, the British government kept these provisions in.[51]

It did this because of the potential for a drug company to abuse the monopoly position created by holding a patent, but there was also recognition that, by providing this reward, drug companies were incentivised to invest in new discoveries. This balance was formally established by the first effort to indirectly control drug prices in Britain, a voluntary scheme introduced in 1957. The scheme, which continues to this day in a somewhat altered form, gave companies freedom to price new drugs however they wished for several years after their launch.[52] After that, profits were pegged to a reasonable return on investment. The idea was to limit companies' ability to grow their profits from older innovations and incentivise them to develop a regular pipeline of new discoveries.[53]

In 1961, Enoch Powell, then the minister of health, announced that the health service would begin importing tetracycline – still a patent-protected drug – and other antibiotics from overseas because of concerns over their high prices. These imported drugs were cheaper because they were sold in countries which did not recognise or grant pharmaceutical patents. Powell's actions were based on invoking the provision in British law which allowed patents to be overridden for 'Crown use' – in this case supplying drugs to British hospitals. The decision prompted a furious reaction but Pfizer lost a legal fight when the House of Lords ruled that the ministry was within its rights.[54]

While Britain took action to impose some controls on the cost of drugs, Kefauver's proposals in the United States failed to gain political traction. In fact, they would likely have been abandoned altogether were it not for a tragedy which was starting to emerge.

Chemie Grünenthal had been founded by Hermann Wirtz, a former Nazi official, in Germany's industrial heartland in 1946. The company developed a sedative called thalidomide in the 1950s and, as was common practice at the time, licensed the drug to other manufacturers. During testing on animals, scientists had been unable to find a dose high enough to kill a rat and as a result the drug was marketed as 'completely safe'. By the end of the decade, it was being sold in nearly fifty countries for a wide range of uses to treat everything from sleeping problems to morning sickness. Unfortunately, what hadn't emerged during testing were the devastating consequences the drug had when taken by pregnant women. Thalidomide was able to penetrate the placenta and reach the foetus, causing severe birth defects. As many as 10,000 would be born with missing or shortened limbs, with half surviving for only a matter of months. The toll could easily have been higher. In the US, 207 pregnant women were given the drug as part of a 20,000-patient trial intended to promote use of the product, but more widespread damage was avoided because a young medical officer at the FDA took issue with the clinical trial evidence presented as proof of the drug's safety and refused to approve it. Frances Kelsey would later receive a medal for service to humanity from President John F. Kennedy for her actions.

The thalidomide scandal led to changes in the clinical testing required to bring a drug to market. In the wake of the tragedy, some of Kefauver's recommendations were revived, although not those relating to patent rights and pricing. The Kefauver–Harris Drug Amendments of 1962 required manufacturers to demonstrate that their products were effective as well as safe before they could be sold. Regulators would now need to be persuaded that drugs offered the therapeutic benefits they claimed to through animal testing and carefully controlled trials in humans. The effects of this were pronounced; when previously launched drugs were subjected to this new level of scrutiny, 600 medicines were branded 'ineffective' and forced off the market within a decade.[55]

It also handed the FDA control over pharmaceutical advertising and required companies to list generic names alongside brand names, emphasising the interchangeability of drugs produced by different manufacturers. In Britain, before the thalidomide scandal drug companies had been 'under no legal obligation to demonstrate the safety or efficacy of their products before marketing them'.[56] A voluntary system of checks on a drug's toxicity data was introduced in the immediate aftermath and was followed by the Medicines Act of 1968, which brought in a licensing system regulating clinical trials, manufacturing and the sale of medicines, including a requirement for drugs to be tested in animals before being given to humans.

These changes in the UK and US were echoed in other major markets and served to significantly increase the hurdles manufacturers needed to clear if they were to bring a product to market. The speed at which discoveries could move from the lab to the pharmacy was slowed, and with that came a reduction in the length of time a product might enjoy the benefits of patent protection in the market-place. Aspirin had gone on sale just months after it was successfully synthesised, but new drugs in the 1960s and 70s would take years to pass through animal and human testing.

The expansion in testing requirements did not, however, change the path by which many new drugs emerged and the respective roles played by publicly funded bodies and commercial scientists. Basic research and key discoveries typically came in academic labs before industry became involved in turning these into something clinically useful. This symbiotic relationship suited drug companies, who were unwilling to fund the pursuit of basic research which might have little direct use and be unsuitable for patenting, as well as govern-ments, which lacked the expertise and the appetite for risking funds on the scale required for large clinical trials and commercial drug development.

The post-war spirit of technological advance saw significant public funds committed to grants for scientists and new research institutes. In the US, a national research institute had been created in 1930 with a brief to carry out 'study, investigation and research in the funda-mental problems of the diseases of man'.[57] After the Second World War, it was reorganised and expanded as the National Institutes of Health, with a budget which expanded twenty-five-fold in a decade and grant-making powers to fund the work of academic and non-profit researchers across the country.[58]

Burgeoning scientific knowledge was crucial to the waves of new drugs which followed and in 1980 a new piece of legislation made it easier for companies to profit from government-funded research. The Bayh–Dole Act meant publicly funded discoveries need no longer remain in the public domain with the rights held by govern-ment. Instead, it allowed academic researchers who had received

federal grants to retain the patent rights to their discoveries and to
license them to drugmakers on an exclusive basis, paving the way
for a generation of scientists to make an entrepreneurial leap into
the commercial sector. In return, the government was granted march-
in rights, meaning it could award licences to other companies in
order to meet public health needs or if a patent wasn't being used.

Legislators would make another significant intervention in the US
pharmaceutical market four years later. After the Second World War,
as many companies began to invest in large research facilities, others
stuck to manufacturing existing drugs.[59] Gradually, this split produced
two distinct industries: large research-led companies concentrated on
developing new drugs while generic manufacturers would sell copycat
versions of off-patent drugs at low prices, with limited research efforts
of their own. While new medicines were given brand names dreamed
up by in-house marketing departments, generics were typically sold
under a shortened version of their chemical names.

Large drug companies bitterly resented the incursions of generic
manufacturers, castigating them as pirates and parasites who made
a fortune from the fruits of their labour. In America, a campaign
was waged to highlight the supposed dangers of generic pills, which
were presented as being of poor quality and dubious origins. The
research-led industry set up the National Pharmaceutical Council,
a body which campaigned against generic substitution and stressed
the importance of sticking with what were portrayed as trustworthy
and reliable brand-name products. The campaign was successful
enough to encourage most US states to pass laws in the 1950s
which prevented pharmacists from dispensing a cheaper copy of
a drug if a patient had a prescription listing a specific brand.[60] Over
time, however, the tide turned. During the Kefauver hearings,
generic drugs were heralded as a means of producing cheaper drugs
for consumers. The publicity generated by the hearings was seen
by some companies as creating a market for generics. McKesson
& Robbins, a large wholesaler which hadn't manufactured drugs
for several decades, announced in 1961 that it would launch a new
generics division to take advantage.[61]

The demand for cheaper generics was growing but their manu-facturers were hindered by the arduous process of securing regulatory approval. It was only in 1984, with the passage of legislation known as the Hatch–Waxman Act, that the US generics industry was given a streamlined application process with a reward for being the first generic to apply. It had previously taken three years after a patent expired for competing versions to hit the market.[62] Now, generic companies could apply in advance and be ready to go on day one. To placate the research-led drug companies, the act allowed drugmakers up to five additional years of patent exclusivity to compensate for delays in receiving regulatory approval.

By the early 1980s, the industry's business model was fully formed. So too was what is, in essence, a social contract between private enterprise and the public for the pursuit and provision of medicines. Public money would fund the basic research with industry then taking up the baton to convert this into practical uses. The compounds that resulted would need to demonstrate their safety and efficacy to regulators before going on sale with a period of exclusivity, usually protected by patents, during which no other companies could make or sell the same drug. This monopoly period gave companies an opportunity to earn a return to compensate for the risk and resources involved in developing a drug. Governments generally gave companies freedom to decide their pricing at this point, retaining some checks and balances to use in case of emergency but trusting the industry to determine a reasonable return on investment, and a reasonable price for their product. When patents ended after what would become by the early 1990s a globally standardised period of twenty years from application, market forces would take over with generics given a straightforward path to regulatory approval which meant they could launch on the very day the underlying patents expired, adding a sharp punctuation point to the end of the monopoly period. Now opened up to generic competition, drugs would fall quickly in price and become cheaply available in perpetuity.

The system was an equilibrium, a balancing act which recognised the need to incentivise innovation and the unusual nature of pharmaceuticals as lifesaving products for which a lack of access for patients can mean death. For years, it seemed to be working. The first four decades after the Second World War saw an extraordinary explosion of scientific advances with corticosteroids, beta blockers, ACE inhibitors and benzos among the major drug classes launched.[63] New technology promised even greater advances. Developed by two Californian professors in the 1970s, recombinant DNA technology allowed scientists to manipulate genetic material, opening the door to a panoply of new possibilities from gene editing to biological medicines. In 1976, the founding of Genentech in San Francisco Valley marked the start of the venture capital-funded biotech industry which sought to translate this new technology into clinically useful products. A US Supreme Court ruling in 1980 confirmed that patents could be granted for man-made living organisms, opening the door for companies to sell products derived from genetically engineered material. The first biologic, a lab-grown version of insulin called Humulin, was approved by the US regulator in 1982.

The pharmaceutical industry had become a major player in the global economy, employing hundreds of thousands of people while their stocks generated returns for millions more. Drug companies were held in high esteem, none more so than MSD, which would soon become the largest drug company in the world.

Under CEO Roy Vagelos, the company prided itself on its investment in science, luring the brightest minds with new, modern labs and sizeable annual increases in its R&D budget. Vagelos, who had joined MSD after two decades in academia and medicine, called his memoir of his time at the company *The Moral Corporation*, boasting of its 'well-deserved reputation for social responsibility'.[64] Central to this was the company's decision to invest in vaccine research even as rivals pulled out. In 1987, MSD scientists searching for compounds that might combat parasites in farm animals had discovered that one, ivermectin, was an effective treatment for onchocerciasis, or river blindness. Spread by black flies, the disease affected millions of people in Africa and Latin America, afflicting those infected with itching, rashes and eye lesions which can ultimately lead to a loss of vision.

MSD initially tried to find someone else to pay for it, but when no government, charitable foundation or international health agency stepped forward, Vagelos told executives: 'We're going to do the right thing' and donated the drug.[65] The company ended up donating more than four billion doses and the programme continues to this day.[66]

In the late 1980s and early 1990s, *Fortune* magazine voted MSD 'America's most admired corporation' for seven years in a row. Yet over the next decade or two, the drug industry's reputation would collapse. Shifting priorities, new technologies, regulatory changes, scientific challenges and a dramatic cultural shift would combine to obliterate the mantra of patients before profits. By late 2019, the industry ranked rock bottom in annual polling of those which were most admired.[67]

This is the story of what changed.

CHAPTER TWO

AZT – the first AIDS drug

I t was September 1989 and the traders lingered in the Tuesday morning sunshine outside the imposing facade of the New York Stock Exchange, enjoying the last drags on their cigarettes before the market opened. As they turned and headed inside, hurrying to make the opening bell, three outsiders slipped unnoticed into their midst. Dressed in suits and ties, and with white passes pinned to their chests, the new arrivals walked through the entrance, turned left and strolled confidently past the lone security guard posted inside. Following the other traders along a route they'd been briefed on in advance, they swung right and climbed a few steps, emerging into the cavernous shrine to American capitalism that was the stock exchange's main hub. Pulling out notepads and pencils, they were quickly subsumed into the chaotic melee of the trading floor.

Peter Staley couldn't believe it had been so easy. A member of the AIDS Coalition to Unleash Power (ACT UP), the twenty-eight-year-old had been told he was HIV-positive four years earlier. Now he was on a reconnaissance mission.

Staley, his boyfriend, a videographer called Robert Hilferty, and another activist, Scott Robbe, made their way among the traders, scoping out the building. Up above, the visitors' gallery was visible behind heavy plexiglass – the legacy of the last incursion into this temple. In 1967 a group of hippie activists led by Abbie Hoffman had thrown dollar bills from the then-open gallery over the trading floor below. Since then it had been safely walled off.

As they completed a circuit, Staley spotted an old wooden balcony with a tiny staircase leading up from the trading floor. Without going up he knew it was the place. There was even a brass railing which would be perfect to hang a banner from. Then a veteran trader stopped him.

'Hey, you're new here.'

'Ah, yeah,' Staley mumbled in response

'Bear Stearns,' the trader said, pointing at the makeshift security badge.

'Yeah, yeah,' the activist said, starting to sweat.

The trader looked confused. He leaned in, peering accusingly at the number on the badge.

'*Five thousand* seven hundred and ninety-four.' He considered it for a moment. 'That's strange. There are only about 1,400 traders here.'

Staley stammered for an answer. 'Uh, must be a new system,' he offered, desperately hoping his interlocutor would be satisfied.

'Oh well, welcome,' the trader said, smiling. 'Good luck.'

As he walked off, Staley turned to Hilferty and took his arm. 'Let's get the fuck out of here,' he said. The trio hurried to the exit and back out into the sunlight.[1]

The plan was hatched. Their target: one of the most expensive drugs in history.

Born in Detroit, Michigan, just two months after the end of the First World War, Jerome Horwitz might have ended up in the family poultry business if it wasn't for Paul de Kruif's *Microbe Hunters*. The book, published in 1926, told a rollicking tale of trailblazing scientists pitting their wits against diseases of all kinds in a race to save millions of lives. The young Horwitz was quickly hooked.[2]

Leaving behind a life of cleaning out chicken coops and collecting eggs, he enrolled in a chemistry degree at the University of Detroit. The United States entered the Second World War while he was still at university, but chronic knee injuries from a youth spent playing American football ruled him out of joining up and he was able to study for a master's degree and then a PhD.

He bounced around between postdoctoral projects, ending up at the Illinois Institute of Technology trying to develop a solid rocket fuel for the US Navy.[3] In the 1950s, test pilots like Chuck Yeager, the first man to fly faster than sound, and the country's nascent space programme had captured the imagination of the American public. But Horwitz's heart wasn't in the work and by the late 1950s the diminutive scientist found himself back in his hometown, happily ensconced in a laboratory in the bowels of what was then called the Detroit Institute for Cancer Research. He won a government grant to search for a cure for the disease.

Horwitz initially followed the established practice of those doing cancer research, testing hundreds of chemical compounds almost at random in the hope that one would prove to be the magic bullet that would selectively kill cancer cells while leaving the normal cells alone. But in 1961 he changed his approach and began to synthesise new compounds, searching for one which would stop cancerous cells from continually dividing.[4] He theorised that he could create 'trick molecules' which would imitate nucleotides, the building blocks of DNA, inserting themselves into the DNA of cancer cells and so preventing them from replicating.[5]

One of the new compounds he synthesised was azidothymidine, known as AZT, and in 1963 he injected it into mice in the hope it would stop the spread of cancer. It soon became clear it hadn't worked. Dispirited by the results, Horwitz wrote up his findings for a short article in the *Journal of Organic Chemistry* the following year and moved on to other compounds.[6]

'It was a terrible disappointment,' he later admitted. 'We found no use for it in cancer research. We dumped it on the junk pile.'[7] He even threw away his notebooks. With no sign of it proving useful, the idea of patenting the compound never crossed his mind.

Two decades later, Horwitz's discovery would seem like manna from heaven.

In the early 1980s, the United States was in the grip of a mysterious new illness. Doctors in New York and San Francisco had noticed a spate of otherwise healthy young men coming down with the distinctive purple skin blotches of Kaposi's sarcoma, a rare skin cancer. It initially seemed to be largely confined to homosexual men and was dubbed gay-related immune deficiency (GRID), or, as some called it, gay cancer. But it swiftly became apparent that the illness did not discriminate on the basis of sexual orientation and a new name was adopted: acquired immunodeficiency syndrome, or AIDS. By the start of 1984, AIDS was killing 2,000 people a year in the United States alone; a figure that was doubling or tripling each year.[8]

Responsibility for tackling this growing public emergency would fall on scientists at the National Institutes of Health (NIH), a collection of more than a dozen government-funded research agencies on a sprawling campus in Bethesda, Maryland.

Dr Sam Broder had joined one of those agencies, the National Cancer Institute (NCI), in the early 1970s and was named the head of clinical oncology at the start of the 1980s. Broder was the hard-scrabbling son of two Jewish diner owners who had moved to Detroit from war-torn Europe shortly after the Second World War. His family did not have much money but he made his way to the top through long hours and hard work, winning scholarships to attend the University of Michigan. The Polish-born scientist brought the same intensity to his work at the NCI.

The successful isolation of the virus which caused AIDS sounded the starting gun on a race for a treatment: hopefully a cure, but at the very least something to buy more time for the thousands who had been given a death sentence. Since the NCI was the only agency within NIH which had traditionally worked on new drugs, it took up the mantle.[9] Broder realised the government would not have the funds and manufacturing capabilities to push a drug through the latter stages of clinical testing so in 1984 he began touring drug companies, urging them to take up AIDS research and offering the services of his team if they did.

'What he found when he spoke to a number of pharmaceutical firms was that they were not interested at that time,' his colleague Robert Yarchoan recalled. 'In effect, they said, "Look, it is an epidemic, but there are only 50,000 people with the disease, and we can't justify a big program to our stockholders for 50,000 people".'[10]

While Broder was drawing a blank at a succession of drug companies, one firm had in fact been quietly working on AIDS research for months.

The previous year, Dr David Barry had joined several colleagues for dinner with a visiting French doctor, Françoise Barré-Sinoussi. Barry was a smooth-talking, chain-smoking virologist at Burroughs Wellcome, a pharmaceutical company with its US headquarters in North Carolina. Born in the prosperous New England town of Nashua, he was educated at Yale and spent his junior year in Paris, studying at the Sorbonne. After leaving college, he was able to take a role in the US Public Health Service Commissioned Corps, thereby avoiding following his brother on deployment to Vietnam. Instead, he worked for the Food and Drug Administration (FDA), trying to help US manufacturers to improve the yellow fever vaccine.

He lasted five years but found himself ill-suited to the internal politics of life as a government scientist. His colleagues were too cut-throat, he thought, too fixated on elbowing their names onto scientific papers. In 1977 he received a job offer from Burroughs Wellcome. Unusually, Burroughs Wellcome was owned by a charitable trust rather than by shareholders, and the collegiate, research-focused atmosphere this helped engender appealed to Barry when he visited. There was a 'very gentlemanly' culture which reminded him of his time as a medical student at Yale, he would later tell an interviewer. 'It was my kind of place . . . it wasn't like I thought of [a] drug company; it was like this research operation and they were doing research in an area that I liked.'[11]

Barry had been asked to take his guest to dinner as a favour to his boss, Pedro Cuatrecasas, whose mother was friends with hers. It proved a fortuitous connection. During the meal, Barré-Sinoussi, who worked at the non-profit Pasteur Institute in Paris, told Barry she and her colleagues had identified the virus that caused AIDS. Her claim was met with scepticism.

'I said fine and I was being nice and polite because between 1981 and 1983 everybody and his brother said I have got the virus that causes it; it's this virus, that virus, hepatitis D, hepatitis this, you know, measles, you name it, and it wasn't it,' Barry said later.[12]

The next day, she came into the company's offices to make a presentation to Barry and other Burroughs Wellcome scientists. Barré-Sinoussi, who would go on to win a Nobel Prize with two colleagues for discovering HIV, began a detailed explanation of her recent work. The virus, she said, looked like swamp fever, or equine infectious anaemia, which was spread by horseflies who latch onto horses and suck their blood. Like swamp fever, it was a specific type of virus called a retrovirus. Retroviruses embed their genome into the DNA of targeted cells, causing these cells to start replicating the virus.

'We looked at it, looked at each other, and said "Jesus, I think she really has it",' Barry would later recall. 'So we sat down afterwards and we said you know [if] it really is a retrovirus, we are the company with the most experience in antivirals, let's work on it!'[13] The company had recently launched an antiviral used to treat herpes virus infections and Barry's work at the FDA had involved trying to eliminate a problematic avian retrovirus from the yellow fever vaccine which was produced in chicken embryos.

Barry and his colleagues decided to start by taking every antiviral drug or candidate off the shelf and testing to see if it worked against the type of retrovirus they had access to, a strain which caused cancer in mice. They held informal weekly meetings to assess the results of the tests but it was slow going and there was internal pressure to focus on other areas.

When Barry mentioned his work on AIDS to the chief executive of the American subsidiary, a gruff former oilman called Bill Sullivan, he was told in no uncertain terms to drop it and focus on something more commercial. Fortunately, Cuatrecasas, the Spanish head of research and development, was more encouraging. 'I'll cover for you,' he said. 'Work on it but be quiet.'[14]

More than a year passed, and although the testing produced some compounds with signs of potential, they were yet to make a real breakthrough.

In October 1984, the government scientist Broder's tour of American pharmaceutical companies brought him to North Carolina for a meeting with Barry. The two scientists were close in age but had very different characters and backgrounds, epitomised by their respective hobbies. Barry loved French literature, while Broder's favourite pastime was collecting old rock-and-roll records: 'Things I liked when I was growing up, but never got on the first go-round because I never could afford them or never had the time to get in the early Sixties.'[15]

Broder flew down with his research colleague Robert Gallo, who opened the afternoon meeting by speaking for two hours about his work on the virus which caused AIDS. Once he was finished, Broder began his pitch.

'I explained what our capacity was in terms of clinical trials and essentially offered a collaboration with them, with the promise that we would, whatever came up, develop drugs as fast as we could and that they would get a product out of it,' Broder later said. 'There was no other way to encourage pharmaceutical companies.'[16]

He had a particularly useful asset to offer. Hiroaki 'Mitch' Mitsuya, a young Japanese scientist on Broder's team, had developed a fast-reacting test, known as an assay, which could tell whether a drug was able to prevent the virus killing human cells within just five days. Barry agreed to send some samples.

The mundane task of testing the compounds being screened at Burroughs Wellcome fell to Marty St Clair, a young scientist with thick, owlish glasses. She would put living cells in Petri dishes, spike them with an animal retrovirus and then add the different drugs being tested. If the drug failed to prevent the virus, holes in the cells known as plaques would be visible within a few days.

A few weeks after Broder's visit, in late October 1984, another Burroughs scientist, Janet Rideout, selected Zidovudine, also known as azidothymidine (AZT), as one of many compounds for St Clair to try. The company had previously worked with AZT in its labs when looking for a treatment for urinary tract infections. The drug hadn't proved sufficiently successful and Burroughs Wellcome's stocks were sent to England where researchers believed it might prove effective at fighting E. coli infections in pigs.[17]

Now, however, AZT seemed to have produced an extraordinary result. 'I was holding them up to the window,' she said. 'I came to sixteen dishes, none of which had any plaques.'[18]

St Clair's first thought was that she had forgotten to add the virus but Barry was confident she was too diligent to have made such a basic mistake. He told her to repeat the experiment to be sure, reducing the concentration of AZT. Two weeks later, the results were in. At the lowest concentration there were a few holes but in higher concentrations the drug had prevented the virus attacking the cells.

Barry pulled a bottle of white wine from his desk drawer and gathered the troops. 'Let's celebrate now,' he told them, 'because I have got a feeling we are going to have to tighten our seatbelts, because we are going for one hell of a ride.'[19] He knew the hopes of tens of thousands of AIDS sufferers were about to crash down on the successful compound and on the company itself. The search for a treatment was 'like the holy grail, literally', Barry later recalled. 'People were dropping like flies, people were taking all kinds of wacky medicines.

'And you would go into Duke [University Hospital] and you would see people, it was pitiful, you know, people our age or younger, a twenty-five-year-old guy dying . . . with an untreatable disease.'[20]

The initial response at the corporate level to news of this breakthrough was less than enthused. The job fell to Cuatrecasas, the head of R&D who later recounted what happened: '[Their] reaction was at first "Oh my God, not another orphan",' a reference to medicines known as orphan drugs which treat rare diseases with relatively small numbers of patients. They viewed it, he said, as 'a scientific curiosity, with no commercial potential. The researchers playing at their game again.'[21]

Despite the celebrations, Marty St Clair's experiment showing that AZT was active against animal retroviruses was not as novel as claimed in the version of events the company would later present to the public. Ten years earlier, Wolfram Ostertag at Germany's Max Planck Institute had demonstrated that AZT could inhibit a mouse retrovirus. He'd even published the results, although they'd received little notice at a time when retroviruses weren't believed to infect humans. Yet when Barry testified before Congress two years later, his account of identifying AZT's use against the 'the replication of certain animal viruses in the test tube' made no mention of Ostertag and presented it as an original discovery.[22]

Back at Burroughs Wellcome it was time to test AZT against the live virus in human cells. That autumn, the company sent a number of compounds for testing against HIV in assays set up by Dr Gerald Quinnan at the FDA and Dr Dani Bolognesi at Duke University. After Broder's visit, Barry also started sending compounds to the NCI but they wouldn't be sent AZT for three months. Instead, it was first dispatched, labelled as compound S, to Quinnan at the FDA in mid-November. His test showed almost no activity against the live virus. Undeterred, it was sent to Bolognesi at Duke a month later. This time it 'popped'.[23]

While the compounds had been sent out for testing, Burroughs Wellcome was already thinking about the commercial potential. They'd discussed patenting the drug as a treatment for AIDS within weeks of the first test result and in February 1985, a draft patent application was completed. Mitsuya's assay soon confirmed that it worked against the live virus in human cells and Broder called Burroughs to report the results. Less than a month later, the patent application was filed.[24]

The drug underwent pre-clinical testing at Burroughs, a process which involves giving the drug to animals, often mice and rats, to check its toxicity, while Broder continued more lab experiments. The company pulled together data from those tests to make an investigational new drug (IND) application to the FDA seeking permission to start the first human clinical trial.

Known as a Phase I trial, the first human trial typically involves a small number of volunteers being given the drug, initially at very low doses, while being monitored for side effects. At this point, scientists are primarily concerned with the safety of the drug. If it clears this hurdle, it moves on to a Phase II trial involving a few hundred patients. Phase II trials continue to check for significant adverse reactions but also look at the efficacy of the drug; whether it is achieving what it set out to do in tackling the symptoms of a disease. This is usually done by dividing up those in the trial, with some unknowingly receiving a placebo (an inactive substance) or the best existing treatment.

Finally, Phase III trials involve a much larger cohort of somewhere between several hundred and several thousand patients. Researchers gather evidence of the safety and the efficacy of the new drug in a larger population, including checking for rare but unwanted side effects. Once this has been completed, the pharmaceutical company puts together a dossier analysing the data generated by the trials and seeks marketing approval from regulators such as the FDA in the US and the Medicines and Healthcare products Regulatory Agency (MHRA) in the United Kingdom. Only when a drug gets approved by the regulator can it go on sale, although testing often continues to take place. These post-approval Phase IV trials are sometimes ordered by the regulator to monitor the safety of a drug or may be part of efforts to find out if it would be useful for other patient groups – potentially expanding the market for the medicine.

The whole process typically takes an average of eight to twelve years, but AZT would take less than two and a half years from when Marty St Clair first added it to the sixteen Petri dishes to its approval for sale in the United States. The incredible speed with which AZT was tested and received regulatory approval owed much to government scientists and administrators and, in particular, to Broder's peerless energy in pushing it through. Barry would acknowledge as much. 'Sam was very enthusiastic,' he said. 'He was doing a bang-up job both in the laboratory and in the clinical centre and from, if you will, the public relations point of view. He was getting the word out, showing people the work, really pushing hard.'[25] The IND application was signed off within a week.

It was agreed that the Phase I trials would take place at the National

Institutes of Health (NIH) and Duke University. Burroughs Wellcome's laboratories were only certified to the P-2 standard of biosafety, a level below what was suitable for working with the live HIV virus, but the company was also apprehensive of the risks involved. Broder's facility similarly lacked a P-3 rating but he felt there was no time to waste.[26]

The level of fear around working with the virus briefly threatened to disrupt the Phase I trial when, just days before it was due to start, Burroughs Wellcome said it wouldn't even accept blood samples from patients. Broder had to reassign members of his team from other tasks to keep it on track.[27]

On July 3, Joseph Rafuse, a furniture salesman from Boston, became the first patient to be injected with AZT. He was seriously ill when he was chosen for the trial, having recently suffered a bout of pneumocystis pneumonia (PCP), and his tests showed an extremely low CD4 cell count of fewer than forty cells per millilitre of blood, far below the normal level of 1,000. Doctors had learnt that a blood test to count the number of CD4 cells, a type of white blood cell called a T-cell which helps recognise foreign particles, could measure the progress of an HIV infection. The virus kills off CD4 cells as it progresses and a low count leaves a patient at higher risk of opportunistic infections.

Broder and Yarchoan watched as Rafuse was injected with the drug at the NIH's hospital facility in Bethesda, on the outskirts of Washington DC. That night, he developed a fever and the doctors returned to the hospital. They had to establish whether he was developing a dangerous allergic reaction to the drug. Fortunately, it appeared to be nothing more serious than a common cold. Although his temperature rose, it wasn't high enough to require them to abandon the research and the trial could continue.

Within two weeks, Rafuse's T-cell count had gone up. 'We did not know what to make of this. We knew that CD4 counts bounced around, but this was a bounce in the right direction,' Yarchoan recalled.[28] Two weeks later, the count was up to 200. That turned out to be the peak, but the patient reported feeling a lot better and skin tests showed white blood cells were not simply increasing in number; they were working, too.[29] Yarchoan likened it to being on lookout on a foggy night: 'You see these patterns and you are never sure whether there is really a ship coming or just eddies in the fog.'[30]

After the first few patients, the dosage was doubled for a new set of six patients and by October Broder and Yarchoan realised the improvement in CD4 counts of all six had reached statistically significant levels. 'We were, at that point, very, very excited that we really had something,' Yarchoan said.[31]

The Phase II trial began in February 1986, shortly before Broder, Barry, Bolognesi and other Burroughs Wellcome and NCI scientists published the results of the Phase I trial in *The Lancet*. By mid-May a total of 282 people had been enrolled across a dozen locations. It was a double-blind placebo trial, meaning that neither the doctors nor the patients knew who was actually getting AZT.

The trial had been due to last until December but on September 10 the data and safety monitoring board met to review some preliminary results. Already there were signs of a significant difference in the survival rates between those on AZT and those receiving a placebo. In all, 137 patients had been administered a placebo and nineteen had died. By contrast, just one of the 145 people receiving AZT had passed away. A week later, after reviewing further data, the board stepped in to halt the placebo arm of the trial. The next day, Dr Robert Windom, the US assistant secretary for health and human services, held a press conference to announce that everyone in the trial was now going to be receiving AZT and the drug would be made available to seriously ill AIDS patients within days. The promised land was here. Doctors who had spent years without a treatment to offer their patients rushed to prescribe the new drug.[32]

A free telephone number set up by the NIH to field calls from those looking to access the drug was inundated. Over the next six months more than 4,000 AIDS patients would receive the drug for free on a compassionate basis while Burroughs Wellcome sought approval from the regulator to be able to sell it. With stock in short supply, desperate patients tried to use any connection they could to get the medicine. Tom Kennedy, a corporate affairs executive at

Burroughs Wellcome, recalled having 'patients screaming and calling, or their agents calling on the phones and at the doorsteps every day'. He said he 'personally took a call . . . from a gentleman who was the Secretary of Defense of the United States of America, trying to get [the] drug for an aide of his'.[33]

In light of the public health emergency that AIDS represented, the FDA waived the usual requirement for a large-scale Phase III trial to have been completed before approval. Ellen Cooper, the regulator in charge of antiviral products, agreed to accept parts of Burroughs Wellcome's application as they were completed in order to speed things up. The full dossier for a New Drug Application (NDA) was in the hands of the FDA shortly before Christmas 1986. On January 16, the FDA's advisory committee met to decide on whether or not to recommend approving the drug. There were initially significant reservations. Not only was there much more limited data than a drug manufacturer would normally have been expected to compile – after all, the drug had gone from the laboratory to a full application within little more than two years, barely a quarter of the usual length of time – but there were also serious concerns about side effects. A significant number of patients in the trials had experienced adverse reactions, with as many as half requiring blood transfusions to combat severe anaemia. The toxically high dose – 1,200mg over twenty-four hours – was the result of concern at Burroughs Wellcome that they 'really only had one shot to show that it was working', one of the government scientists recalled. 'Burroughs thought that it was better to be a little toxic but to have the drug work than not to have the drug work.'[34]

Jean McGuire, who was executive director of the AIDS Action Council in the late 1980s, recalls attending a hearing on AZT with a Texan colleague who had been diagnosed with AIDS and was taking the drug. 'We're walking up the congressional steps on a hot July day. I put my hand on his white shirt and he bleeds through his shirt to my hand. Because that was the level of the anaemia that AZT was inducing.'[35]

In the January FDA committee meeting, however, the urgent need to offer patients some kind of treatment ultimately won the day. The panel voted to approve the drug by a margin of ten to one. Meanwhile, inside Wellcome Plc, the British parent company of Burroughs Wellcome, the decision facing executives was coming to a crunch: what price to set for this revolutionary new medicine which faced no competition and which would be the only treatment for an epidemic killing thousands. Then, as now, the drug company making and selling a new medicine in the United States faced no regulatory or government restraints on the price it set.

In some ways, Wellcome's research-oriented ethos made it an unlikely company to find itself in the role of public villain it would soon be cast in. Founded in 1880 by two American pharmacists and headquartered in a grand building on Euston Road in central London, it was owned by a charitable trust and traditionally sold cures for rare tropical diseases with little commercial appeal. But by this time it was undergoing a dramatic culture shift. In the early 1980s, after several fallow years without major new drug launches, research budgets had been squeezed. Bill Sullivan, the former oilman who spent years as a company lawyer, moved across to the business side of the American business with a remit to shake things up. He brought in management consultants to look for cost savings and scrutinise researchers' priorities and applied a harder commercial stance to some of the company's existing drugs. A heart medication saw sales of $8–10 million dollars a year rise to $45 million a year 'simply by raising the price'.[36]

Sullivan thought the company was soft, taking the view that 'we're making money, very respectably, so we're not going to try to squeeze the last dollar out of what we could get'.[37] He blamed the lack of 'market discipline' on the fact that it was privately owned. That all changed in 1986 when, buoyed by the promise of AZT and a recently launched herpes drug, the charitable trust which owned the business decided to sell off around a quarter of its shareholding, making Wellcome, for the first time, a public company. Now the company had a share price to protect and external stockholders to please.

From the moment the results of the Phase II clinical trial emerged, analysts and media reports had speculated that AZT, as the company's new golden goose, would be expensive – perhaps even as much as $5,000 per patient per year.[38] The business was well aware of the value of the drug to patients, offering, as chief executive Ted Haigler put it during a congressional hearing in March 1987, 'the only hope for patients suffering from this deadly disease'.[39] Executives faced a quandary – how to balance the life-saving potential of the drug with the company's desire to make a profit?

By mid-February, the company had its answer: a price of $188 for a bottle of 100 pills of 100mg strength. By way of explanation, a press release issued by Wellcome Plc in London offered only a vague and terse comment: 'In establishing the price, Wellcome has taken into account a number of social and economic factors.'[40] A spokeswoman acknowledged that, with patients taking two capsules every four hours, the retail price of the medicine would be up to $10,000 dollars a year, double analysts' steepest predictions. It was one of the highest-priced prescription drugs in history.[41]

The stock market had no complaints, with investors pushing the company's share price up by 24 per cent on the day of the announcement. Elsewhere, however, the backlash was almost immediate. Less than a month after the pricing of the drug had been unveiled, David Barry and Ted Haigler, Bill Sullivan's successor as chief executive of Burroughs Wellcome USA, were summoned to Washington to appear before a committee led by congressman Henry Waxman, a Democrat from California. Room 2322 in the Rayburn Building was packed with TV cameras and reporters for the hearing on the 'cost and availability of AZT'. 'Everyone in the world who thought they had an interest in AIDS, including AIDS patients, [were] jamming the place,' Tom Kennedy recalled. 'It was a zoo.'[42]

During questioning, Waxman outlined the conundrum at the heart of the matter. 'What is an adequate profit when you've got a drug that, if you set it at a price that's going to be too high, some people are going to have to . . . go without this lifesaving drug,' he asked. Burroughs had 'monopoly control', Waxman added, and the government had no means of second-guessing 'your evaluation of a reasonable return on your investment' because the drugmaker wouldn't provide the figures. Later, a frustrated Representative Ron Wyden would put it more bluntly, suggesting that the price had been plucked out of thin air and asking Haigler: 'Why didn't you set the price at $100,000 per patient?'[43]

Both men were referring to the implicit agreement, the social contract balancing private profit and public benefit, which existed between drug companies and the public. The pricing of AZT exposed just how fragile this fundamental deal was in relying, as it does, on the behaviour and fair-mindedness of for-profit entities. Burroughs Wellcome had done significant work on developing AZT and bringing it to market, but the drug they were about to start selling was far from the fruit of their own research. The chemical compound had been synthesised years earlier by Jerome Horwitz, funded by a government grant. Its use against animal retroviruses had been discovered by a German scientist in 1974 and merely repeated by Burroughs Wellcome a decade later. The company had relied on Duke University and the NCI to demonstrate it could suppress live HIV and to carry out the Phase I trial and accompanying studies. Government scientists had been crucial to its discovery and government officials had been crucial to pushing it through testing in record time. Yet, it was Burroughs Wellcome alone that was free to set a price of its choosing and reap the financial rewards.

An economist called Peter Arno summed it up when giving testimony during a Senate hearing in February 1993. Taxpayers, he said, would end up paying for AZT five times over: for Horwitz's discovery, Broder and Mitsuya's testing, the NIH's role in the Phase I trial, through tax credits under the Orphan Drug Act, and in meeting the cost of prescriptions through Medicaid and the Ryan White CARE Act, a federal programme introduced in 1990 to pay for AZT and other AIDS treatments for the poor and uninsured.

The price of AZT was not just seen as unconscionable. For many activists, it meant that this soon-to-be-approved first treatment for AIDS, a long-awaited glimmer of light in the darkness of a plague, would be out of reach. Some insurance plans wouldn't cover the drug and those without insurance faced an unwelcome choice. In order to be eligible for the government's Medicaid programme, many states required patients to go into poverty paying for AZT before they would qualify on a 'spend down' basis. In other states, tight limits on the total spend on prescription drugs would effectively mean it wasn't covered anyway. In Florida this cap was just $22 a month, far below the price of AZT. 'A lot of the young people that got sick weren't insured,' recalls Jean McGuire, head of the AIDS Action Council. 'They weren't insured, they weren't eligible for Medicaid. Even rich or relatively well-off gay men couldn't carry the cost.'[44]

The drug was so expensive Congress voted to set up a new scheme called the AIDS Drug Assistance Program, providing $30 million towards the cost of AZT for patients who weren't covered by Medicaid.[45] In 1989, the government would take $100 million allocated to the AIDS research programme at NIH to cover the emergency purchase of AZT for those who couldn't afford it. 'The high price of AZT . . . became an active barrier to research on newer and better drugs because they took that money right out of research and used it to pay the company for the drug,' says Mark Harrington, an ACT UP activist.[46] For those whose lives were being defined by the disease, leaving them scrabbling for black-market drugs or forced to watch friends and lovers suffer and die, it went far beyond an argument about the ethics of pricing a life-saving drug with a captive market. They decided they had to act.

ACT UP had been birthed in a fiery speech by the famous playwright Larry Kramer at the Gay and Lesbian Community Center in lower Manhattan in March 1987. At the next meeting, a vote was taken on possible targets for direct action and, by a show of hands, the financial district was the clear winner.[47] So it was that on the morning of March 24 several hundred young gay activists made their way to Wall Street. Among those passing through the area were Peter Staley, who was on his way to work nearby. Staley had been diagnosed with what was then called AIDS-related complex – he was infected with HIV but the disease had not yet progressed – in November 1985.

'I had this newish gay boyfriend . . . visiting from Amsterdam and he was in my apartment and we sat down to watch the very first TV movie about AIDS called *An Early Frost*,' he says. In the film, the actor Aidan Quinn played a closeted gay man who is diagnosed with AIDS after developing a previously rare type of pneumonia called PCP 'which was the number one killer of people with AIDS back then. His first signs are a bad cough. And as it went to a commercial break this Dutch boyfriend turns to me and said, "He sounds like you",' Staley says. 'I was hacking away coughing and I said, "I know, I know. I'll go to my doctor."'[48] Tests on Staley's white blood cells confirmed that he was HIV-positive.

The following summer, Staley worked up the courage to attend one of the support groups for those affected by AIDS which he had read about in gay newspapers. 'I finally said well, you know, I'm learning all this medical stuff but I still haven't met another person with HIV.' He found his first meeting at Gay Men's Health Crisis in New York's West Village a depressing affair, full of guys 'wallowing in fear and stigma' who said they felt toxic and would never have sex again. But one of the two dozen or so attendees drew his eye. 'He had this crazy spiked white and blond hair and pale, very pale skin, [a] black leather jacket and a whole goth outfit and multiple earrings coming out of his ears,' Staley recalls. 'So he had this kind of intense scary look, but he was also a flaming queen. I found him fascinating.'[49]

The goth was Griffin Gold, one of the co-founders of the People With AIDS Coalition and Staley's introduction to the world of AIDS activism. Staley, a buttoned-up banker who kept his sexuality hidden from his colleagues, wasn't yet ready to be seen in public playing an active role but he began offering financial support. Gold, who would die of AIDS three years later, put him in touch with leading activists. When Staley read about a group calling themselves the Lavender Hill mob – named after the 1951 Alec Guinness crime caper – who had heckled President Reagan's health and human services secretary, Gold led him to the guys behind it and Staley duly set up a dinner and wrote a cheque.

The protestors from ACT UP had given out flyers, complaining about the government's alleged failure to push ahead with the testing of a string of experimental drugs. It included a reprint of an op-ed by Kramer which declared that 'AIDS sufferers, who have nothing to lose, are more than willing to be guinea pigs', as well as attacking AZT's 'unconscionable' price.[50] Several traders had brought them into the office, prompting, for the first time, a conversation among Staley's colleagues about AIDS. It came to an abrupt end with an intervention from one of his mentors.

'Well, if you ask me, they all deserve to die because they took it up the butt,' his fellow trader said.

'Everybody's eyes widened and they just put their hands up and kind of walked away. And I sat there just fuming, you know. It was like someone had stabbed me. And I couldn't say anything.'[51]

That night Staley went home and turned on the evening news. Dan Rather, the CBS news anchor, was reporting on the demonstration he had walked into earlier, and there was the head of the FDA, Frank Young, making a small concession on clinical trial access. This group was getting results, Staley thought, and he wanted to be part of it.

In trying to justify the price of AZT, Burroughs Wellcome offered a number of different public explanations. One of the most commonly advanced arguments was that the drug had only a small market and very limited time in which to recoup costs, given the likelihood of other AIDS treatments being discovered. Haigler, the US chief executive, was particularly keen to play up the huge uncertainty the company supposedly faced.

It was a line that grew more tenuous each time it was rolled out. While AZT was being developed, AIDS patients numbered only in the tens of thousands, but that figure was growing at a rapid rate. Scientists working on the disease knew the numbers would soon be enormous. Robert Yarchoan, at the NCI, recalled his own personal reckoning when he read papers written by his colleague Robert Gallo on the virus that would be called HIV in 1984. Yarchoan described 'doing a rough mental calculation of the number of gays in the country and the percentage who were likely to be HIV-infected, and estimating that there were half a million to a million people infected with this lethal virus who did not know it'.[52]

When the drug was approved in early 1987, Burroughs said it expected to be able to produce enough for 30,000 patients in the first year. Those figures alone would translate into sales of $300 million. The company also knew that trials were being launched into the drug's usefulness as a preventative medicine for those who were HIV-positive but did not yet have AIDS – something which would hugely increase the size of the market. No one at Burroughs could seriously have believed this would remain a niche product.

The validity of other explanations were hard to gauge because Burroughs steadfastly refused to open their books or reveal how much had been spent developing the drug. Under grilling from Representatives Waxman, Wyden and others in March 1987, Haigler said he believed 'we have balanced our concern for patients with the development and production costs involved and the risks we have assumed'.[53] But he repeatedly declined to say how much it had cost to take it through two clinical trials. The only figure he floated – $80 million – was an outlay on the raw materials for producing the drug rather than development costs. A later explanation Barry gave to a newspaper reporter as to why he couldn't provide the figure gives little confidence that it would have been seen as an adequate explanation. 'Whatever number you give out, it'll be used to mislead,' he said.[54]

Although Burroughs Wellcome had strongly implied that the company had established a specific figure for the cost of developing the drug but couldn't give it out for commercial reasons, executives later interviewed for an internal oral history project admitted there was no such number. They said that research and development was simply treated as an overhead and they were not able to break down costs for specific projects. Given this, it is hard to see how much development costs could have influenced the chosen price.

Analyst estimates of the likely costs were modest. Samuel Isaly, who ran an investment firm focusing on drug companies, told *Fortune* magazine in 1990 that AZT 'probably cost less than $50 million for direct development before it was approved'.[55] AZT's clinical trials had been much smaller and shorter than normal, although Barry would protest that this had made little difference to the cost because the seriously ill volunteers required close medical attention. Burroughs hadn't even needed to complete the most expensive, large-scale trial normally required because AZT was approved without a Phase III trial. It is also hard to argue that Burroughs Wellcome needed to subsidise enormous losses from its research work. The antiviral research programme which worked on AIDS treatments had been in place for years and had produced the company's most profitable drug, the blockbuster herpes treatment Zovirax, which launched in 1982.

Another argument advanced by the under-fire business was that it represented great value for taxpayers and the government because of the savings healthy AIDS patients would bring in vacated hospital beds and the economic value they generated by returning to the workforce. 'I have no compunction about charging this price,' Barry once told a reporter from the *Wall Street Journal*. 'No one flinches at hundreds of dollars a day in hospital costs, but everyone expects a drug that prevents hospitalisation to be much less.'[56] By this logic, the sky was the limit for what constituted good value. After all, if a patient might die if they didn't receive a medicine, anything less than whatever could be calculated to be the economic worth of the rest of their life could be presented as representing good value.

Finally, the company's patient access programme was also offered as justification for the pricing because no patients, it was argued, would have to pay this price if they couldn't afford it. This spared little thought for those burning through their life savings to meet the cost, nor for the enormous burden that fell on taxpayers through Medicaid and other government programmes. By 1992, the US government had spent at least $325 million buying the drug.[57] Meanwhile, the patient access programme, which activists believed had helped just 300 people by late 1989, failed to prevent doctors and patients being unable to get hold of the drug. A reporter for the *Wall Street Journal* interviewed Joseph Wilber, medical director of Georgia's public health AIDS programme in September 1989. 'Many patients still can't get AZT,' Wilber said. 'We have 18 patients in Savannah who doctors think should get AZT but there's no source. We've used up all our federal money.'[58]

The public explanations offered by Burroughs, to the extent that they were offered at all, would be echoed by industry executives seeking to explain countless pricing decisions in the years to come. But it was all smoke and mirrors. The truth about Burroughs Wellcome's pricing decision is that the company charged as much as it thought it could get away with.

Bill Sullivan, who had been president of Burroughs Wellcome in the United States until shortly before AZT launched, gave a frank summary in 2001 when asked about pricing drugs. 'You basically price a drug the same way you price any other commodity: what you think the customer will pay for it. An automobile, a suit, fruit, whatever it is . . . You obviously have to charge more than it costs you to make them, but beyond that, you're going to charge as much as you can.'[59] His predecessor, Fred Coe, echoed Sullivan's appraisal, saying you 'find out how much it's going to cost to make . . . and then you add on whatever you think you can get away with'.[60]

Of course, consumer products like cars or clothing are not the same as medicines in two key ways. Other products must compete in an open market with other companies making more or less the same product, and they must compete for consumers' attention with a myriad of potential purchases. By contrast, new medicines are sold with a legally enforced monopoly to a captive market of, in this case, patients with a potentially fatal disease for which there was no other treatment.

For all the blustering attempts to impress upon Congress and the public how complicated and carefully weighted the pricing decision had been, senior employees at Burroughs Wellcome would later admit that it had been nothing more sophisticated than, as Sir Alfred Shepperd, chairman at the time of AZT's launch, put it, a 'finger in the wind decision'.

'We didn't know the demand, how to produce it in large quantities, or what competing drugs would come on the market. There was no way we could stop to find out,' he said.[61] In another interview he agreed with the suggestion that it was a gut decision where 'it's almost like, you put your finger in the air . . . and you say, what would the market take?'

'Exactly, yes. That's right,' Shepperd replied.[62]

During the 1987 congressional hearing, Haigler, the chief executive of the US company, said the ability of patients to afford the
medicine hadn't been a consideration. Burroughs had simply assumed
the government would step in if necessary. 'We didn't make any
calculations as to how many patients could or couldn't afford the
drug,' Haigler said.[63] In a prepared statement for the hearing, he
added: 'As we determined the price of the drug . . . we alerted those
responsible for public and private policy and financing to the difficulties that some patients might face in purchasing the drug.'[64]
Burroughs cut the price of AZT by 20 per cent shortly before
Christmas in 1987, citing a reduction in production costs, but the
new price tag of $8,000 remained out of reach for many.

Shortly before the price cut, Staley, who enjoyed a generous medical
insurance package through his Wall Street role, had decided to start
taking AZT. He lasted no more than a couple of months before the
side effects became intolerable; he was so fatigued he even fell asleep
at his trading desk.

Staley struggled through the winter but in March 1988 his T-cell
count dropped below 200 and he decided to draw a line. 'The very
next morning I go into my boss's office first thing and I tell him
everything.' He left the office and was signed off on long-term disability. The news rippled around offices in London and Tokyo. 'I was
the first person to come out as HIV-positive on the US government
bond market, the first person to come out as gay. But I was out the
door as well.'

With time on his hands, Staley threw himself into full-time
activism. A few weeks earlier he had watched with admiration news
reports of protestors being arrested for scaling the roof of a
Burroughs Wellcome warehouse near San Francisco in an effort to
draw attention to the company's 'profiteering'. Patients were being
arrested over the price of a drug. 'It was basically saying, "Sorry,
$8,000 is still way too high,"' Staley says. 'And I loved that. I was
like, yes, we are angry and are hard to satisfy – as we should be.'[65]

In March, ACT UP repeated the protest outside the New York

Stock Exchange which had drawn Staley's attention a year earlier, blocking traffic and holding up placards. More than 100 people were arrested. The activists were becoming well acquainted with the power of media coverage. When they had a sit-in in the lobby of a Japanese pharmaceutical company which was stopping groups of patients known as buyers' clubs from going to Tokyo and buying up stocks of an over-the-counter blood thinner called dextran sulphate which was seen as a potential anti-HIV drug, three of the country's television networks were tipped off. A week later a deal was struck between the company and the Japanese government, reopening the tap.

By October 1988, ACT UP was launching its largest and most spectacular action yet, bussing more than 1,000 people to Maryland to hold a 'die in' which shut down the Food and Drug Administration for a day. The protest, accompanied by a banner reading 'SILENCE=DEATH', was over the lack of access to experimental drugs. The FDA changed its policy within a couple of months.

One morning, Staley decided to telephone Burroughs Wellcome and ask for a meeting. To his surprise, Barry agreed to speak with him. 'He was a brilliant, brilliant scientist,' Staley says. 'But his brilliance was matched by arrogance. And he was so arrogant that he thought he would love to debate these stupid AIDS activists from New York so he agreed to meet with us.'[66]

Staley and another activist, Mark Harrington, flew down to Raleigh-Durham airport on January 23, 1989 to meet with executives from Burroughs Wellcome. Harrington was there to discuss the science, Staley the financial side. They were met at the airport by Lisa Behrens, the public affairs officer who served as a 'peppy tour guide' for the day, and driven to the company's futuristic new headquarters.[67] Harrington thought that the striking modernist building with its concrete sloping walls and angular design looked like something from the film *2001: A Space Odyssey*.[68] Inside, they sat down for lunch with Barry, Behrens and Tom Kennedy, another PR executive. Harrington produced a tape recorder and asked to record the meeting.

He began by questioning the high dosage prescribed for AZT. Why hadn't Burroughs done more work on the effectiveness of a lower dose, given how toxic it was proving, he asked. And why hadn't the recommendation been lowered when a French study published in *The Lancet* the previous month had shown that it was effective at half the dose, something which would significantly reduce the cost for patients? Barry dismissed the French study but said the NIH was running a trial that looked at lower doses anyway. The conversation moved on to price.

'People are being driven into poverty to pay for your drug,' Harrington told Barry and his colleagues. 'People who lack access are dying because they can't get your drug.'[69] Barry brought up Burroughs Wellcome's patient assistance programme but Harrington said no one knew about it. 'It seems to me that you've gone to great efforts to keep this programme from being more well-known,' he said. Staley questioned why Wellcome wasn't paying for the 4,000 people who received the drug through a government assistance programme.

Barry said the company had spent $330 million on research during the previous year in the US and UK and repeatedly referenced Wellcome's stock price as proof the profits being made weren't excessive. 'If people thought we were going to make a huge amount of money, an excessive amount of money, the stock would be way above what it is,' he said.[70] In fact the stock had soared since Wellcome went public three years earlier, up from $1.69 a share to around $7.

What the activists didn't know when Barry talked about the company stock price was that in late 1985, shortly before the flotation, he had tried to put together a management buyout of the US company; something which would have made him a multi-millionaire.[71] Every time the stock went up, it was a reminder of the fortune he had missed out on.

Staley asked Barry about analysts' estimates that improvements in lowering production costs meant the profit margin on the drug was as high as 80 per cent. The Yale-educated scientist wouldn't give a direct answer but remained adamant that he needed every penny that was coming in from AZT. The pair went back and forth. Barry said any price cut would require price increases for other drugs, cuts to research budgets or cuts to the dividend paid to shareholders. He talked about the importance of researching better drugs for the future.

Finally, Harrington couldn't bite his tongue any longer. 'In the meantime, although you don't realise it, because you're far from the scene of the actual battles, people are dying, all the time. People are dying because they do not have access to the drug which is priced beyond the range of most of them, and which in many states is not available. And you're totally washing your hands of responsibility for it.'[72]

The price remained unchanged after the meeting, but it wasn't a complete loss for Staley, who had used the opportunity to scout out the layout of Burroughs Wellcome's headquarters. In April, he and eight other activists piled into a hired minibus and drove to Durham, North Carolina, where they spent the night at a motel. The next day, Staley and three others dressed in business suits and packed their briefcases with walkie-talkies, a banner and electric drills.[73] They made it past security by pretending to have an appointment and asking to use the toilet before dashing into a lift and heading upstairs. Walking into an office, they told the secretary working there that there was a 'security emergency' and she had to leave. Once she was gone, they went to work with the drills, bolting the door closed with metal plates and quick-drying screws. Their plan to display a banner was thwarted, however, when they discovered how strong the reinforced windows were. Even taking a chair to them had little effect.

The activists had brought food, water and medications to last several days but the local police smashed through the thin internal walls and had them out within half an hour. It didn't matter. As the television cameras whirred, the activists were led out, still attached to the chain they'd handcuffed themselves to. It made for a powerful image on the evening news. Staley had hoped that Burroughs would press charges, leading to an attention-grabbing court appearance, but the company saw the trap and declined to do so. The drugmaker did, however, take up ACT UP's offer of paying for the damage and a bill for around $9,000 was settled by the activists.

By the late summer of 1989, pressure on Burroughs Wellcome to reduce the price of AZT had reached a crescendo. The company was under attack from all sides. In August, Dr Tony Fauci, who led the US government's AIDS research effort as director of the National Institute of Allergy and Infectious Diseases (another of the NIH agencies), gave a press conference to announce the results of two government-run clinical trials. They showed that AZT appeared to work as a preventative for patients who were HIV-positive but for whom the disease hadn't progressed to AIDS. Once this use was approved by the FDA, Burroughs Wellcome would have more than half a million patients to sell AZT to who had the virus but no symptoms.

The news sent shares in the company soaring and blew away the remnants of the already threadbare argument that AZT would have only a small market of potential patients. Despite this, Burroughs remained resolute and said it had no plans to change the price.

In late August, Fauci spoke at a conference in San Francisco and urged doctors to 'pressure' Burroughs into reducing the price of the drug.[74] The *New York Times* followed with a hard-hitting editorial under the headline 'AZT's Inhuman Cost'. It described the price of the drug as 'extraordinary' and noted that the company was 75 per cent owned by the Wellcome Trust, a charitable foundation.[75] The editorial criticised the 'strange kind of charity that cordons off people already suffering from a terrifying disease'.

A few days later, sixteen US groups working with AIDS sufferers wrote to Burroughs Wellcome pleading with the company to cut the price of AZT. Dr Sid Wolfe of the pressure group Public Citizen suggested a fair price would be a reduction to around $1,000 a year.[76] Meanwhile, government lawyers were considering invoking a 1910 law which would allow them to override Wellcome's patents and license the drug out for other companies to manufacture and sell for a cheaper price.[77]

On September 7, Staley and other activists including Jean McGuire of the AIDS Action Council met with Barry and several Burroughs Wellcome flacks. Unwilling to let the ACT UP boys back on the company's Research Triangle Park campus, a conference room was booked in an airport hotel in nearby Raleigh. With news vans waiting outside, the activists repeated their complaints. They argued that government-funded scientists had played a huge role in the drug's development and that the market was about to expand hugely. Surely, they pleaded, the price must come down.

It all fell on deaf ears. Congress hadn't yet been persuaded to extend the government's AIDS Assistance Program for low-income patients, which was due to end in September, and activists felt time was running out.[78] During a break in the meeting, Staley pulled Lisa Behrens, the Burroughs PR executive, aside. 'Just so you know, ACT UP is going to have a massive demonstration in front of the New York Stock Exchange in a couple of weeks,' he warned her.[79]

In fact, the activists had something even more spectacular planned.

On the morning of September 14, 1989, seven members of ACT UP gathered at a McDonald's close to Wall Street. The security badges which had nearly led to Staley's undoing during the trial run two days earlier had been hastily remade with lower numbers. They'd told the man behind the counter at the Greenwich Village print shop that they were bankers planning a skit during a forthcoming corporate retreat and he seemed happy to ask no further questions.

Shortly before 9.30 a.m., they walked into the stock exchange, once again passing the security guard unchallenged despite the building having been warned of a planned ACT UP protest on the street outside later that morning.

Five of the activists walked rapidly up the steep staircase leading to the old VIP balcony that Staley had earmarked during the practice run. Once there, they crouched down and began unloading the items they'd smuggled in. Two others, Robert Hilferty and Richard Elovich, blended into the trading floor crowd and got into position to take photographs, fingers fidgeting nervously over the cameras in their pockets.

Up above, the crouching activists pulled out a banner urging traders to 'Sell Wellcome' and put it in position to be unfurled over the balcony. Staley took a large chain from a bum bag strapped to his stomach and wrapped it around the railing, padlocking it in place for the protestors to lock themselves to with handcuffs. Finally, each of the activists took from their pocket a miniature marine foghorn, devices so loud they carried a warning about the risk of ear damage if held too close. On Staley's command, they sounded them in unison.

The effect was instantaneous. 'It's like the world stops,' Staley says. 'The New York Stock Exchange has never heard this sound before and everything just slows down. All eyes are on us.'[80] The noise was so loud no one could hear the opening bell. From their other pockets, the activists pulled out fake bills and threw them over the side of the balcony. As they hit the floor, the traders began reading the message inscribed on one side: 'FUCK YOUR PROFITEERING – people are dying while you play business'.

'I've got this shit-eating grin on my face because I know at that moment that we've totally succeeded,' Staley recalls. The two photographers had captured the protest and gone straight outside to hand their cameras over to a runner who would take the film up to the offices of Associated Press to be developed. The story would be running on news wires within minutes.

Back inside, the traders below were furious. 'They start picking up these dollar bills . . . and they go into rabid mode,' Staley says. 'They start rolling these bills up and throwing them at us. Cans are being thrown at us. We're hearing the f-word. We're hearing "die faggots".' Security rushed to the balcony and had to form a human chain between the protestors and the traders to prevent scuffles breaking out.

As he was eventually led outside to a waiting police van, Staley looked up across the street. He could see his old J.P. Morgan office. 'Our view was the pillars of the New York Stock Exchange – it's what I looked out at for five years.' He knew his former colleagues would be watching, faces pressed to the glass.

The stunt drew huge news coverage, with the activists' actions making the front page of the next day's *Wall Street Journal*. Three days later, Ted Haigler and David Barry walked into Representative Waxman's office and announced they were cutting the price of AZT by 20 per cent.[81]

Those arrested declined the offer of agreeing to community service in exchange for the charges being dropped and appeared in court the following spring. Once there, the judge made a remarkable and highly unusual decision, dropping the charges on the grounds that they had acted in the 'interests of justice'. Judge Richard Braun said that the defendants had tried to 'encourage Burroughs to lower the price of AZT in the hopes that the drug would become accessible to more people in order to prevent possible grave illness to, and the deaths of, great numbers of people'. He concluded that the 'broader community would likely approve of the defendants' fight to bring down the cost of AZT and help AIDS sufferers' and 'most likely condemn Burroughs for charging such a high price for AZT'.[82]

At the start of the year, during their meeting with Barry in Burroughs Wellcome's North Carolina offices, Staley and Harrington had questioned why the company wasn't more vigorously investigating evidence that AZT could be as effective at a much lower dose than the toxic levels being prescribed. It's unclear when exactly the company had become aware of this but in an interview for a Burroughs Wellcome oral history project in 2001, a year before he died, Barry, acknowledging that the 'price was very high', suggested the company had known 'that the dose of the drug was likely to be lowered by half', resulting in a significantly lower price.[83] The results of the large government-funded studies announced by Fauci that August had established the efficacy of lower doses, but months later nothing had been done to secure FDA approval for the change in dosage. It was only in mid-December, two days after receiving a memo from ACT UP demanding a lowering of the dose, that Burroughs Wellcome sent data on the change to the FDA, the *New York Times* reported.[84] A spokeswoman for Burroughs insisted the timing was not connected to ACT UP's action. The following month, the government approved a new recommended dose of 600mg, effectively halving the price of the drug to around $3,000 a year, a far cry from its original price tag.

The dispute over the government's role in developing the medicine didn't end with the new lower price. Shortly after the stock exchange protest, Burroughs Wellcome's American chief executive, Ted Haigler, had a letter published in the *New York Times* defending the 'research risks' the company had taken and all but dismissing the role of the National Cancer Institute team in developing the drug, seeking to portray them as nothing more than a useful pair of hands.[85]

It served to finally push Broder into responding publicly. In an angry rebuttal published in the same newspaper, scientists from the NCI and Duke University, including Broder, wrote that 'there are few drugs approved in this country that owe more to Government-sponsored research.

'We believe that the development of this drug in a record two years, start to finish, would have been impossible without the substantive commitment of Government scientists and Government technology,' they concluded. 'It does not serve anyone's interests to nullify the importance of Government-sponsored research in solving problems of American public health.'[86]

That year, in the wake of what had happened with AZT, the NIH introduced a 'reasonable pricing' clause which would be applied when it licensed drugs it had discovered to pharmaceutical companies. Under the terms of the clause, the government could revoke licences in the case of 'excessive pricing'. Meanwhile, legal challenges to Burroughs Wellcome's patents for AZT were launched by generic companies who wanted to make a cheaper version of the medicine. One, Barr Laboratories, said that if it succeeded with a legal challenge, it would price the drug at half the figure charged by Burroughs, as well as paying the NIH a royalty fee for a non-exclusive licence to use their patent. The cases dragged on for years but the courts ultimately ruled in Burroughs Wellcome's favour, concluding that five of the six patents for AZT were rightfully attributed to Burroughs scientists. The sixth was sent back to a lower court but never pursued.

The fight over AZT placed drug companies on warning that when pricing a drug they couldn't necessarily have things all their own way. There might not be any regulatory or legal restrictions on the price, but companies didn't have complete impunity, particularly when they came up against a well organised and angry patient group. A company's spin on why a price was justified wouldn't just be meekly accepted and the role of public funds in generating private profits became a key topic of debate.

For companies looking to avoid a similar furore in future, it also pointed towards some of the tools the industry could deploy. Patient assistance schemes to give a drug away for free to those in poverty who fell into the cracks between insurance and government safety nets would become an important means of distancing patients from the true price of a drug, and thereby discouraging dissent. Another method was for the industry to begin funding patient groups in the therapeutic areas in which it worked in the hope of exercising an element of control over them. Just as Burroughs began giving thousands of dollars to groups such as the National AIDS Network and the National Association of People with AIDS, companies didn't want to be caught out again by the power of their own patients organising together.[87] Researchers have found that groups with industry funding are more likely to hold positions that benefit their sponsoring companies.[88] Advocacy groups reliant on funding from large drugmakers also have strong financial incentives to avoid criticising their benefactors on pricing and other matters.

More positively, the actions of ACT UP and other groups such as Jean McGuire's AIDS Action Council improved access to promising but experimental drugs while they were still being tested and helped establish the principle that patient groups should be involved in research decisions. Eventually, prices for AIDS treatments would once again spiral but the battle over AZT had an effect for several years. When Bristol-Myers introduced didanosine, known as ddI, a reverse transcriptase inhibitor like AZT, in August 1991, it was cheaper, costing patients just under $2,000 a year.[89] DdI had been discovered by Broder's team at the NCI and licensed to Bristol-Myers, meaning the company was subject to the new 'reasonable pricing' clause and had to pay a royalty of 5 per cent of sales. A third treatment, ddC, was approved for use in conjunction with AZT in 1992 and was slightly cheaper again, with a price tag of around $1,800 a year.[90] Even several years later, in 1996, when breakthrough protease inhibitor drugs came onto the market, companies wary of repeating Burroughs Wellcome's experience steered well clear of the $10,000 price point and kept them to $4,500 to $6,000 a year.

For all the political pressure it came under, the pricing of AZT proved lucrative for Wellcome Plc. When the price cut and the lower dosage brought the price of AZT down, Burroughs quietly raised the price of other drugs, including its herpes drug Zovirax, which was often used by AIDS patients. Between 1985 and 1989 it rose in price by nearly one-third.[91]

Global sales of AZT had reached $1.4 billion by 1992, with estimated profits of almost $600 million, according to a Senate report the following year. Its success helped make the company an attractive target for a takeover by the British giant Glaxo in a £9 billion deal in 1995.

AZT did all this despite a decidedly mixed legacy as a clinical treatment. By the early 1990s it was apparent it offered no benefit as a preventative taken before the onset of AIDS. Tens of thousands of patients had endured severe toxic side effects for no purpose. The drug would still find new life as part of the combination therapies that began emerging a few years later. By the time the patent on AZT in the United States finally expired in 2005, the drug had generated sales of more than $4 billion.[92]

The battle over the price of AZT illustrated the struggle at the heart of the business of selling medicines. It forced the public to consider the central question of how to reward innovation without leaving those who needed the drugs without them, and to confront the issue of who gets to decide what a fair price is. But if activists hoped it might prove to be an object lesson for drug company executives in why they should act reasonably and conservatively when pricing treatments across a broader range of therapy areas, they would prove to be sadly mistaken. Instead, even as Burroughs Wellcome was licking its wounds, a lightning bolt had struck the industry; one which would completely change expectations of what it meant to have a successful drug.

CHAPTER THREE

The hunt for blockbusters

The announcement finally came in February 1987, a month before AZT hit the market. For the first time, a single drug had notched up annual global sales of more than $1 billion. The trophy belonged to Tagamet, a groundbreaking stomach ulcer medication which had gone on sale a decade earlier. The moment was a bittersweet one for the drug's manufacturer, SmithKline Beckman, which had expected to reach that summit several years earlier and was now expending its energies trying, with only fleeting success, to keep a rival product at bay. For the industry, however, it was nothing short of revolutionary.

A drug had previously been considered a top seller if it brought in revenues of $100 million a year. With Tagamet came a new benchmark: the billion-dollar blockbuster. It fired the starting gun on a race to find others. At the end of the 1980s, a handful of drugs had achieved the milestone. By 2006, there would be more than 110.[1] Among them were drugs like Lipitor, Plavix, Nexium, Diovan and Prozac, products which would secure their place among the biggest-selling drugs in the industry's history. There were drugs like Tagamet which meant stomach ulcers no longer required surgery and a hospital stay, but could be treated at home with a simple course of tablets. Others were once-daily pills which lowered cholesterol levels or blood pressure, reducing the risk of a heart attack or stroke. Or anti-depressants which one leading psychiatrist memorably claimed could make you 'better than well'. A panoply of treatments sold to tens of millions of patients.

The industry became fixated on what Jürgen Drews, a former head of global research at Roche, called the 'blockbuster religion'. A large portfolio of drugs, each producing modest profits, was no longer enough. Companies and investors wanted huge, transformative bestsellers: mass-market drugs which would single-handedly send the stock price soaring and provide vast profits and growth for years to come.[2]

The profits of this new age flowed freely. Historically, in the 1970s and early 1980s, profit margins had hovered at around 8 or 9 per cent of revenue. By the end of the 1990s, they had more than doubled. Soon, the ten drug companies on the Fortune 500 list of America's largest companies made more money than all of the other 490 companies combined.[3]

As drug companies hired tens of thousands more employees, their headquarters and research facilities grew into vast campuses: gleaming temples of concrete, glass and chrome built on sites the size of dozens of football pitches complete with employee-only gymnasiums and libraries. Drug industry executives, consistently among the best paid of any industry, flew between offices in luxurious company-owned private jets and helicopters. Meanwhile, the huge profits left those paying for the drugs with soaring bills. In Canada, expenditure on drugs doubled between 1996 and 2003.[4] In Europe, the value of the pharmaceuticals market tripled between 1990 and 2005.[5]

It was no coincidence that top-selling drugs became known, like bestselling films, as blockbusters. As the 1980s progressed, the business models of drug companies and big Hollywood movie studios became more and more alike. Both would rely on a few mega-selling blockbusters to provide the majority of revenues and make up for the flops. As at the cinema, it was very difficult to predict which new drugs would succeed while they were still being developed. The largest revenues didn't necessarily go to films lauded as the critics' choice or the most innovative drugs. But companies gave themselves the best chance with the loud, mass-market approach or with a sequel which tweaked the original formula and hoped to deliver another success.

At the heart of this new direction was the power of marketing: television adverts beamed to American consumers, ghostwritten articles in medical journals and thousands of sharply-dressed sales reps beating their way to the doors of doctors' surgeries across the United States and other key drug markets. Blockbusters, so the mantra went, were made not discovered. Similar drugs from different companies could have radically different revenues on the strength of a manufacturer's ability to market it effectively.

Tagamet's success had prompted only muted celebrations for its manufacturer because the Philadelphia-based drugmaker was in the midst of a struggle for market dominance with another anti-ulcer drug. Glaxo's Zantac was, like Tagamet, an H2-histamine antagonist, which had launched six years after its rival but quickly gained ground as a result of an exemplary marketing campaign. Zantac only needed to be taken twice a day, unlike Tagamet's four-times-a-day regimen, and a promotional campaign hammered home the results of studies which suggested patients would suffer fewer side effects.

By the end of 1987, just ten months after confirmation that Tagamet had reached $1 billion in annual sales, Zantac became the world's biggest selling drug, a position it would hold for nearly a decade. Its success had been secured by the tools which would dominate this new era. It wasn't about a cheap price – at launch, Zantac was 50 per cent more expensive than the already established Tagamet.[6] It was about marketing.

For those who grasped this, the blockbuster age offered the opportunity to transform a previously middling company into a global behemoth. Over the course of the 1990s, Pfizer upended Merck Sharp & Dohme as the largest drug company in the world, driven by its mastery of the dark arts of pharmaceutical marketing. The company was so adept at selling drugs that rivals beat a path to its door, offering up a share of their profits on promising new drug launches if Pfizer would lend its marketing muscle. One such deal, reached with the American company Warner–Lambert, helped turn Lipitor into the first ever $10 billion-a-year drug.

The foot soldiers of these victories, from Zantac's triumph over

Tagamet to Lipitor's over a host of rival statins, were the travelling reps sent out to persuade doctors to prescribe a particular company's drugs. Drug reps were employed across Europe, Israel, Australia and Japan, amongst other markets, but it was in the United States where the idea that any medical problem could be solved with a pill was truly in full swing.

In the autumn of 1998, Shahram Ahari was looking for a job. His mother had returned to their native Iran, he'd just finished his degree, and he wasn't sure what exactly it was he wanted to do with his life. Starting a PhD in molecular genetics was a possibility, but the idea of spending all day stuck in a lab wasn't very enticing. Besides, after four years of paying his own way through university, he was tired of being broke.

Then his roommate's brother mentioned he could get him a job interview at Eli Lilly. The company had an opening for a pharmaceutical rep in its neuroscience division. He'd be selling the company's two cash cows – the antidepressant Prozac and the antipsychotic Zyprexa – which together made up half of the company's sales. When he found out it came with a starting salary of more than $50,000 plus bonuses, a company car, stock options and a large expense account, Ahari was sold.

A couple of months later, he was among two dozen would-be reps who were flown to Indianapolis and put up in well-appointed condos while they attended six weeks of sales training on Lilly's expansive campus.

Ostensibly, the role of a drug rep is to educate doctors and provide samples of a company's medicines. Ahari thought the new job would allow him to put his molecular biology and biochemistry degree to good use, spending his time talking to doctors about 'the merits of one molecule versus another in the language of hard science'.[7] But as he took a seat in the windowless room, one of several where training would take place, what seemed to be the true requirements for the job began to become apparent.

The other reps included a used-car salesman, an elementary school teacher and a physical fitness instructor, all retraining in a new field. What they had in common, Ahari realised, was that they 'were all engaging, charismatic, and very attractive'. They were there to sell a product; the fact that this particular product was a drug made no real difference.[8]

Lilly wasn't alone in this; the practice of recruiting athletic and good-looking sales reps was commonplace. 'That was the culture across the board,' Ahari says. 'Pfizer was notorious for hiring these statuesque former athletes or models, just beautiful people – they looked like they belong on a magazine cover rather than ploughing the streets of New York with drugs in their bag.' Former cheerleaders proved such popular recruits as drug reps that, for a few years in the mid-2000s, a Tennessee-based recruitment company built a business which helped graduates who had been on cheer teams find jobs at drugmakers.[9]

The pharmaceutical industry has employed people to go out and talk to doctors about their wares since the middle of the twentieth century. Back then, the well-spoken 'detail men' who toured physicians' offices with a clutch of scientific articles were expected to have a degree in science and some companies, including Lilly, employed registered pharmacists to do the work.[10]

These 'sober, conservatively-dressed gentlemen' were a different breed to the recruits of the 1990s.[11] As training started, it quickly became apparent that Ahari was the only rep with a scientific background. Even the trainers, one of whom was a former basketball player who'd briefly made it to the NBA, didn't seem to Ahari to have any detailed knowledge.

'On the first day of sales school, I had to explain to my instructors and to my classmates how a neuron works,' Ahari says.[12] 'And that was when I realised that no one in that room had any college-level science education.' As time went on, he came to understand that it 'wasn't the science which sold the drugs, it was the personality of the drug reps and the relationship [with doctors]'.

Ahari and his fellow trainees spent six weeks learning how to persuade doctors to buy the company's drugs. There were science lessons, but from what he called the 'Eli Lilly perspective, meaning you know all the benefits of your medication and you know all the flaws of your competitors'. The reps were taught psychological analysis techniques to allow them to 'deconstruct your target . . . and figure out how to motivate them'. And, again and again, they practised what they would say when out in the field talking to doctors, taking it in turns to play the rep or the physician and adjusting for everything from a sixty-second elevator pitch to a lengthy directed conversation over a meal.

There was, Ahari says, a win-at-all-costs mentality. Flirting or any sexual interest was 'seen as a weapon in your arsenal – use it when you can'. The official limits on expenses were there to be worked around. If doctors brought up the side effects of a drug, reps were told to play them down or change the topic.

When sales school was finished, Ahari was partnered with another new rep – a pretty, young former sorority member who, like him, had recently left college – and equipped with the key tools of the trade: free samples, a large expense account and, the rep's secret weapon, a laptop. Along with a senior colleague, they were assigned around 300 doctors across Brooklyn and Staten Island.

Ahari and other reps were instructed not to let doctors see their laptops. They didn't want to give physicians any inkling of the huge amount of information they had on them. New technology enabled drug companies to buy data showing exactly how many prescriptions individual doctors had written for specific drugs each month. The laptops also allowed reps to maintain a company-wide database carefully recording everything they had gleaned about a doctor.

'So we would write things like, "I spoke with Dr Smith, he's in the throes of a divorce, he's very upset, can't talk today, we left samples. But he does want to go to dinner at this restaurant next week – use that as leverage." And if my partner writes that [then] I come into the office and say, "Hey, Dr Smith, we've got reservations at this restaurant you wanted to go to if that's OK. I'm very sorry for your personal difficulties. We'll go out there, we'll have a good time, we won't talk medicine. It will just be our way of saying thank you for all your loyalty."'

The granular prescription data allowed reps to assign each doctor a number from one to ten depending on how many prescriptions for the company's drugs they were writing. Anyone below five didn't warrant a visit, while the best prescribers were lavished with attention.

Ahari aimed to visit nine different surgeries or doctors' offices each day. If a doctor didn't want to meet, he would look to ingratiate himself with other members of staff, including receptionists, nurses and pharmacists.

He might show up every Friday morning with coffee and bagels, establishing a routine which meant that if a doctor wanted him to leave he or she would have to contend with staff unhappy that they were no longer getting a free breakfast.

If he made it into a doctor's office, every piece of information was weaponised: 'I look for magazines, I look for pictures of family, I look for degrees on the wall, postcards, music they listen to, anything, any personalising aspect in the office. I try to find a bridge where I can find a relationship with the doctor or find a bridge that maybe my partner can capitalise on.'

As soon as he left the office, he would go back to his car and type up everything he'd memorised in a 'call report'. Any observation or titbit, even gossip, could ultimately help to push prescription numbers up.

During his frequent office calls, Ahari would hand over free samples of the company's drugs. He said drug reps view samples 'in the same way that the free bag of crack cocaine is given on the street. The first one is free and then you're hooked.' As well as the visits and samples, Ahari, like other Lilly reps, had an annual expenses budget of $100,000 – and he was expected to use it.

Dinners were commonplace, with drug reps dining out with doctors several nights a week, frequently at fancy Manhattan restaurants where, even two decades ago, the $100 per head cap on expenses wouldn't go far. Fortunately, Ahari says, 'our instructors would teach us ways to work around that approach'. He knew of colleagues who were 'spending over $1,000 a night with certain clients, some of whom were taken to strip clubs after dinner, drinks, things like that'.

If a doctor liked a sports team, they would be taken to a baseball or basketball game, with the drug company covering the cost. If they were a fan of musicals, here was a pair of the hottest tickets on Broadway, free of charge. Gifts, even cheap ones like branded pens or clipboards, were used to engender a sense of 'reciprocity'.

'You want to cultivate a sense of gratitude and rather counter-intuitively . . . little gifts tend to create a disproportionate amount of reciprocity,' Ahari explains. These cheap gifts were handed out so frequently that when, in 2008, the industry adopted a voluntary ban on the practice, a trade association for promotional products suggested its members would lose $1 billion a year.[13]

The events were designed to create a personal relationship between the drug rep and the doctor which could be leveraged later. As one Lilly instructor told Ahari: 'When you're at dinner with a doctor, they're sitting with a friend, but you're sitting with a client.'

For some doctors, larger rewards were available. 'At the time we also had unconditional grants, which were basically a blank cheque. Ostensibly it was for the physician's research or a consulting fee but it could just as well have been arranged that it was going to lay the foundation for their swimming pool.' Lilly paid for doctors to attend conferences in the Caribbean, while those with the right credentials – meaning 'a degree from the right school [and] proper drug loyalty' – could be put on the speaker circuit. They'd start small, perhaps joining a dinner with other local doctors, but if they proved to be good speakers who could 'handle objections in a seemingly neutral manner' they could be elevated to the national circuit, earning thousands of dollars per speech.

With their years of training and specialist knowledge, the doctors Ahari targeted didn't believe that a few nice dinners or inexpensive gifts could change their prescribing behaviour. But the figures the reps had access to for each doctor told a different story.[14]

'This is not a logic process, this is a social process,' Ahari says. 'And the drug reps vastly outnumber and outgun the physicians. We have money to spend, we have time to burn, we're engaging and charismatic people that were selected based on those natural talents and the training takes it to an escalated level.' With some doctors, friendly contact with reps who would, at the right moment, talk up the benefits of their drugs was enough to drive up prescriptions. Others needed more of a push.

'You could say, "Hey, doctor, I've been giving you free samples of Prozac for the past six months. You haven't told me of any new patients you've put on Prozac, my boss is concerned that I'm just giving you these free samples and he doesn't think that you really want to use our drug. I told him that wasn't the case but do you think you can give me three new patients on Prozac between now and the next time I visit? Otherwise my boss is going to tell me I'm not allowed to give you samples any more",' Ahari explains.

The tactics he'd been taught were very effective but they didn't need to be. 'Prozac and Zyprexa practically sold themselves,' he says. 'Our goal was not just to command market share, but to expand the market and encourage their use in patients who might be depressed, who might be in the grey diagnostic field for depression.'

When some doctors raised concerns that Zyprexa was causing significant weight gain in some patients, he was told by Lilly's marketing department to allay their concerns by suggesting patients be instructed to drink water before and after taking the drug in order to reduce their appetite. If that didn't work, he would ask doctors: 'Would you rather have a fat, sane patient, or a skinny, psychotic patient?'

'The overarching concept as a rep is that you minimise side effects, redirect the conversation elsewhere where you can or offer suggestions that might manage it,' Ahari says. Over the next decade, Lilly would spend more than $1.2 billion settling thousands of lawsuits from people who claimed they developed diabetes or other diseases after taking Zyprexa. The company agreed to pay another $1.4 billion to settle claims it had instructed sales reps to market the drug 'off-label' for non-approved uses including as a dementia treatment.

Ahari stuck at it for the best part of two years, but he eventually became disillusioned. He says it had become clear that 'the marketing isn't there to benefit the physician'.

'This doesn't help physicians make the best clinical decision, it just helps promote a product.'

Nevertheless, the experience left him with some clarity about what he wanted to do with his life. He moved into public health and later went to medical school. Ahari now works as an accident and emergency doctor in a hospital in Rochester, New York. 'All of it after Eli Lilly was this notion of public service.' Having left Iran during the cultural revolution, he found he 'really appreciated any opportunity I had to feel I was a contributing member of the community'.[15]

Ahari had joined Eli Lilly in the midst of a huge recruitment boom for drug reps. While he was at the company, it opened an $18 million training centre and increased its US sales force from 3,600 to 6,000 reps.[16] Across the industry, the number of drug reps increased from 38,000 in 1995 to 100,000 in 2005, amounting to one drug rep for every six doctors.[17] Marketing and administrative costs, by the industry's own estimates, outstripped the amount being spent on researching and developing new drugs. Even then, industry figures are likely to underplay the amount spent on promoting drugs because they exclude the cost of some promotional exercises, such as meetings or talks paid for by a pharmaceutical company or post-approval Phase IV clinical trials, many of which are designed to generate data which can be used to promote the prescribing of a particular drug.[18] At one point, as many as three-quarters of these trials were managed by a company's commercial side rather than the clinical division, an indication of the true purpose of the exercise.[19]

Despite periodic bouts of public concern over their activities – as long ago as 1974, Senate hearings had revealed that doctors were being awarded points for prescribing drugs; points which could then be exchanged for colour televisions, watches and golf clubs – drug reps at the time were unregulated.[20] In 2002, an industry body introduced a voluntary code of conduct, but Ahari believes it made little difference because reps were already being encouraged to circumvent their companies' own expenses rules.

The growth in sales reps in the 1990s was accompanied by an explosion in advertising targeted directly at potential patients in the United States. Most developed countries had long prohibited drug companies from placing adverts for prescription medicines aimed at the general public, driven by concerns that supposed efforts to educate patients were in fact designed to get patients to pressure their doctor to prescribe expensive brand-name drugs.

In the US, companies had been placing direct-to-consumer adverts in the 1980s but were obliged to include an often lengthy list of side effects in any advert which made claims about the benefits of a drug. This was just about tenable in magazine inserts or other print ads, but it proved impossible to include in a relatively short TV advert and pressure grew on the FDA to revise the onerous requirement.

In 1997, in a landmark decision, the industry got its way. The FDA decided that TV adverts for drugs needed only to disclose major risks, with patients directed to a toll-free phone number or website for a fuller list of side effects. With the new guidance, the US joined New Zealand as the only countries in which direct-to-consumer adverts for prescription drugs could include claims about the clinical value of the medicine and the floodgates were opened for flashy drug adverts to be beamed directly into American homes. A former presidential candidate was hired to sell an erectile dysfunction treatment while American football stars touted the benefits of hypertension and cholesterol drugs.

Soon, some of the most advertised drugs in the world's largest pharmaceuticals market were also the most successful, with three of the ten most heavily advertised drugs also making it onto a list of 2001's ten most-prescribed drugs.[21] The industry's spending on direct marketing to consumers in the US rocketed from $47 million a year in 1990 to $1.2 billion in 1998.[22] Prescription drug adverts remain a mainstay of daytime television in the US to this day, with more than 770,000 a year recorded.[23]

Television adverts and the thousands of new sales reps stalking the floors in doctors' surgeries and hospitals were necessary because achieving the vaunted blockbuster status often required drugs to elbow their way there through crowded markets. When a new drug hits the market as the first of its kind in a new drug class, the first statin for example, or the first SSRI antidepressant, it is often followed by a multitude of competitors with a similar chemical structure. These follow-on drugs became known as 'me-toos', and with little difference in clinical value, the competition for market share they created was fierce. Throughout the late 1980s and 1990s, around half of new drugs hitting the market were deemed to offer little or no therapeutic benefit over existing options, according to the designations applied by the American regulator.[24] Only just over one in four drugs launched each year were deemed to be significant improvements.[25]

'Me-too drugs' prompted criticism that the pharmaceutical industry was deliberately going after easier, duplicate drugs rather than investing in the riskier environs of cutting-edge science and untapped therapeutic areas. Ahari, the ex-Lilly sales rep, believes some companies took the view: 'Why make it complicated for yourself? Why find a novel pathological mechanism for treating depression? Why find an alternative target for reducing blood pressure or cholesterol? The blockbuster period showed that you can reinvent the wheel and still make a profit,' he says.[26]

Given how long it typically takes to bring a drug from the laboratory to the market, drug companies couldn't simply watch a rival successfully launch a drug and then seek to ape it. If they started from scratch, by the time they came to market the original drug would likely have gone off patent and they would now be competing with cheap generics. Instead, 'me-too' drugs often reflect the clustering caused by rival companies following the same advances in science and the same target markets – those chronic diseases with large numbers of patients. Novel ideas for new drug targets in the body, or advances in the understanding of a particular disease, would generally originate in academia. Multiple companies would pick up on the same ideas and begin trying to identify new compounds to hit those targets. In the competitive race to market that followed, the companies who were slower might be left with 'me-too' drugs which they had hoped would be an entirely novel therapy. In other cases, compounds which had been put on a shelf or projects which had not been prioritised could be given a new impetus by news that a competing company had successfully completed an expensive clinical trial with a similar drug. These rival companies could now rush their own versions to market without having to shoulder the same level of risk the original company had in funding an expensive clinical trial for a drug with a previously unproven mechanism of action. By the late 1990s, the average time the first drug in a new class had in the market without competition was down to just over fourteen months and in almost all cases a rival was already in clinical trials when the first drug went on sale.[27]

A flock of new drugs in the same class didn't necessarily result in a winner-takes-all situation; several drug classes were large enough to contain multiple blockbuster drugs. But generally only one or two drugs would reap the majority of the sales. These winners were likely to be determined by the success or failure of marketing efforts aimed at demonstrating that company's product was better or more convenient than its rivals. In a normal market, an increase in supply should result in price competition and lower prices. However, the launch of new on-patent 'me-too' drugs did not generally lead to significant price reductions.[28] As we shall see in the next chapter, even with three or four competing versions, drugmakers found it far more effective to rely on marketing which emphasised differences in side effects or toxicity rather than cutting prices.

With a strong marketing campaign, a late arrival could still out-muscle competing drugs to dominate a new field. Tagamet, the first blockbuster drug, responded to the launch of other stomach ulcer drugs by raising rather than cutting its price.[29] Although Tagamet had been first to go on sale, it was subsequently out-marketed by a competitor, Glaxo's Zantac, and rapidly lost market share. By the end of the decade, Zantac was being prescribed twice as much and the failure forced Tagamet's manufacturer SmithKline Beckman to merge with another company, Beecham.[30] Ultimately this new company would itself merge with Glaxo.

When the cholesterol-reducing drug Lipitor was launched in 1997, there were already four types of statins on the market. Atorvastatin, the generic name of Lipitor, appeared to have an advantage over the existing drugs because clinical trials had shown it was more effective at lowering bad cholesterol and so could be taken in lower doses.[31] Nevertheless, Warner–Lambert, who decided to partner with Pfizer to promote the drug so they could focus their in-house sale efforts on a new diabetes pill, did not expect a huge success, believing the statins market was simply too saturated. Surveys showed that doctors were happy with the statins they were already prescribing and were unlikely to change their habits. 'I wish someday you guys could make us a drug we could sell,' the drug's inventor, Bruce D. Roth, recalled being told by the company's marketing division.[32]

Warner–Lambert expected peak sales of no more than $300 million a year. Instead, bolstered by Pfizer's sales force, the initial demand was so high stocks ran out. In the first year alone, sales reps promoting Lipitor made nearly one million visits to doctors, highlighting how effective the drug was at a lower dose than rivals, while millions of free samples had been given out to patients who it was hoped would remain on the drug for years.[33] Unusually for a new drug, Lipitor was priced significantly below its rivals and the price, coupled with its potency, which appealed to doctors who might feel uncomfortable giving patients higher doses, made it a runaway success. Barely twelve months after it had launched, Lipitor had already captured 20 per cent of the market.

Lipitor's success led to a battle for control of Warner–Lambert which was won by Pfizer in a $90 billion takeover bid. It had already benefited from the promotion other firms had done to raise consumer awareness of the dangers of high cholesterol levels, and to suggest this was treatable with pharmaceuticals, but Pfizer's strategy now was to change the parameters of when a statin was needed. To do so, *Fortune* magazine reported, Pfizer and Warner–Lambert took advantage of the relaxation in television advertising rules to launch a campaign 'aimed at conveying two simple messages. The first: You don't have to be visibly unhealthy to have dangerously high cholesterol. The second: "Know your number" – that is, the level of bad cholesterol in your blood. A reading above 160 milligrams per deciliter of blood is considered risky, while a reading below 100 is optimal.'[34] The ad breaks on the hugely popular George Clooney medical drama *ER* were frequently punctuated with Lipitor ads repeating this 'know your number' refrain.

Lipitor's advertising didn't always stay on the right side of the line. The FDA ordered the withdrawal of adverts for the drug which had either falsely claimed it was safer than competing statins or given the misleading impression it could reduce heart disease.[35] But these citations had no impact on the success of Pfizer's marketing push. Lipitor became the bestselling drug of all time, bringing in a peak of nearly $13 billion in revenue in 2006 and racking up global sales to date of more than $150 billion.

Pfizer, like other statin manufacturers, benefited from changes in guidelines on what were deemed to be acceptable levels of LDL, or bad cholesterol. This shifting definition of what was considered healthy, and therefore how large a market for a drug might be, was not unique to anti-cholesterol drugs. Common conditions, everything from depression to diabetes, saw expanding benchmarks and new categories of 'pre-disease', often pushed through by panels where the majority of members had financial ties to drugmakers who stood to benefit from their new guidance. One study looking at fourteen new clinical guidelines issued in the 2000s found that, on average, 75 per cent of the authors had financial ties to the industry.[36] A 2004 decision to lower the threshold of acceptable LDL levels was taken by a nine-person panel, eight of whom had financial ties with statin manufacturers.[37]

The changes led to accusations that drug companies became adept at 'selling illness' or 'disease mongering', packaging up a normal characteristic as something treatable, or encouraging patients with even relatively low risks of developing a condition to take a preventative pill.[38] The charge is perhaps most associated with so-called lifestyle drugs which recast pharmaceuticals as enhancements for the well, rather than merely cures for the sick. None are better known than the diamond-shaped blue sildenafil citrate pills sold by Pfizer: Viagra.

Viagra was initially developed as a possible treatment for the heart condition angina before patients in clinical trials began reporting an unexpected side effect: frequent and lasting erections. Brought to market as a cure for impotence, Pfizer's marketing machinery soon broadened it out into a 'lifestyle accessory' which could enhance the sex lives of ordinary men.[39] Male impotence had previously been seen as a specific issue arising from other underlying medical problems, such as a spinal injury or diabetes.[40] But with high-profile television adverts fronted by former Republican presidential candidate Bob Dole, and later by a retired baseball star, Rafael Palmeiro, the blue pill was promoted to the mass market. Pfizer's advertising and promotional materials raised awareness of erectile dysfunction, but it also expanded the definition of who might warrant treatment to include younger men and those with only mild or occasional issues. They too, the marketing suggested, could enjoy improved sex lives by taking a pill. Viagra became, in the words of a Canadian professor who studied Pfizer's tactics, 'a drug that "normal" men could use to enhance their ability to achieve an erection and to maintain it (in a "harder" state)'.[41] Clinical trial data showed that only around half of patients taking the drug in two trials had reported their attempts at having sex as having been successful. Pfizer, however, emphasised more subjective measures of success, namely the more than 80 per cent of men who believed it had improved their erections.

The pursuit of blockbuster drugs had wide-reaching consequences for the industry. It contributed to an expansion in R&D spending as companies lured scientists away from academia and into for-profit research, but it also shaped the focus of that R&D. The best route to a mass market and windfall profits was a new drug for a chronic illness which had to be taken daily for patients' entire lives, so investment in 'lifestyle drugs' soared: drugs like Viagra and Prozac which could be sold to the masses as pills which would make them happier and improve their sex lives. By the early 2000s, more than $20 billion had been invested in research into drugs which promised to reverse life's gradual atrophy: improving mental function, making patients thinner or reversing hair loss.[42]

Companies became more ruthless at nixing development projects which didn't appear to have a big enough market, even though the industry showed a resolute inability to accurately predict which drugs would become blockbusters. The balance of power within companies began to shift away from scientists and towards the marketers. At the US drug company Merck & Co., long held up as the most research-oriented of the industry giants, employees in the marketing department were given a role in even the earliest stages of drug development.[43]

Jürgen Drews, the former Roche executive, complained in 2003 that scientists and the 'rigour and discipline of good science' were losing control in favour of 'a marketing dogma in which R&D is degraded to a tool for generating medicines that qualify as block-busters'.[44] He believed scientists needed freedom to roam, to take creative approaches and have the time for serendipitous discoveries. Everything, in short, this new era appeared to be turning away from.

Bernard Munos held similar views. Born in Morocco to French and Spanish parents, Munos has retained a Gallic insouciance and accent despite spending most of his career in America. Much of that – some thirty years – was spent working for the company which had employed Ahari as a sales rep, Eli Lilly. Munos, who holds three degrees, joined Lilly, one of the great American drugmakers, fresh out of business school in 1980. One of his earlier degrees had been in animal science and so he started in the animal health division, working his way through a variety of marketing and business oper-ations roles. It was an exciting time to be working at the company. 'The first decade for me was exhilarating. Going to work was a blast every day,' he says. 'You'd rub shoulders with people who were truly innovative scientists. They'd have fresh perspective on everything. They'd blow your mind every day. I couldn't get enough of it.'

When he joined, a public-spirited ethos remained firmly entrenched. He recalled sitting on a monthly committee reviewing inventory levels of the company's products in different areas of the business. It was around 1984 and Munos, who had received his MBA from Stanford a few years earlier, was keen to show his aptitude for finding money-saving efficiencies.

Sitting in the meeting, Munos, who was there to represent the animal health division, noticed that the main pharmaceutical business had a large amount of one of the company's drugs, the hormone replacement insulin, sitting in warehouses.

'And so I brought up and I said, "We're trying to be efficient . . . and it seems to me that we're really out of line with insulin, that we could do ourselves a lot of good if we can whittle down those inventories",' Munos says. 'And I remember an old timer, a Vice President, sitting across a table from me and really getting unhinged with that.'

The executive pointed at Munos. 'Insulin is a life-saving drug,' he told him, weighing each word. 'And yes, we have a lot of it around this company, because no patient should be unable to access it for whatever reason, earthquake, calamities, whatever. And you know what, it may not make sense to an MBA like you, but it makes a lot of sense for patients. And this is the way it has been, and this is the way it's going to be.'

'That was the culture of the industry at the time,' Munos says. 'We're going to do the right thing, and if we do the right thing, we'll be successful.'

In 1986, he accepted a move to Europe, first a year in Lisbon and then other roles in Vienna, helping with the company's business in central and eastern Europe, and in Paris, where he was tasked with kicking French operations into shape. When he returned to Indianapolis in 1993, he sensed something had changed. Many of his former colleagues were still around, but they seemed different now. 'Somehow the dynamic had changed, the culture was not the same,' he says.[45] It took him several years to realise what was happening, something he saw close-up when he moved to the pharmaceutical side in 1998 as a strategy advisor on R&D.

Middle management was changing. Scientists were being replaced by business executives and with them came a more disciplined approach. These new managers lacked a detailed understanding of the science behind drug discovery and 'frankly, were uncomfortable with the risk that is inherent in science', Munos says. They wanted researchers to commit to specific targets and to focus on developing new drugs which were within the 'marketing franchises' each company had built – the therapeutic areas where the company already had a blockbuster drug, accompanied by a formidable sales and marketing infrastructure which had built relationships with the doctors working in that field.

Researchers were put to work to come up with replacements for these key blockbuster drugs, improved versions which could be sold to the same patients. So when Prozac's patent life was running out, 'the CEO demanded a replacement [neuroscience drug] and in doing so overlooked the fact that science was not really ready to provide anything much better than Prozac'.

In that situation, 'at best you would get a "me-too" kind of replacement that really doesn't do much to improve public health', Munos says.

The hunt for blockbusters also created an urgency to get a new drug on the market and prescribed to as many people as possible. 'The blockbuster era [philosophy] was every quarter's profits needs to be greater than the last,' Ahari, the former Lilly drug rep, says. This could have calamitous consequences. For all the data companies have to generate to satisfy regulators before they can enter the market, significant and unexpected side effects can still emerge within the first years after launch.

If Pfizer's ascent up the rankings of the world's largest drug companies marked it out as the biggest winner of the blockbuster age, Merck & Co., for years America's most respected company, was high on the list of losers. After Roy Vagelos reached retirement age and had to stand down as CEO in 1994, the company's reputation and profits slumped as his successor struggled to find new drugs to replace the previous bestsellers as their patents expired. Vioxx, a

treatment for acute pain and arthritis, was touted as the drug that
would finally halt the slide when it hit the market in 1999 and it
quickly reached $1 billion in US sales. Within five years of its launch,
however, it was pulled from pharmacy shelves amid growing evidence
that the painkiller increased the risk of a heart attack or stroke. It
subsequently emerged that concerns about these risks had been raised
within MSD years earlier.[46] A US official estimated that between
30,000 and 55,000 people could have died prematurely as a result of
taking the drug.[47] The company ended up spending $5 billion to
resolve legal claims brought by tens of thousands of patients and
paid another $1 billion in a settlement with the US Justice Department
over the illegal marketing of the drug.

   The pursuit of billion-dollar drugs which consumed the pharmaceutical industry placed marketing departments, and the businessmen
and women who led them, at the forefront of driving up profits.
Their focus on trying to cajole more and more doctors to write more
and more prescriptions, and the sort of drugs that flourished with
this approach, pushed aside some of the old norms governing how
drugmakers could be expected to behave. Alongside this development
in the late 1980s came another major cultural shift: the arrival of the
biotechs and, with them, a newly aggressive and less inhibited
approach to setting prices. It had its roots in an unlikely source.

CHAPTER FOUR

How to price a drug

Abbey Meyers sat in the waiting room with the torn-out section of *Parade* magazine placed carefully in her purse.[1] She had known there was something different about her nine-year-old son David since he was an infant, but no one could explain exactly what was causing the twitching, flailing arms and strange noises. Finally, she thought she had found the answer.

The article was about a teenager with a rare neurological condition, Tourette's syndrome, and the description of his symptoms seemed to match David's. She handed it to the paediatrician and told him to read it. 'The doctor was amazed because he said "I've never heard of this disease",' Meyers recalls.[2] He went away and did some research and came back with a number for a specialist: Dr Arthur Shapiro in New York City.

Dr Shapiro put David onto the only approved treatment for the disease, but the heavy-duty tranquilliser had severe side effects and they moved on to trying drugs intended for other conditions. 'We went through a series of drugs, most of which put him to sleep so he couldn't stay awake in class,' Meyers says. 'Finally the doctor said he was doing a small clinical trial on a drug that was approved in Europe but not in the United States and maybe we should try David on that.'

The drug was Pimozide and the effect on David proved miraculous. Meyers remembers thinking that 'this is the drug that I will keep him on for the rest of his life'. A year or so later, however, there was a shock. When they went to the doctor's office to collect the latest three-month supply, Dr Shapiro had some bad news: this would be the last time he could give them the drug. The small investigational study he had been running had been of little interest to the company which held the drug's American rights, a subsidiary of Johnson & Johnson called McNeil Laboratories. They were applying for approval to sell the drug as a treatment for schizophrenia but this had hit complications and McNeil Laboratories had decided it wasn't worth launching the medication in the US after all.

'What about people with Tourette's syndrome?' Meyers asked.

'There aren't enough people with Tourette's syndrome in the United States to convince the company that the drug could be profitable,' the doctor replied.[3] He said it was known as an orphan drug.

At the time Meyers's son's Pimozide ran out in 1979, the pharmaceutical industry viewed research into rare conditions as a backwater. There were thousands of serious illnesses and conditions which each afflicted only a relatively small number of people so even a successful treatment promised small financial rewards. Once the costs of paying scientists' wages, setting up a new manufacturing facility and advertising to try and locate patients who might benefit were taken into account, it just didn't seem worth doing.

The term 'orphan drug' was first coined in 1963 by Harry C. Shirkey, an American paediatrician, to describe medications which had been approved to treat adults but whose manufacturers had avoided the additional expense of seeking approval as a treatment for children.[4] The definition subsequently expanded to include any drug which a company wasn't making because they felt the market wasn't big enough. Among them was a host of medicines which had proved effective at treating a rare disease but were of no interest to manufacturers. Drugmakers had once been prepared to make these 'public service drugs' at a small financial loss but times had changed and this was no longer the case.[5]

With the failure of the clinical trial, Pimozide had been orphaned and was no longer available in the United States. David came off the drug once the last batch ran out but other Tourette's patients found ways to buy it overseas, where it was still available, and bring it back into the country. Muriel Seligman, the mother of a Californian teenager with Tourette's syndrome, was one of those who managed to get the drug from Canada. Seligman, whom Meyers had met through Tourette's support groups, had a friend who would fly north on business with a prescription from her son Adam's doctor, collecting Pimozide from a Canadian pharmacy and bringing it back in his suitcase.

Like David Meyers, Adam Seligman had tried a series of other medicines – nearly thirty in his case – and struggled with their severe side effects before trying Pimozide on a friend's recommendation.[6] He had been on the drug for several months when, one autumnal morning in 1979, his mother's friend flew into San Francisco airport and was stopped by customs officers. They confiscated the drug. As it wasn't licensed in the US, it was illegal for anyone to bring the drug into the country unless it was for their own personal use. After the drug was seized as contraband, Seligman's mother rang Meyers in a panic and was advised to ring her local congressman.

'They took the drug that my son needs,' she told a member of Henry Waxman's staff who answered her call. 'What are you going to do about it?'[7] Waxman was already a well-known Democratic congressman with significant clout and an interest in health policy. The phone call led to a hearing on Capitol Hill in June 1980 to highlight the problem of drugs and diseases which the pharmaceutical industry didn't deem sufficiently profitable. Adam, then eighteen, appeared before the subcommittee to describe how Pimozide had enabled him to graduate from high school, while the alternative drug, which he would now have to return to, 'brought fatigue, depression [and] blurred vision'.[8] Waxman also heard from Melvin Van Woert, a doctor at Mount Sinai Hospital in New York, who was treating patients with a neurological disorder called myoclonus with an experimental drug called L-5-HTP. Patients who were 'bedridden or completely incapacitated are able to take care of themselves and walk while on L-5-HTP therapy', Dr Van Woert said.[9] He had tried to interest a pharmaceutical company in producing the drug in pill form but was repeatedly rebuffed; the market was too small and L-5-HTP is an amino acid which is naturally present in the body, meaning it was not patentable. Instead, Dr Van Woert was making the 'miracle powder' himself, buying the chemical in its raw form and relying on recovered patients volunteering to help purify and pack it into capsules in his laboratory.[10]

The cause picked up more steam after a newspaper report of the hearing caught the eye of Maurice Klugman, a writer and producer who was himself suffering from a rare form of cancer. Klugman's brother, Jack, was the star of a popular American television show, *Quincy, M.E.*, in which he played a medical examiner solving unusual cases. After speaking to Meyers, they decided to write an episode to push for an Act of Congress to address the problem.

In the episode, which was broadcast in 1981, a character called Tony Ciotti, who has Tourette's, appears before Congress. A spirited Ciotti tells the assembled politicians he is there to speak on behalf of 'anyone who is unlucky enough to have a disease that never made it to the top forty'. He bemoans the lack of interest in rare diseases while 'all the drug companies are tripping over one another, trying to come up with a better diet pill or a better sleeping pill . . . The truth is that the only real chance of research money going to these diseases is if you the Congress make the orphan drug bill a reality,' Ciotti concludes.[11]

In the meantime, Meyers, who was involved with a group for parents of children with Tourette's syndrome, had picked up the phone and talked to those representing other rare diseases. 'I realised, boy, we could put together a nice coalition and instead of me fighting for Tourette's syndrome, we could be fighting for all of us,' she says. What started as ten or twenty other groups soon became a hundred, all pushing for legislation which would create financial incentives for drugmakers to start manufacturing existing treatments for rare diseases which were being left on the shelf and to pursue the development of new ones.

By now Meyers had found another drug for her son, David. Several months after his Pimozide supply ran out, she reached a doctor at Yale who was studying Tourette's and asked him if he knew of any other treatments. As it happened, he was just starting a new clinical trial for a blood pressure drug which was thought to help people with Tourette's. 'David was the second one to go on it and he's still on it now, he's almost fifty years old,' Meyers says.[12] Her commitment to the wider cause was unwavering, however, fuelled by a sense of injustice that people were being treated as second-class citizens because they had a rare disease.

Jack Klugman brought his star power to Washington, testifying at a hearing on the proposed Orphan Drug Act. By 1982, a draft bill was ready to be put to a vote. To incentivise new orphan drugs, the legislation granted manufacturers a tax credit worth 50 per cent of research and development spending and access to grants for clinical trials.[13] The first manufacturer to bring each orphan drug to market was also guaranteed seven years of exclusivity during which no other companies could sell a similar drug to patients with the same rare disease. Crucially, the clock on the seven-year exclusivity period would only begin when a drug was approved for sale and ready to hit the market, meaning it would often last longer than a patent granted while the drug was being developed.[14] If a manufacturer found a new indication, meaning a new group of patients the drug benefited, it could also get a new exclusivity period for the same drug.

These financial rewards were designed to encourage investment in an area in which manufacturers could have 'no reasonable expectation' of a drug generating a profit. Lawmakers initially required drug companies to demonstrate that they wouldn't expect to be able to recoup the cost of developing the drug without the benefits provided by the 'orphan' designation. This was quickly amended, however, allowing potential treatments to qualify simply on the basis of the disease being targeted having a patient population of less than 200,000.[15]

The Orphan Drug Act was passed unanimously by the US House of Representatives but was then held up by a dispute with the Senate, which had amended the bill to remove the tax credit element.

Supporters believed that this change, tabled by Orrin Hatch, the Republican senator from Utah, would effectively neuter the bill and so efforts focused on persuading him to back down. In response, the Klugmans wrote another episode of *Quincy* in which a fictionalised senator was blocking similar legislation. The episode's pivotal scene depicts Klugman confronting the senator, who insists that no one cares about the Act.[16] Klugman tells him to look out of the window. Down below, a crowd of 500 people have gathered to demand an orphan drug bill. The extras hired for the scene, which was shot in a Pasadena street standing in for Washington DC, were all people who suffered from rare diseases.[17] A deal was duly reached on the tax credit and the bill passed both houses of Congress within little more than a month of the episode's broadcast. It was signed into law in 1983.

The pharmaceutical industry had publicly opposed the Orphan Drug Act when it was first proposed, arguing that there was no need for legislation to solve the issue. Some had privately indicated they were supportive of the proposal, but Meyers was under no illusions when the Act finally passed: persuading large drug companies to invest in rare diseases was going to be an uphill struggle. Now installed as the first president of the National Organization for Rare Disorders (NORD), a new non-profit which formalised the established coalition of support groups for different diseases, Meyers made her first priority finding manufacturers for those drugs which were known to work. Fearful of adverse publicity, McNeil Laboratories had agreed to begin manufacturing Pimozide again before the Orphan Drug Act was even passed, but convincing other companies to take up the mantle proved difficult. That was until Meyers turned to small generic drug manufacturers. 'They didn't mind making a drug that only brings in $10 million a year,' she says. 'The big companies say no, $10 million dollars, that's [not good] enough.'

One of the most challenging tasks was finding someone to manufacture L-5-HTP, the myoclonus treatment that Dr Van Woert was making in his own lab. In order to be able to sell the drug, expensive clinical trials would need to be funded, something which was complicated by the fact that one of the treatment's side effects – severe diarrhoea – made a double-blind trial all but impossible. There was one other option: it could be manufactured as an experimental drug and offered to patients, but regulators prohibited companies from charging for these.

Shortly after establishing NORD, Meyers was put in touch with a small generic manufacturer in Long Island called Bolar Pharmaceuticals. On a visit to the company's factory with Dr Van Woert, she explained the pressing need for someone to make the drug despite its poor commercial prospects. Bolar's chief executive was unfazed by the lack of profitability. 'I have just the machine to do it,' he told his visitors, taking them to the back of the factory to point out a machine which could put the capsules together with the medicine in it. 'For several years he manufactured that drug so that each capsule would be equivalent. And after a while, four or five years, we were able to stop manufacturing it because better drugs for myoclonus were developed,' Meyers says.

Around eighteen months after the passage of the Orphan Drug Act, Margaret M. Heckler, the US health and human services secretary, held a press conference to laud its success in encouraging manufacturers to bring nearly a dozen therapies to market. These orphan drugs, she said, 'will make nobody rich, but will help treat a small group of tragically handicapped people'.[18] Given that rare diseases, by definition, have small potential markets, it was anticipated that the prices charged for orphan drugs would be higher than mass-market medications. But Meyers and the other activists had never anticipated just how much higher those would prove to be.

While the pharmaceutical establishment was initially sceptical of going after markets with only small numbers of patients, the fledgling biotechnology industry was quicker to recognise the potential value of treatments for rare diseases.

One of the early orphan drugs was developed by Genentech, the biotechnology company co-founded by Dr Herbert Boyer to commercialise his work in the new field of genetic engineering. In 1979, with the company needing to demonstrate to investors that they could successfully take a new medicine to market, it decided to try and develop a synthetic version of human growth hormone (HGH). The hormone was used to treat dwarfism in children but was in short supply because the only way to obtain the natural version was by harvesting it from the pituitary glands of cadavers. This method also had its dangers, as would be tragically demonstrated a few years later when, in an incident unconnected to Genentech, several children died after receiving a batch taken from glands which turned out to be infected with Creutzfeldt-Jakob disease, a fatal brain disorder.

Genentech's attempt to create a genetically engineered version of HGH was a success and, after clinical trials, the treatment was approved for sale in 1985 under the brand name Protropin. Two years later another synthetic HGH, this time made by the pharmaceutical giant Eli Lilly, also hit the market. Unusually, both received orphan drug status, granting them separate seven-year exclusivity windows, after the regulator decided that Eli Lilly's was sufficiently different to constitute a new product. A lengthy legal battle between the two companies followed the decision, but when it came to pricing their new treatments Eli Lilly followed its rival's lead and the cost to patients of each drug came to between $10,000 and $30,000 a year, depending on the quantity needed. Genentech claimed it was 25 per cent cheaper than the previous human version, ignoring the fact that its product had to be administered in much higher quantities, resulting in an annual cost that was up to six times higher.[19]

The price of the therapy quickly attracted criticism, as did the fact that Genentech had seemingly applied for orphan drug status only as an afterthought, filing its application shortly before the drug was approved for sale rather than in the early stages of development as was the norm. The company openly admitted in court that the Orphan Drug Act had played no role in incentivising the development of recombinant HGH.[20] It was the amount of money the drug was soon bringing in, however, which most significantly raised hackles among those who had fought for the legislation.

The drug had been developed to treat a market of just a few thousand Americans with a pituitary gland disorder. However, Genentech was likely aware that HGH had other uses, too. Bodybuilders had discovered that growth hormone helped build muscle tissue and reduce fat. Dan Duchaine, known as 'The Steroid Guru', described the benefits in his 1982 publication, *The Underground Steroid Handbook*. 'Wow, is this great stuff!' he wrote. 'It is the best for permanent muscle gains . . . People who use it can expect to gain 30 to 40 pounds in muscle in ten weeks'. Duchaine said it was the 'most expensive' and 'most fashionable' athletic drug which 'has firmly established itself in power-lifting and within a few years will be a commonly used drug in all strength athletics'.[21] A black market for the new synthetic versions sprang up, with vials resold in gyms and athletic training centres across the country.

The use of HGH by drugs cheats was thrust into the public eye when Ben Johnson, the Canadian sprinter, was stripped of his Olympic gold medal after failing a drug test in the wake of the 100 metres final in Seoul in 1988. It later emerged that he'd taken Genentech's Protropin along with a banned steroid and nutritional supplements during a training camp before the race. The bottle of synthetic HGH supplied by a Canadian doctor had cost $1,000, more than four times its usual price.[22]

The makers of any drug can only advertise it as a treatment for the uses for which it has received marketing approval. However, doctors are legally entitled to prescribe a medication for any use they see fit. HGH, in a mark of its illicit popularity, became so widely abused that a 1990 law overrode the normal 'off-label' rules to prohibit its prescription for strength building and other non-approved uses. The change had little practical effect, and while Genentech and Eli Lilly also took their own measures to try to tightly control the medication's distribution, its use as a performance-enhancing drug nevertheless helped boost sales and pad the companies' bottom line. By 1990, HGH was bringing in up to $200 million a year in sales and Genentech had established itself as the prototypical biotech company.

Those 1990 revenue figures were matched by another orphan drug,

Epogen, which had been launched just a year earlier by Amgen, another Californian biotech firm then in its infancy. The drug, a genetically-engineered protein, helped prevent anaemia in kidney patients by boosting red blood cells, allowing patients on dialysis to avoid having to endure repeated blood transfusions. The protein was grown in hamster cells and cost Amgen just $140 to make a year's supply for a single patient.[23] Amgen priced the treatment at $8,000 a year. With 100,000 kidney patients in the US alone, and additional markets for cancer and AIDS patients added to the label within a few years, it became a licence to print money and Epogen would go on to become the first biotech blockbuster. Like HGH, it also enjoyed popularity among athletes as a performance enhancer and was among the disgraced cyclist Lance Armstrong's medications of choice as he later cheated his way to a succession of Tour de France titles.

These prices, and the profits that followed, prompted a 1990 congressional hearing which focused on HGH, Epogen and a third drug called aerosol pentamidine. Pentamidine was a treatment for AIDS-related pneumonia which, like AZT, had been eligible for orphan drug status despite the fast-growing epidemic because at the time of the application fewer than 200,000 Americans had been diagnosed with the disease. These were not drugs with realistic doubts about a route to profitability of the sort the Act had been intended to foster, but they were nevertheless able to enjoy the benefits the legislation conferred.

The congressional hearing considered whether the Orphan Drug Act needed to be reformed. 'We need a kinder and gentler pharmaceutical industry,' Abbey Meyers told the hearing, saying that she personally had 'begged Eli Lilly and Genentech several times to lower their prices on human growth hormone and they both say that they can't do it'.[24] An amendment was later produced which would have curtailed the exclusivity window offered to orphan drugs if their sales exceeded $200 million but was vetoed by President George H.W. Bush.

Then, in April 1991, came a development which would reshape the limits of what most in the industry had thought possible when it came to the pricing of drugs. That month, US regulators approved a new treatment for type 1 Gaucher's disease, an inherited condition which left many adult patients confined to wheelchairs. The treatment was an enzyme replacement therapy, pioneered by a biochemist called Dr Roscoe Brady. Dr Brady worked at the US National Institutes of Health and the government had funded most of the drug's early development, leaving Genzyme, the company he'd partnered with, to spend less than $30 million on the drug's discovery.[25]

The treatment, however, came with an unusual and highly expensive manufacturing process. In order to get even a small amount of the modified enzyme which was injected into patients, dozens of fresh human placentas had to be collected and processed to extract the desired protein. It was a complex and time-intensive process, requiring as many as 22,000 human placentas to make enough of the enzyme for a year's supply for one patient.[26] The cost of this labour-intensive work, along with distributing and marketing the drug, pushed Genzyme to contemplate an unheard-of price, far above those charged for other orphan drugs. Ceredase would cost an average of $150,000 per patient, with more than half of that the result of just how expensive it was to make.[27] For some patients needing larger doses the bill would be $300,000 a year or more.

When it launched, the price, predictably, provoked a backlash. One of the company's co-founders, the medical researcher Dr Henry Blair, would later admit: 'I never thought we could charge that much.'[28] Non-profit organisations complained it prevented people from getting the drug and Genzyme's chief executive was summoned to Washington to appear before a congressional committee. Yet, despite the outcry, insurers, Medicare and Medicaid paid up and the drug generated sales of nearly $100 million in 1992. There were complaints, but they paled in comparison to the outrage AZT had stirred up just four years earlier despite a price tag fifteen times higher. Out of the limelight, with just a small number of patients, you could get away with a lot more. Even with a high price, these drugs barely registered on national health budgets.

As president of the National Organization for Rare Disorders,

Meyers was soon to hear from patients who were unable to get Ceredase because of its price. During her frequent attempts to pressure the company into reducing it, Meyers became friendly with a Genzyme lobbyist in Washington called Lisa Reines. Reines assured her that the high cost was simply the result of a complicated manufacturing process which involved buying large numbers of human placentas from African hospitals and shipping them to France for processing at a cosmetics factory. When they could instead make the drug through biotechnology, the price would come down, Reines declared. The company estimated that the cost of the raw material alone would fall to one-seventh of what it was paying when using placentas.[29]

Within a couple of years of Ceredase's launch, Genzyme had used recombinant technology to successfully create a genetically-engineered version of the same protein as promised. Reines called Meyers to tell her the price that had been set for Cerezyme, the new therapy. 'Well, I have good news for you,' Reines began. 'The FDA has approved the biotechnology version and I convinced Henri Termeer, the CEO, not to charge any more for it.'[30] Reines was expecting a grateful response. She didn't get one.

'How dare you,' Meyers bellowed. 'You've been telling me for how many years that as soon as the biotech version is approved [it's] going to be much less expensive, and yet you still are charging as much as buying a new house every year.'

Cerezyme was much cheaper to make but Genzyme had crossed the Rubicon; Ceredase had shown what was possible, so why price it any lower?

When questioned by reporters about the decision, Genzyme executives said they needed to pay for the new manufacturing facility. Once that was up and running, they said, the price would finally fall. These cost savings were never passed on to patients. Instead the drug, which must be taken for a lifetime, has actually seen its price rise and the typical annual cost of treating a US patient is now between $200,000 and $300,000.

In a repeat of the impact of AZT''s high price 'they were charging so much people were spending themselves into poverty so that they qualified for Medicaid,' Meyers says. In her view, Genzyme 'just saw how much profit they could make and they really didn't care about the welfare of patients'.[31]

Orphan drugs helped to turn the biotechnology industry from an idea into a reality. As the first biotech blockbuster, Epogen became known as the 'biotech drug that launched a thousand companies'.[32] The promise of using new technologies to make therapies from biological material which had sent scientists west in search of venture capital was finally starting to be realised. The successes of Amgen, Genentech and others showed, after years of product-free public offerings and inflated valuations, that biotechs could deliver products with tangible benefits and genuine commercial prospects. In the process, these drugs helped to shepherd in a new attitude towards the pricing of drugs.

For decades, when pharmaceutical companies wanted advice on how to price a new drug, Mick Kolassa was the man they hired. Over a forty-year career in the drug industry, Kolassa helped to revolutionise drug pricing. When he started in a job at Upjohn in 1980, the biggest barrier to higher prices came from drug companies themselves. They were the 'most price-sensitive segment of the pharmaceutical market', he says, and it would drive him crazy. 'You had products that could have easily had very reasonable prices twice as high as they were. But the companies, out of caution, chose not to do that.'[33]

At that point, pricing wasn't a specialist job and it was left to marketing executives who 'always saw price as an impediment to a sale'. Back then the calculation was simple, Kolassa says: 'It was basically this. Is my product a therapeutic advance? And if the answer is no, then I price it at or below the competition.

'If it is an advance, do I expect a significant competitor within two years? If I do expect a competitor within two years, I price it low. If I don't, I price it at a premium . . . to what's already out there, and then a premium was 10 or 12 per cent.'

The result was only modest increases in the price of drugs during the preceding decades, with sales growth driven by increased prescription volumes rather than price rises. In 1975, the average US prescription was just eleven cents more expensive than it had been in 1960, once adjusted for prescription size.[34] Over 40 per cent of new drugs in the preceding two decades had been introduced at lower prices than rival treatments in an attempt to capture market share.[35] The Kefauver hearings which began at the end of the 1950s lingered long in the industry's institutional memory and the large companies wanted a 'safe price' for new drugs. Few executives wanted to end up like Dr David Barry or Sir Alfred Shepperd during the controversy over Burroughs Wellcome's pricing of AZT, with protestors outside the office and their faces across the newspapers for all the wrong reasons. Sir Alfred and his wife, Lady Shepperd, had even had to have the windows at their country home reinforced after being told they were at risk of being personally attacked.[36]

Biotechnology companies, with their disruptive Californian spirit, lacked the reticence of staid pharmaceutical giants in the Midwest and on the East Coast. Perhaps as importantly, they also didn't have a portfolio of existing drugs or a reputation they needed to protect. 'They were the first to realise that they could push past those barriers in the market and not hurt themselves,' Kolassa says. 'There were kind of these rules. The biotech companies didn't know the rules [so] they didn't follow them. And it kind of changed everything.'[37]

The high manufacturing costs and small markets for the orphan drugs which made up the biotech industry's first offerings meant health systems and insurers were ultimately prepared to accept the prices charged.[38] With few patients, the prices might have been high but overall costs remained relatively low. Soon, however, these drugs would add new markets and larger groups of patients to sell to and still no major push back on prices came. Drugs like human growth hormone (HGH), which became a sought-after drug after acquiring a dubious reputation as an anti-ageing treatment, helped create the expectation that biological drugs would be more expensive than traditional pills. In turn, the biotechnology companies would show the way for the wider pharmaceutical industry to begin charging higher prices.

'I think the biotechnology companies with their pricing showed the big companies that they can put those ridiculous prices on [orphan] drugs,' Meyers says. 'The more serious the disease, the more that people will feel that they absolutely have to pay for that drug because they don't want those people to die.'

'The pharma companies were horrified at those prices, they didn't see how they were sustainable,' Kolassa says. But Genzyme's success in selling Ceredase and Cerezyme had broken through a barrier, setting price precedents which insurers and health services appeared willing to pay. In time, the market had become inured to six-figure price tags; when a new orphan drug launched, that just became what was expected. Any push back was minimal. 'Reimbursement has never been a problem,' the chief executive of the biotech BioMarin would tell attendees at a healthcare conference a full decade later as he discussed launching a drug with an average cost of $200,000. 'Genzyme has never had a problem with Ceredase or Cerezyme.'[39]

'It was the first drug that really proved you could charge what you want and you'll be able to make big profits from orphan drugs,' Meyers says. 'And there was a psychology that changed at that point where other companies said. "Well, if Genzyme did it, we could do it." And we started seeing very, very expensive drugs.'[40]

In political science, there is a concept called the Overton window, which contends that there are a range of policies considered to have mainstream acceptability. Politicians and their followers can shift the window, meaning that policies that were once considered extreme become something the public are prepared to accept, or at least contemplate. Cerezyme, HGH, Epogen and the other high-priced orphan drugs launched in their collective slipstream started to shift the pharmaceutical pricing equivalent of the Overton window. In certain circumstances, insurers and healthcare systems seemed willing to contemplate prices that those setting them had previously considered unthinkable. And if they could charge that much for these drugs, the thinking went, surely, further down the pricing scale, we can push things a bit further for non-orphan drugs.

The prices of Ceredase and Cerezyme didn't change things overnight. In the immediate aftermath of their launch, the threat of President Clinton implementing major healthcare reforms in the United States – the engine room of the global drug industry – left the industry wary of provoking a confrontation over pricing and few other treatments would match the cost of those for Gaucher's disease for many years. But the biotech companies who built their businesses on the success of orphan drugs like HGH and EPO became major players as the 1990s progressed. Large drug companies started to take notice, buying significant stakes in successful biotechs, partnering on product launches, and gradually learning from this new industry's approach. While mass-market treatments couldn't command prices anywhere close to Cerezyme's, companies were beginning to wake up to the realisation that they could push prices much further than they had been doing. They were 'seeing the prices that other companies were getting when they weren't following those [old] rules', Kolassa says. The huge growth in insurance coverage in the US from the late 1980s and into the 1990s also helped, with insured patients typically using more drugs – and particularly more expensive drugs – than those forced to pay for medicines out-of-pocket.[41]

At the same time as the biotech industry was demonstrating the true extent of manufacturers' pricing power, a new approach was pushing the argument that drugs were underpriced. Burroughs Wellcome's approach to setting the price of AZT was characterised by Sir Alfred as a 'finger in the wind decision', but by the 1990s specialist pricing departments were commonplace and setting a price was becoming increasingly central to the development of any new drug. This change came as a discipline called pharmacoeconomics grew in popularity. It offered drug manufacturers a way of using economic analysis to calculate and understand the value of their product to patients, doctors and health systems.

Alongside this was the idea of 'value-based rather than cost-based pricing' coined by the pricing strategist Dan Nimer. Nimer, who died in 2015 at the age of ninety-three, was working for Zenith, an American manufacturer of television sets, and Canteen Corp, which sold hot dogs at baseball stadiums, when he developed the idea that a price should try to capture the value of a product to a customer, rather than being set to recover costs.[42] A higher price could serve as a marketing tool to communicate the perceived value of the product, he argued.[43]

Kolassa became a prominent advocate of value-based pricing, believing drug companies were unwittingly leaving money on the table because they didn't understand the true value of their product to consumers and society. 'What is it worth not to have a cold?' Kolassa asked in an American television interview in 1993, explaining the philosophy. That's what people would pay and so that should be the price, he said. 'If people buy it, the price is justified.'[44]

The first companies to try this approach had found it difficult. Nimer worked with Sandoz in the 1980s as they prepared to launch Sandimmune, an immunosuppressant drug which became the main treatment used to prevent organ rejection after a transplant. The drug cost between $3,000 and $5,000 for a year's supply when it went on sale, which was so far above ordinary drug prices at the time it was deemed 'horrendously expensive'.[45] A few years later, Kolassa, who by now had moved from Upjohn to Sandoz, was involved with the launch of the schizophrenia drug Clozaril. While previous treatments had cost hundreds of dollars, Clozaril launched in 1988 with a price-tag close to AZT's at nearly $9,000 a year, including a patient monitoring system needed because of a potentially fatal side effect in a small number of those taking the drug.[46] 'That was priced based on value,' Kolassa says. 'The average patient cost between $20,000 and $30,000 a year [while] institutionalised, and this drug could get people out of that setting very quickly.' The market wasn't yet ready for such prices, though, and Sandoz ended up disassembling the monitoring and selling it at a lower price. The company, however, held firm on the price of Sandimmune and it subsequently spent many years as Sandoz's highest-earning drug.

The success of orphan drugs in breaking through pricing barriers helped to pave the way for drug companies to adopt the 'value-based pricing' approach to justify the higher prices they now realised they could get away with charging. Kolassa, who spends his time these days as a blues musician performing in the Deep South, insists that 'value-based pricing' wasn't simply about charging the highest price possible and that 'part of it is not being greedy – don't try to take it all'.

But following in the path of highly priced biotech drugs, pharmaceutical companies became more and more willing to take an aggressive approach to pricing. He pinpoints the turn of the millennium as the point at which companies started to take the handbrake off the prices they were willing to charge.

'What happened over time is that the blockbuster became the target that everybody was going for and if you couldn't get there with the value of the product then you could get there with the price,' Kolassa says. '[Companies] went from trying to find out what their products were worth, to finding out how much they could get for them . . . I saw companies that we worked hard to get them to understand they had a $15,000 drug and once they found out it was fifteen they said, "Well, can I get twenty-five?" "Well, maybe." "Well, if I can get twenty-five, can I get thirty-five?"'

In early 2000, Eli Lilly, the US drug company based in Indianapolis, was under pressure. Prozac, the money-spinning antidepressant which had powered the business through the 1990s, was expected to lose its patent protection within a few years. At the same time, Zyprexa, another of its most lucrative drugs, was under threat from competing products. If nothing could be found to fill the impending revenue collapse, those inside the company feared it would be vulnerable to an unwanted takeover by a larger rival.

Fran Leath, the daughter of a schoolteacher and a Ford factory worker, had gone to college in Indiana and joined Lilly straight after finishing her degree in the summer of 1987. The economics graduate moved between various roles but ended up as a manager in the business development and strategic planning team. Among other responsibilities, the role meant she had a front-row seat during pricing discussions.

Lilly was contemplating what price to set for a new biological medicine which it was hoped would treat sepsis, a life-threatening condition caused by bacteria entering the bloodstream. For acute medicines used for a short time like this one, the company would commission research on the price of other drugs in the same area, with the view that 'we needed to be within a reasonable range of what the market is currently bearing, otherwise they won't pick up our drug', Leath says.[47] With no sepsis treatments on the market, analysts examined other drugs which were administered in emergency situations. They ended up using 'models [that] were really based on cardiovascular or stroke drugs that were on the market at the time', Leath recalls. The figures that emerged would give the new treatment, which was then called Zovant but would be renamed Xigris, a price tag of between $500 and $700 for a four-day course of treatment.

Then, in June 2000, the company received some unexpected news which injected a new urgency into the decision. Xigris had proved so successful during a Phase III trial that an independent panel of doctors had stepped in to halt it. It was no longer ethical to give patients suffering from septicaemia a placebo pill instead of the new treatment.

The news was a huge boon for Lilly at a crucial time. Just two months later, a court in New York would hand down a ruling which meant that generic competition for Prozac could hit the market the following year, rather than in 2003 as had been expected, potentially costing the company $2 billion. The pipeline looked so bare that there seemed to be nothing that could be launched and have time to grow before the company's other bestseller, Zyprexa, came off patent a few years later. Here, in a gift from the science gods, appeared to be a new blockbuster drug ready to launch in just a few months.

Within a week of the announcement, Lilly's approach to pricing Xigris had changed. 'All the old models went out of the window and then it just became a discussion about what can we get away with,' Leath says. The new price floated by a marketing executive in an internal meeting was $10,000.

Sepsis causes a rapid deterioration in patients, meaning the drug would be used in emergency situations where there was no time for discussion. 'You put that drug into the person, you have the opportunity to save someone from death. So it felt like the perfect drug where you could play with the price,' Leath says. The proposed price tag was so high that Leath decided to speak to her boss, questioning whether it would be accepted by patients and insurers. 'His response was "Hey, you know, if grandma's on the table, you're not gonna ask about the price".'[48] It was a mantra which characterised a transformation in Eli Lilly's culture.

There was also a feeling inside the company that Prozac, which cost around $2.50 a pill, or around $2,000 a year for patients who took it twice-daily, had been underpriced and even larger profits could have been made. Executives didn't want to repeat the mistake with Xigris. 'The $10,000 was not model-based at all. It was what will the market bear, and what do we need to tell Wall Street,' Leath says. 'It felt like we had moved from being a company that was getting a very healthy return for its original research to a company that was gouging.' She felt the company wasn't considering patients, and the risk that someone without insurance might be unable to afford the drug, because it was so fixated on keeping shareholders happy.

In her early days at Eli Lilly, patient care had been frequently raised in meetings. 'Now I'm sitting in senior management meetings and our conversations are always about Wall Street and what return do we need to have,' she says. 'The focus was on what will the Street require, what are the returns we need.'

The drug eventually launched with a price of $6,800 per treatment course, far above the $500 to $700 range. Charles Gordon, the chief financial officer, told a reporter that, with no other treatment available for sepsis, 'you could define this drug as having infinite value, but if we priced it too high, it wouldn't be used too much'. Gordon used the language of value-based pricing to justify Lilly's approach to Xigris and other medicines, claiming that 'the price of the drugs is minuscule compared with the economic cost of the disease'.[49]

Analysts had named Xigris the most anticipated drug launch of the year, predicting profits of up to $2 billion a year. The drug was given a big sales push. The *Wall Street Journal* reported that Lilly paid 250 doctors up to $1,500 per talk to tell colleagues about Xigris and paid for promotional events including a concert by the Grammy Award-winning jazz musician George Benson during a San Diego conference.[50]

Despite all this, the 'sure-fire blockbuster' would ultimately flop. The sales efforts were never able to overcome doctors' reticence to prescribe it, with data suggesting it significantly heightened the risk of brain haemorrhages in patients. When it was withdrawn from the market in 2011, lifetime sales of Xigris had not topped $1.5 billion.[51] By the time Fran Leath left Lilly in 2003, she had become very jaded about the industry. She felt executives were now putting all of their energy into 'performing for Wall Street'. Employees were rewarded with much larger bonuses under a new compensation scheme but Leath was left embarrassed by the size of the cheque. 'It felt like we were looking for new ways to milk cash out of the company on the compensation side while at the same time milking patients,' she says.

The approach to drug pricing formed in the 1990s largely remains the approach today and the reality is a far cry from the rhetoric used to explain high prices. Until relatively recently, the favoured explanation of drug executives and pharmaceutical lobbyists was that drugs were expensive because R&D is expensive. In truth, research and development costs play little role when setting the price of a new drug. They are, as one former chief executive of a major pharmaceutical company put it in the jargon of business, 'a sunk cost'. 'Even though the industry justifies the high cost of drugs by the high cost of research, I've been through twenty or thirty of those worldwide decisions of how to price a drug [and] the research cost never came up,' he says.[52]

R&D expenditure across the industry gives an advantageously high figure with which to make the general case that one high figure leads to another one when determining the cost of an individual drug, but in truth executives rarely know exactly how much was spent developing one particular product. Disentangling spending on different research strands is too complicated and, even when possible, it makes little difference. The argument that insurers and health services should accept a high price for a stomach-acid drug just because the company wasted a lot of money chasing a cure for cancer which didn't work is unlikely to prove very persuasive. It's up to individual companies to budget for drug discovery as they see fit and to make enough money across all the successes and failures to keep the show on the road.

Manufacturing costs, on the other hand, are a known amount which, once established, set a clear pricing floor, although this is usually only a small proportion of the final price. From there, companies will turn to extensive market research. Work on the likely size and value of the market for a new treatment takes place throughout its development in order to secure the sign-off to keep it moving forward. Analysts collect information on competing products and model the likely behaviour of those buying and paying for the drug at different price points. Hundreds of doctors and other medical practitioners will be interviewed and asked what they make of the current treatments and what sort of value they might place on the new drug's benefits. Consultants hired by the drug company will likely speak to insurers and healthcare officials too, trying to get a sense of how the market might react.

Ultimately it comes down to a judgement call, with consultants presenting the pros and cons of a range of pricing levels. At that point everything from earnings estimates to corporate bonuses are geared towards higher prices. In fact, under the value-based approach, executives worry that a lower price would simply mean that their drug would be perceived as inferior.[53]

'You're not rewarded for having a low price and for the most part, the market doesn't punish a high price,' Kolassa has said.[54] As he put it in his 2009 book, *The Strategic Pricing of Pharmaceuticals*: 'With few exceptions, we have found that the specific price charged for a medicine has little effect on its unit sales.' Demand, he argued, was driven by the 'underlying epidemiology of the disease and the utility of the product in treating it'.[55]

While new drugs might once have tried to undercut the price of existing treatments to build market share, from the late 1980s drugmakers started to learn that this was rarely the most profitable approach. Instead, existing prices served simply to set a floor above which the new product would push prices higher still, with the scale of that premium depending on how much better the manufacturer believed their product to be, or even just how willing they were to weather criticism.

In many therapy areas, this remains the approach. 'You look at the advantage over existing therapy, cost savings and benefits to patients, you look at the price of competing drugs, and you make a decision,' the former drug industry chief executive says.[56] If it's a totally new therapy area without obvious benchmarks or a transformationally better medicine – a cure, for example, rather than a treatment for a disease's symptoms – a drugmaker has even more freedom to inflate the price it will seek to charge.[57]

Kolassa's outlook, that 'if we can get customers to understand the value of our products, price won't matter', sat hand-in-hand with the role of sales reps like Shahram Ahari whose effectiveness meant it was far more profitable for a company to set a high price and persuade doctors that their drug was the best rather than offer it as simply a cheaper alternative.[58] When the copycat drug Zantac launched at a price that made it 50 per cent more expensive than Tagamet it was a huge commercial success. After initially attempting deep discounting to try and further undermine its new rival, Tagamet's manufacturer eventually ended up increasing its price because there was no advantage to be found from its cheaper price – doctors were prescribing what they thought was best.

Beginning in earnest in the 1990s, health insurers in the US used managed care networks – which specified which hospitals and doctors insured patients could use – and pharmacy benefit managers (PBMs) to try and manage their drug spending more proactively. Over time, this led to significant discounts from list prices in therapeutic areas where there were several branded drugs which were sufficiently similar, among them statins, antidepressants and rheumatoid arthritis drugs.[59] But even with this approach, there were limited incentives for price competition. PBMs tended to choose one or two drugs in a category to offer to patients and then exclude the rest. The winners would invariably be those who had already captured large market shares because their vast revenue meant they could offer the largest rebates.

In this situation, launching a new drug into a crowded category at a cheaper price simply didn't work, as Bayer's statin drug Baycol demonstrated.[60] 'You could come in at a significant discount with a superior product and still not get on the formulary,' Kolassa says. Doctors wouldn't prescribe something just because it was cheaper and PBMs wouldn't give it preferred status because these products, with their tiny market share, could offer only small sums in rebates even if they were high as a percentage of that drug's price. Instead, for drugs likely to win only a modest proportion of prescriptions, it made sense to set a high price and take whatever revenue could be brought in that way. For many key products, among them cancer drugs administered in hospitals and treatments for rare diseases, there remains little effective competitive pressure and so for drug-makers the equation remains simple: the higher the price, the higher the profits.

As the millennium dawned, the large drugmakers of Big Pharma had fully embraced the pricing and marketing revolutions. But even as they harnessed these changes to record phenomenal profits, attention turned to a part of the industry which acted as a brake on even more riches: the generic drugmakers who were poised, as soon as patent protection ended, to claim their own rewards by selling the same drugs at far lower prices.

CHAPTER FIVE

Dirty pharma

In July 2006, Pfizer, the largest drug company in the world, announced that Jeff Kindler, a pugnacious fifty-one-year-old former trial lawyer, would be its new chief executive. Kindler, who beat two other internal candidates, was something of a surprise choice. While his rivals were industry veterans, the well-tanned Kindler had only been working for Pfizer for four years, his first job in the sector. Instead, he'd spent most of his career in legal and corporate roles at the industrial giant General Electric, which sells everything from light bulbs to aircraft engines, and at McDonald's, where he oversaw pizza and Mexican-themed fast food brands.[1] 'I went from being a hamburger lawyer to being a drug dealer,' he would quip, joking that his time at Pfizer was penance for six years spent raising global cholesterol levels.[2]

A year later, another large drugmaker, the Swiss firm Novartis, tapped Joe Jimenez to head its pharmaceuticals division. Jimenez, too, had no scientific or medical background. He'd worked for the baked beans and tomato ketchup manufacturer Heinz and advised the private equity firm Blackstone Group before joining Novartis. For the first twelve months after he started his new job, he received hour-long morning tutorials on the biology of diseases and how the company's drugs worked in order to get up to speed.[3] Within a few years, Jimenez would ascend to the top job at Novartis, months before a corporate litigator, Ken Frazier, who had spent time in the trenches defending lawsuits as well as heading marketing and sales efforts, was named as the next chief executive of Merck & Co.[4]

Drug companies had once been helmed by medically-trained doctors or research scientists, before business executives clutching MBAs from Harvard, Wharton and Columbia began to fill the ranks of middle management. As the blockbuster era progressed in the 1990s and on into the new millennium, Kindler, Jimenez and Frazier embodied the ascent of lawyers and salesmen to the top jobs as the new kings of pharma. They reflected the changing priorities of an industry in which the key to success, and the power balance within many firms, had shifted firmly from clinical research to the commercial side. It was in courtrooms and television adverts and sales visits to doctors that the riches shareholders demanded would be won.

William Lazonick, a Canadian economist living in Boston, has coined the term 'financialisation' to describe the shift that took place in the pharmaceutical industry and in the wider US economy. Lazonick, who is in his mid-seventies favours open-necked shirts and has grown his remaining hair long, giving him the appearance of an ageing hippie. He credits the changes in how companies approached the business of selling drugs to the widespread adoption of a new philosophy. Its genesis, he says, can be traced back to the leafy, tree-lined squares and imposing neo-Georgian buildings of Harvard Business School, where he joined the faculty in 1984.

'In 1984, no one at Harvard Business School was saying that companies should be run to maximise shareholder value. And by 1986, this was something that was quickly becoming the dominant point of view,' Lazonick says. 'And I saw it happen.'[5]

What changed was the arrival of a new professor, an economist from Minnesota called Michael Jensen. Jensen, then in his mid-forties, was a leading proponent of an approach first put forward by Milton Friedman in 1970 which held that company executives should only follow their shareholders' interests, and that these interests were to maximise profits. The mantra was 'maximising shareholder value'. It replaced any sense of balancing the interests of employees, customers and the public with a singular focus on driving the share price up and giving money back to those who had bought the company's stocks. Jensen believed that simply investing profits back into a company often meant wasting money on inefficient or unprofitable projects and what he called 'organisational inefficiencies'. Instead, he called for businesses to 'disgorge' this cash back to shareholders, to whom, he reminded his students, it ultimately belonged. At a time when President Reagan's free-market approach had unleashed corporate raiders and the swashbuckling, testosterone-fuelled Wall Street financiers immortalised by Tom Wolfe as the 'Masters of the Universe', these ideas soon caught light.

By the 1990s it had become firmly entrenched on Wall Street as the dominant corporate ideology and in 1997 the concept of maximising shareholder value was formally adopted by the US Business Roundtable, an influential body made up of the chief executives of America's largest companies, which declared that the purpose of a company was to serve shareholders.[6] Companies began to return more money, either directly, by paying higher dividends, or, increasingly, through a new form of financial manoeuvring known as stock buybacks whereby a company buys some of its own shares back from shareholders. These buybacks typically serve to drive up the company's stock price, at least initially, because they increase earnings per share, a measure used by investors in valuing stocks.

More generally, critics argue, maximising shareholder value fostered a short-termist approach which prioritised immediate growth over all else. Jensen urged companies to reward chief executives with large stock options, giving them even more of a personal incentive to focus on keeping the share price moving in the right direction.

Lazonick says he began to sense a problem in the late 1980s with this 'ideology of value extraction' when he read newspaper headlines reporting 'company lays off 10,000 people, stock price soars'. By the turn of the century, some inside the industry had also recognised that a profound shift had occurred. Jürgen Drews, the former head of global research at Roche, wrote a journal article in May 2003 in which he decried how 'the ethics of successful business have replaced those of medicine'. 'The supreme loyalty of today's companies is not primarily directed at patients and their physicians but at shareholders', he wrote.[7] In a previous book, he had bemoaned how research departments, which should be the 'contributor of ideas', had become a 'receiver of instructions' following 'strategies determined by market forces'.[8]

Mick Kolassa says he saw the same shift in mentality first-hand: 'In the early 2000s pharmaceutical companies went from being healthcare companies to being banks. And so they acted more like any other purely financial organisation, and a drug just happened to be the way they made their money . . . The fundamental nature of the industry changed.' The desire to see 'how much can I get?' for a drug would ultimately cause patients to suffer but 'companies don't see that', he says. It is a change which lies at the heart of the drug pricing crisis. 'The industry now pays much more attention to Wall Street, they just care how the stock markets treat them.'[9]

He said he had been in meetings discussing the price of new drugs where 'stock analysts are pushing for higher and higher prices. The price will never be low enough to make customers happy and it will never be high enough to make Wall Street happy. But Wall Street will be a lot more loud at a price they see as too low than anybody will be at a price that's too high.'

In this financialised model, growth is all-important since a company's share price reflects investors' expectations of future profits. The profits brought in by blockbuster drugs are underpinned by patents, the intellectual property which gave drug companies a legal monopoly. But patents only last for twenty years from filing and a significant portion is lost to the clinical trials and regulatory approval process required before a drug hits the market.[10] Once on sale, a drug typically has seven to twelve years of patent protection remaining before generic manufacturers are free to launch their own cut-price versions.[11]

Since the US reforms of the 1980s, the generics industry had grown rapidly and by the late 1990s it was looking with covetous anticipation at the huge markets that statins, antidepressants, heart drugs and other blockbusters had managed to carve out. By then, half of all prescriptions were fulfilled with generic drugs and this would reach 75 per cent by 2010 and over 90 per cent a decade after that.[12] In Europe, the uptake of generics was more varied, but in key markets including Germany and the UK, health systems were implementing measures to encourage doctors and pharmacists to dispense more cheap generics.

When the system works, generic drugs are a key part of the equilibrium between private profit and public benefit, ensuring that the innovations of previous decades subsequently become cheap, mass-manufactured drugs available to all. They also serve as an incentive for drug companies to develop new, innovative products to replace the lost revenue.

For Big Pharma, however, the end of patent protection for a key blockbuster drug could carve an ugly hole in a previously sparkling balance sheet, creating a drop so precipitous that it became known in some companies as the 'shark fin' – named after the feared shape of a sales graph when a drug lost patent protection. To try to avoid this calamity, drug companies devoted vast resources to developing an entire toolkit of strategies to keep generic competition at bay for as long as possible, methods which remain central to the drug industry to this day. These tactics became so commonplace there was even a neutral-sounding name for it – lifecycle management.

For drug companies the most straightforward solution to an impending patent expiry was to find a way to tweak the molecular structure of the existing drug just enough that it would qualify for a new patent. Never mind how much of a clinical advance the tweaked version truly represented, the pharmaceutical company just needed something to work with and its marketing department could do the rest. Clinical trials would be set up to show favourable results – however minor the advantage over the older drug – and sales reps could be sent out to persuade doctors to move their patients across. If timed right, the loss of patent protection on the old drug would be no more than a glancing blow.

AstraZeneca took this approach when contemplating what to do about its bestselling stomach ulcer drug, omeprazole, a protein pump inhibitor sold under the brand names Prilosec and Losec. In the mid-1990s, with patent protection on the basic compound due to expire in the US and other markets in 2001, the company put together a team to tackle the impending cliff edge. The Shark Fin project started work in 1995 and considered dozens of different options, from developing a faster-acting treatment to combining it with an old ulcer medication to create something new.[13] In the end, however, AstraZeneca ended up with something very simple: omeprazole is composed of two molecules known as enantiomers, which are mirror images of one another. One was thought to be biologically inactive so the company isolated the other one and repackaged it as a new drug: Nexium.

Those working on the project believed Nexium was no better than Prilosec, but AstraZeneca needed to run head-to-head trials between the two pills in order to market it to doctors as an improved product. It tackled this problem by comparing 20mg of Prilosec with a higher 40mg dose of Nexium in three studies. AstraZeneca justified the use of a higher dose of Nexium because it was testing for erosive esophagitis, a serious but rare condition. Results for acid-reflux disease, 'a far more common cause of heartburn' and the main way in which the drug would be used in practice, were unequivocal, however, showing that 'Nexium offered no significant advantage over Prilosec even at higher doses'.[14] In a fourth study, the only one which compared 20mg of Nexium with 20mg of Prilosec, the new drug showed a 90 per cent healing rate for erosive esophagitis after eight weeks, compared with 87 per cent for Prilosec.[15] Nevertheless, it was enough. Nexium, packaged up like its predecessor as a distinctive purple pill, could be touted as an improved version of Prilosec. It was launched in 2001 and brought in $2 billion in 2002 and $3.3 billion in 2003, more than offsetting the loss in US sales of Prilosec which followed.

'You can keep the franchise alive,' says Josh Krieger, an assistant professor at Harvard Business School who describes Prilosec and Nexium as 'the classic example' of this behaviour. 'They are chemically quite similar drugs. Prilosec consists of two isomers – essentially mirror images – of the same molecule, while Nexium contains just one of those isomers. [Although] the clinical evidence suggests that Nexium is only marginally better than Prilosec, AstraZeneca . . . was able to get a separate set of patents on Nexium. It made a big marketing push to convert customers to the new drug.'[16] Other companies pursued the same approach of creating a copycat drug and presenting it as new and improved. Forest Laboratories' Lexapro was marketed as a better version of its antidepressant Celexa and Schering-Plough brought out Clarinex as an improvement on its existing allergy pill Claritin, which happened to be facing imminent patent expiry. Several European countries including the British National Health Service refused to toe the line, pointing to the lack of evidence that Clarinex offered an advantage for patients, but it didn't stop Schering-Plough sending sales reps to British doctors' surgeries offering to help change patients' prescriptions over to the new drug.[17] Clarinex quickly built global sales of $600 million a year, only one-quarter of what Claritin had once brought in but still a significant revenue stream.

If a company's scientists couldn't find a way to change an existing product enough to call it a new drug at a molecular level, delivering the medicine in a different form could also provide a route to extending its revenue-generating life. Fran Leath's final position at Eli Lilly before she left in 2003 was as one of three global lifecycle managers for the anti-psychotic Zyprexa. Eli Lilly had experienced a vivid demonstration of the importance of a strategic approach to patent expiry in 2000 when a shock US court ruling meant that patent protection for the antidepressant Prozac ended in 2001, two years earlier than expected. On the day of the ruling, the company's stock price fell by more than 30 per cent.[18]

Zyprexa wasn't due to go off patent in the United States until 2011 but strategising the planned lifecycle of a drug began even before it went on sale for the first time. What's more, Prozac's patent expiry led to an immediate collapse in sales, down 70 per cent within six months, meaning Zyprexa was now the company's most important product. The pressure was on to squeeze as much revenue from the drug as possible.

'My job was to facilitate the creation of line extensions and new formulations and whatever we could figure out we could throw at it to extend the life of that drug,' Leath says.[19] Eli Lilly had already had some success with new indications for the original drugs and with a new formulation, a fast-dissolving tablet which it called Zyprexa Zydis. 'Zyprexa is for people who are in high hallucinations and if you give them a pill they will spit it out, but if you can get a tablet in their mouth and have it basically fizz and swallow you're getting something in there without actually having to physically restrain to deliver a shot or trying to force a pill down someone,' Leath says. That alteration had its uses, 'but a lot of the extensions were about how do you play with manufacturing just to extend the life of the drug', she admits.

The company funded trials into putting Zyprexa and Prozac into one combination tablet and launched the resulting drug Symbyax in 2003 but sales never took off. Another avenue, which Leath helped to oversee, was the development of a long-acting injectable version of Zyprexa, Relprevv, which would only need to be administered every two to four weeks, replacing a daily tablet. A rival antipsychotic, Johnson & Johnson's Risperdal, had launched its own long-acting depot injection, Risperdal Consta, in the UK in 2002 and Eli Lilly wanted to compete in the same market. An injectable version was better suited for cases where doctors might be concerned about patients complying with instructions to take a daily pill, but there was also a more nakedly commercial motive. Eli Lilly was able to obtain a new patent on the delivery device which lasted until 2018, seven years after its patent on Zyprexa would expire. 'The pill may be generic but if you still have the depot, you're still reaping the benefits,' Leath says.

In the event, when Zyprexa went generic in 2011, long after Leath had left the company, its long-planned strategies were ineffective. The injectable version didn't get market approval until 2009 because of concerns it caused 'excessive sedation' and was subsequently hit by further problems when the deaths of two patients prompted an FDA safety probe. Two years after Zyprexa's patent expiry, Relprevv was generating revenues of less than $60 million.[20] By then, the entire Zyprexa franchise, which had once brought in $5 billion in annual sales, was worth $1.2 billion and falling fast. Nevertheless, when reformulations worked, they could bring in extensive revenues for drugmakers, keeping patients on expensive patent-protected medicines rather than the cheap generics they would otherwise be taking. In 2007, AstraZeneca launched an extended-release version of its antipsychotic Seroquel. The new formulation, Seroquel XR, had an extra five years of patent protection and its annual sales of $1.5 billion helped to soften the blow when generic versions of the original drug launched in 2012.

As well as trying to use scientific tools to extend a franchise, drug companies became increasingly adept at using legal filings to defend existing monopolies for as long as possible. One study found that between 2005 and 2015 nearly 80 per cent of new patents were for existing drugs. The same research looked at the hundred top-selling drugs and found that more than 70 per cent had been able to extend their market monopoly by obtaining additional patents, with more than 50 per cent doing it more than once. Around one in eight of these bestsellers added four or more extensions.[21]

The multitude of patents protecting a single product was possible because there are several different types which can apply to the production of pharmaceuticals. The core patent for a new chemical entity is known as the compound or composition of matter patent and covers the active ingredient itself. This offers the greatest protection but drug companies have been able to buttress it with secondary patents for different formulations, created by combining the active ingredient with other ingredients or delivering the drug in a different way, or specific methods of use. Patents covering manufacturing processes can also be sought to bolster the legal protections around a product.

Industry efforts to widen the scope of intellectual property rights and use them to protect their products pitched them into perpetual legal battles with generic manufacturers with vast sums at stake. When AstraZeneca was facing patent expiry on Prilosec, a legal battle with generic manufacturers allowed it to delay the launch of generics. With Prilosec bringing in $10 million a day, even a few months was worth a fortune as well as giving more time to switch patients onto its successor, Nexium.

Generic drug companies would challenge patents of all kinds, asserting that compounds or processes didn't meet the requirements of being sufficiently novel, 'non-obvious' and useful enough to merit protection. In the US market generic manufacturers were incentivised by an extra prize: under legislation passed in the early 1980s, the first one to file for regulatory approval and risk a patent infringement lawsuit is rewarded with a 180-day period in which no other generic companies can launch their products. On the other side, research-led companies, with their burgeoning legal departments, would lodge their own infringement claims, dragging generic companies through the courts to force them to prove they weren't violating patents. By suing for patent infringement, a manufacturer places an automatic thirty-month pause on the US regulator approving the generic.

The pharmaceutical industry had looked for ways to extend the patent life of its drugs for decades. Before changes to patent law in the early 1980s, it had been common for a company to ensure it was the first to file a patent and then to follow this with a barrage of modifications to delay when the clock started running. A patent for the tranquilliser Valium was first filed in 1959 but further applications meant it wasn't issued until 1968, five years after it had gone on sale.[22] It was in the 1990s, however, that this 'evergreening' became increasingly central to the drug industry's model, creating pressure to find more and more creative ways of extending a franchise for as long as possible.

Tahir Amin, a forty-nine-year-old Yorkshire-born intellectual property lawyer, has spent years exposing the ways in which pharmaceutical companies game the patent system. He gave up a corporate job in London in the early 2000s to move to India and challenge pharmaceutical patents after becoming disillusioned with the way the IP system had developed. 'Often I would be acting for big clients where I would be squashing a lot of smaller businesses and it wouldn't be because I had a great legal case, it was because I had deep pockets and I had a litany of IP rights,' he says.[1] 'A lot of them weren't really properly formed and should never have been granted, but that's the way the system works and you can just threaten people with lots of IP rights.' He subsequently co-founded the New York-based Initiative for Medicines, Access and Knowledge (I-MAK), which highlights how drug companies weaponise intellectual property rights.

Applications for patents covering a new drug would typically be staggered in the hope of extending protection over many years. After securing a twenty-year patent on the active ingredient, 'what companies do then is two or three years later they might file a formulation patent, or five years later they might file a different form of that compound, what we call a crystalline form, because small molecule compounds can exist in different crystal structures and have different properties', Amin says. 'They're overlapping with the original patent so they add on two or three extra years and they keep building these out.' Even if some of the patents wouldn't hold up under legal challenge, they can serve as a deterrent to generics. 'So I file as many patents as I can, create this huge wall and make it hard for my competitors to get over. And even though many of the patents I don't use . . . you can think about it in terms of property and building my fence as far out as possible so no one can encroach on my land.'

The practice of building up 'patent thickets' – interlocking webs of legal protection which any potential generic manufacturer would have to try and unpick – became more pronounced as large molecule biologics grew in prominence. These complex products, grown in living cells rather than chemically synthesised, have allowed their manufacturers to seek far more patents than those surrounding a typical drug. Amin's organisation I-MAK has tallied almost 250 US

patent applications filed on AbbVie's $20 billion-a-year biologic
Humira, with at least seventy of those also filed in Europe. The
cancer drug Imbruvica, which was launched by the same company
in 2013, had accumulated eighty-eight patents by the end of 2019.[24]
Not all of the patents are likely to withstand a legal challenge, but
their presence makes the process of being able to sell a copycat
'biosimilar' without being deemed to infringe one or more of these
patents much harder.

The cost and risk of litigation for both sides led to the phenomenon of 'pay-for-delay' settlements whereby a research-led drug
company strikes a deal with the generic manufacturer challenging a
patent. Under a typical deal, the generic company would agree to
stay out of the market for a set period in exchange for a cut of the
profits or the right to enter the market early, giving it a head-start
on other generic versions. Some included an agreement by the original manufacturer not to introduce a generic version of their own
drug – a so-called 'authorised generic' – which could threaten the
generic manufacturer's eventual profits.

David Maris, a former analyst who began covering the pharmaceutical industry in 1994, blames the 180-day exclusivity period given
to the first generic for exacerbating the problem. 'By giving such a
long incentive, you make it valuable for people to settle,' he says.
'And that goes against the idea of getting generics to market faster.'[25]
The 180-day prize has been interpreted to give exclusivity to the first
generic competitor to file for regulatory approval regardless of
'whether or not that company succeeds in invalidating the patent or
finding a way to avoid infringement'.[26] By striking a deal without
allowing a court to decide on the validity of the patents being challenged, the innovator company removes the risk of an immediate
end of its monopoly while the generic manufacturer can still enjoy
its 180-day reward at a future date. Such deals can therefore be in
the interests of both companies, though they help to maintain higher
costs for consumers by delaying generic entry.[27] Other generic companies who might be seeking regulatory approval for their own versions
must wait until 180 days after the first generic has hit the market.

Pay-for-delay deals became commonplace during the 2000s, with dozens of agreements each year.[28] In 2005, AstraZeneca reached a settlement with Ranbaxy involving its protein pump inhibitor Nexium. Under the deal, the Indian manufacturer agreed to delay the launch of its generic product until May 2014, while AstraZeneca agreed not to launch an authorised generic during Ranbaxy's 180-day exclusivity window. AstraZeneca also reached deals with two other generic manufacturers. The US drug company Cephalon, which was later bought by Teva, boasted of securing six more years of patent protection for its sleep drug Provigil by entering into settlements with four generic manufacturers which kept them out of the market until 2012, generating '$4 billion in sales that no one expected'.[29]

By 2010, the Federal Trade Commission estimated that the delays created by these types of agreement were costing the public $3.5 billion a year in the United States alone. Amid criticism from academics and policymakers, the legality of the agreements became hotly contested. In 2011, the British competition watchdog opened a case against GlaxoSmithKline investigating agreements it had struck to pay generic drug manufacturers £50 million to delay the release of competing versions of its antidepressant Seroxat. A seemingly major breakthrough came in June 2013, when the US Supreme Court ruled in *FTC* v. *Actavis* that pay-for-delay agreements were subject to antitrust laws. However, whilst there have been a number of large settlements – in 2015, Cephalon paid $1.2 billion to settle an FTC case over Provigil – the tactic has not been stamped out altogether.[30]

The law professor and author Robin Feldman has argued that companies have simply found more complicated ways to structure deals which have the same anti-competitive effect but have left regulators struggling to keep up. Feldman has highlighted how, in three-quarters of settlements where a generic company has agreed to delay market entry, the FTC has admitted being unable to identify an obvious form of compensation received in return. In what she calls the 'modern era of pay-for-delay agreements . . . [they] may be more cleverly disguised, and they often incorporate complex side-deals that are difficult for courts and antitrust authorities to unravel'.[31]

The practice has also spread to biologics. AbbVie reached licensing deals with three biosimilar manufacturers over its blockbuster arthritis drug Humira under which they were permitted to launch in European countries from 2018 but would stay out of the US market until 2023.[32] A lawsuit challenging the deals was rejected on the grounds that the Supreme Court's 2013 decision only covered cash payments in exchange for delayed entry.[33]

With the vast sums of money blockbuster drugs brought in, even short delays became hugely valuable and drug companies looked for every edge they could get. The FDA had long run a 'citizen petition' scheme to allow members of the public to raise concerns about drugs being considered for approval, but from the early 2000s drug companies began using this to try and disrupt the approval of rival products.

An analysis of citizen petitions filed between 2000 and 2012 by Feldman found that drug companies were routinely using the petitions 'as an 11th-hour effort to prevent generic competitors from gaining FDA approval and entering the market'.[34] Even if the concerns raised were dismissed, they could still benefit from the time it took the regulator to consider them.

Some of the frivolous reasons drugmakers cited in trying to persuade the regulator to delay approval of generics included the fact that the original drug had two lines scored onto the tablets and the proposed generic only had one. It just so happened that the drug company, Warner Chilcott, had recently added the second score line to its own tablets. On another occasion, a company making generics tried to delay rival generic manufacturers from launching by citing concerns over different types of orange juice used in a study. Both petitions were rejected, but Feldman's research suggested drugmakers had succeeded in delaying other generics.[35]

Drug companies were routinely prepared to play dirty in an effort to keep rival drugs off the market. In the mid-2010s, with the patents protecting AstraZeneca's statin Crestor fast approaching their expiry date, the company tested the drug on fourteen children with a rare inherited condition called homozygous familial hyper-cholesterolemia (HoFH). HoFH patients have a high risk of heart attacks because of high cholesterol levels, the same problem addressed by Crestor's existing mass-market use so it was no surprise that the trial showed favourable results. Orphan designation was duly granted for this use and it received market approval to be sold to HoFH patients in May 2016. This was just two months before Crestor was due to go off patent, opening the $5 billion-a-year drug to competition from several cheap generics which would dramatically reduce AstraZeneca's market share.[36]

The drugmaker then used Crestor's orphan designation for a small group of patients with a rare condition to try and delay the launch of eight generics until 2023, arguing that there would be safety concerns if the generic drug labels did not include data on the medicine's potential use for paediatric HoFH patients. This data was protected by the exclusivity rights attached to orphan drugs.[37] On this occasion, AstraZeneca's tactic was not successful. 'This case is not about the medical needs of a small population of paediatric patients with a rare disease,' lawyers for the FDA and US government wrote in response to the lawsuit. 'It is about AstraZeneca's profit-driven desire to substantially extend its virtual monopoly on one of the world's most popular medicines.'[38] A judge agreed and the generic versions were able to launch.

Allergan, a drug company based in Dublin, where it benefits from Ireland's low corporation tax rates, is among the latest to demonstrate the lengths the industry will go to in efforts to protect the revenues from bestselling drugs. In 2012, the US introduced a new patent review tribunal to adjudicate on challenges to drug companies' patents brought by manufacturers looking to sell generic versions. Four years later, the generic drug companies Teva and Mylan asked the board to throw out the patents protecting Allergan's second biggest-selling drug, a dry eye treatment called Restasis. Revenues of $1.5 billion a year were at stake.

The following year, Allergan did something that no drug company had tried before: it transferred six patents for the drug to the St

Regis Mohawk Tribe in upstate New York. The idea, which had come
from Michael Shore, a Texan intellectual property lawyer, was that
the tribe's status as a sovereign entity meant it was exempt from the
US Patent and Trademark Office adjudicating on cases it was involved
in.[39] Instead of having to contest the case in front of the patent
review board which had been set up to make faster determinations,
any challenge, it was believed, would need to come through the
slower-paced federal courts.

Shore, negotiating on behalf of the tribe, struck a deal under
which Allergan paid the tribe $13.75 million and agreed to pay annual
royalties of $15 million for as long as the patents remained active.
The tactic was heavily criticised and was ultimately unsuccessful, with
the tribunal rejecting the idea that the tribe's sovereign immunity
applied to patent reviews. That decision was upheld by the US
Supreme Court.[40] In the meantime, a federal judge had already ruled
against Allergan.

The win-at-all-costs mentality which started to govern so many
aspects of how drug companies operated in this financialised model
helped push some businesses over the line into illegality as executives
laboured to boost their numbers. The US non-profit Public Citizen
has published several reports cataloguing the number and size of
civil and criminal penalties paid by the pharmaceutical industry to
settle allegations of law breaking. The picture they paint is an ugly
one. Between 1991 and 2017 drug companies handed over $38.6
billion to federal and state authorities in the US to settle claims, an
enormous sum, albeit one that pales in comparison to annual pharmaceutical sales in America of more than $350 billion.[41]

The misdeeds run the gamut from deceptive marketing and illegally
promoting a drug for off-label use to overcharging government health
programmes, paying kickbacks, concealing clinical trial data and selling
substandard products. One of the most egregious examples of
malfeasance came when the British company GSK was caught in the
early 2010s paying bribes to doctors in China. GSK paid fines totalling nearly half a billion dollars after a whistleblower revealed that
employees had been paying kickbacks as well as pushing drugs for

uses for which they hadn't been approved. The payments were routed through travel agencies, with GSK reportedly paying for fake 'conference services' to hide bribes designed to boost sales and allow the company to raise prices.[42] Claims about alleged bribes paid by GSK in Eastern Europe and the Middle East followed, with the company accused of paying doctors for speeches which never took place and making payments to doctors for prescribing Parkinson's disease and prostate cancer drugs.[43]

GSK is not alone in having paid kickbacks. A few years earlier, Johnson & Johnson paid $70 million to settle a criminal complaint filed by the US government. The charges included employees of a Romanian subsidiary bribing 'publicly-employed doctors and pharmacists to prescribe J&J products' during the 2000s.[44] Doctors were paid a cut of the cost of the drugs they prescribed. When an internal audit began investigating these cash payments in 2007, the scheme switched to paying for doctors' travel to medical conferences, with employees arranging for the company to be overcharged in order to give the doctors 'pocket money' or cash to allow their families to join them on the trips. More recently, in December 2016, the generic manufacturer Teva paid more than $500 million after admitting to bribing senior government officials in Russian and Ukraine and doctors in Mexico to boost sales of Copaxone, a multiple sclerosis drug, and other products.[45] At least eleven drug companies have paid settlements over bribery claims.

The playbook of techniques for extending the lifespan of a blockbuster drug franchise was only one part of the equation for ensuring longer exclusivity periods in which drugs could be sold at high prices. Drug executives remained mindful of other major threats to their profits: it wasn't just cheap copycat drugs which could bring prices crashing down; politicians and organised patient groups speaking out through protests and in the media also posed a high risk. As lifecycle management became more and more important, so too did the ways in which the industry managed these other risks. The pharmaceutical industry has always been a lobbying powerhouse; the long legacy of failed efforts to impose significant US drug pricing reforms since the 1990s is testament to that, as are the political contributions and donated private jet flights which help to keep politicians on side.

'They're notorious,' says Donald Macarthur, a retired British pharmaceutical industry consultant. 'If there's any development on pricing that they don't like, in any state of the union, or any individual city in the [United States], they'll fly about 50 lawyers to absolutely kill it off. And they have 100 per cent success rate.'[46] Over the twenty years from 1999, drug companies spent at least $4.7 billion on campaign contributions and political lobbying, amounting to more than $230 million a year. Whenever key drug-pricing reforms and regulations were due to be voted on, 'there were large spikes in contributions to groups that opposed or supported the reforms', a study found.[47]

In the United States the industry enjoys a unique advantage purely as a result of its geographical spread. Drug companies can count on the support of free-market Republicans for ideological reasons, but powerful Democrats also tend to be supportive because many drug companies happen to be based in reliably blue states – either on the East Coast in Massachusetts, New Jersey or Pennsylvania, or in California. Of the money given to individual candidates, 59 per cent went to Republicans and 41 per cent to Democrats.[48] In Europe, the industry's influence takes subtler forms, but lobbying groups in Brussels, London and elsewhere remain powerful voices in political debates and keep a close watch on proposed regulatory and intellectual property changes.

'It's a dirty business, I'm afraid,' Macarthur says. 'They always like to think they have the high moral ground but they don't, it's the same as tobacco or an oil company – basically they're just trying to make as much money as they can.'

Away from the corridors of power, the AZT debacle had shown the sort of noise a small, determined group could whip up if they considered a price to be exploitative. So it is little surprise that in the wake of this encounter, managing potential dissent from patients also became an important consideration.

Patient advocacy groups were not in themselves a bad thing for pharmaceutical companies. In fact, they could prove extremely beneficial, as Abbey Meyers and other patient leaders had demonstrated in the early 1980s. As well as helping to push through the Orphan Drug Act, the flurry of patient groups for those suffering rare diseases helped companies with a promising drug compound to easily find patients for clinical trials. If a successful treatment was developed, these groups allowed a manufacturer to avoid the need for considerable outlays to identify who might benefit from the drug and to market it to them.

By the 1990s, drug companies were routinely providing significant funding to patient groups and in 2017 a study found that more than 80 per cent of large advocacy organisations had received industry money.[49] There were shared interests in pushing for the uptake of new drugs, even if they had relatively minor benefits for the sums charged, and for increased government funding for research into the basic science in that therapy area. The financial support didn't necessarily buy complete silence on pricing issues but at the very least it ensured that disagreements were much more likely to be raised in private meetings rather than aired in public. Patient groups have been notably muted in recent drug-pricing debates and are far more likely to focus their criticisms on insurers and government officials for refusing to pay for treatments rather than manufacturers for setting excessively high prices.[50]

Some patient groups have even raised funds for drug research and partnered with pharmaceutical companies to try and develop treatments. The Cystic Fibrosis Foundation played a critical role in funding the early development of what later became several breakthrough treatments for cystic fibrosis which were brought to market by Vertex. The charity was able to sell its royalty rights to the drugs for more than $3 billion, but faced criticism for not doing more to try and tackle the high cost of the treatments, which, as we shall see, were launched with price tags of up to $300,000 a year.[51]

Alongside this, industry-funded patient assistance programmes helped to undermine measures used by insurers to dissuade their customers from using higher-priced drugs. In countries like the US where private health insurance plays a key role, insurance companies often require patients to make higher contributions, known as co-pays, towards the cost of more expensive drugs and can use increased co-pays to reduce demand in the event of a price hike. To circumvent this, it became commonplace for drug companies to fund assistance programmes for the less well-off or offer coupons which covered these costs.

Drugmakers are banned from offering direct financial assistance to US Medicare patients under federal bribery laws, but have found a workaround as they can donate to independent charities which in turn help people access their drugs. As well as helping to boost sales and serving as a useful PR tool in the face of pricing criticism, drugmakers' contributions to patient assistance programmes can qualify as charitable giving, making them tax-deductible.[52] In 2001, the industry spent less than $400,000 on patient assistance programmes. By 2014, that had topped $7 billion.[53]

The combined impact of all these efforts, in tandem with the changes in marketing and pricing, was to smash the delicate equilibrium that defined the industry's social contract. The industry wasn't so much putting its finger on the scales as dumping billions of dollars a year on them – funds that paid for lobbyists and lawyers, for coupons so patients wouldn't notice as their drugs rocketed in price, and for clinical trials to herald a mildly tweaked bestseller as a new and improved drug which could keep the cash train rolling. It didn't always work, but when it did the results of these new strategies could be spectacular, allowing single drugs to remain patent-protected long past their original shelf life. Companies were able to extend one discovery into franchises which brought in billions in annual sales for decades.

On the other side of the equation were generic drugmakers, viewed by research-led firms as parasites and pirates. With no patent protection, generics are traditionally a low-margin industry, with manufacturers needing to shift vast quantities to make a reasonable profit from these cheap drugs. These old drugs are meant to serve as an important check on the ability of drugmakers to profit from their discoveries, ensuring that drugs become significantly cheaper over time. Only here too the desire to make money could distort the market, with those selling generic drugs not necessarily averse to dirty tricks of their own. By the 2010s the cultural changes and financialisation which had barrelled through the pharmaceutical industry had created the conditions for a new kind of drug company: one which took the ethos of drugs being nothing more than financial assets to the extreme.

CHAPTER SIX

The trick

Marc Cohodes likes to collect trophies. An axe engraved with the words 'THE FRAUD SLAYER', six pinball machines, a framed share certificate for a long-bankrupt Belgian software company: they are all monuments to vanquished foes.

The arcade games are a nod to his initiation into the world of short selling. Cohodes, then a fresh-faced twenty-one-year-old, was working at a Chicago bank when, one day in 1982, an analyst named Paul Landini asked if he wanted to join him on a trip to an arcade that evening to count the number of people pushing coins into pinball machines.

'Why are we doing that?' Cohodes recalls asking him.

'Because video games have just come out and I want to see how coin-operated pinball machines are doing,' was the reply. 'Because if video games become the rage, this company called Bally Manufacturing, which makes pinball machines, could have a huge problem.'[1]

That night, and again one night a week for several months, they worked their way around Chicago's arcades, talking to staff and trying to get a gauge on the weekly takings.

'Over a couple months, the coin drop kept going down, which meant people weren't going to these arcades, they were playing games at home,' Cohodes says. 'So we shorted Bally Manufacturing which I recall was a high $20, low $30 stock at the time. And the stock ended up going for $3.

'That was the first time I ever shorted anything, and I said, "This is kind of cool."'

He's been hooked ever since. Short-sellers, unlike typical 'long' investors, bet against companies. They hope shares will fall, rather than rise, and place bets by selling borrowed shares which they have to buy back at an agreed later date. If the share price has fallen, they can make huge profits. Depending on who you ask, short-sellers are either fulfilling an important public service, popping bubbles and keeping markets rational, or they are the cynics, sitting comfortably outside the fray and taking potshots which destroy the value of hard-working companies.

Both sides agree there is something different about short-sellers in their desire to stand apart from the herd and flout conventional wisdom. 'I always say that if you short stocks, there's something genetically wrong with you,' Cohodes says. 'You see the world differently.' He views himself as a 'champion of the common man', helping to protect unsuspecting investors by sniffing out what he calls 'fads, frauds and failures'.

Cohodes, who is in his late fifties, has been chewed up by the financial system. During the global financial crisis in the late noughties, amid market conditions that should have been perfect for short-sellers, he had to liquidate Copper River Management, once a billion-dollar hedge fund. He blamed Goldman Sachs for mishandling trades and forcing the fund's demise, charges the bank has denied. Now he bets with his own money, rising each morning at 4 a.m. to brew a cup of coffee and check on the chickens who graze on his twenty-acre farm in Sonoma County, California. From there, he heads to his office, an esoteric den with a bright pink sofa, ping-pong table and a large collection of lava lamps sharing space with stacks of books, a Bloomberg terminal and piles of research. It is here, dressed in a bright shirt and shorts, that he hunts for his next target.

'I always refer to myself as a stalker,' he explains. 'At any point in time, I probably have three to five hundred names in my head that I'm aware of, you know, what the companies do, how they do it, where they are in the cycle, things like that.'[2]

In the summer of 2015, he'd already been persuaded to bet against one Canadian drug company after one of his protégés, Fahmi Quadir, convinced him to short Valeant. Now a friend in Canada, the prominent investor Roland Keiper, was drawing his attention to another firm in the same industry: Concordia.

'He kept calling me up and saying, "Are you watching this Concordia?" The thing was going up and up and up,' Cohodes recalls.

'And I said, "Yeah, I'm watching Concordia." He goes, "Are you involved yet?" I said, "No, I'm not involved yet." And he said, "Why?" I said, "Because the thing's crazy."'

Cohodes was interested. 'I always say bet the jockey not the horse,' he says, and in Concordia's chief executive, Mark Thompson, he saw someone who he thought was 'a career failure'.

But with the stock rising so fast, Cohodes feared being caught out by a large margin call – the requirement for short-sellers to post a proportion of the value of potential losses – and having to liquidate the position.

So for now, he told Keiper, he was prepared to wait. 'I say never go after the jaguar in the tree,' Cohodes says. ''Cause if you're a hunter, and you go after, [or] climb a tree to wrestle the jaguar out of the tree . . . the jaguar will bite you, scratch you, push you, do whatever, and you'll fall out of the tree and you'll be dead and the jaguar will be looking at you and laughing.

'So I wait for someone to shoot the jaguar out of the tree, and then once the thing's on the ground, I'll then jump on the jaguar and carve the thing up.'

Like Cohodes, Dimitry Khmelnitsky had always been an outsider. Born in Moscow before the fall of the Soviet Union, he moved with his family to Israel at the age of thirteen to escape the food shortages and petty crime.

'Everything was in short supply,' he says. 'You had to line up for bread. Meat was in short supply. In order to buy sausages, a very poor quality sausage, you literally had to stand in line for two hours to get it.'

After three years of military service in Israel, Khmelnitsky flew to Toronto to visit his best friend from high school and decided to stay. He enrolled in a computer science degree, dutifully following his father's wishes. 'I studied for one year in computer science and then I figured I just can't do it,' he says. A classmate suggested he try accounting instead. 'What attracted me to accounting was not boring accounting rules, because accounting could be extremely boring. But it's really how companies could play games with their accounting,' he says, his words still carrying the staccato Slavic accent of his youth.

He loved discovering the things large companies didn't want you to know. 'It involves a lot of investigative work, a lot of detailed work. You've got to read the whole bunch of documents, like a puzzle, and it's all over the place and you've got to try and put it together in a coherent picture.'[3] The instructor who sparked his interest was Anthony Scilipoti, one of the founders of an equity research firm called Veritas Investment Research. After Khmelnitsky had completed his training as a chartered accountant, his former teacher offered him a job.

Equity research analysts like Khmelnitsky usually work at banks or other large financial institutions; companies which may have a corporate finance division loaning money to the company being covered, or investment bankers trying to sell its shares. 'The analysts that followed Concordia, they weren't hard critics because their firms benefited from a lot of investment banking and underwriting fees,' one investor says. Indeed, one analyst who covered Concordia admitted he was directed by bosses to abandon a planned 'sell' rating which would have recommended investors dispose of their shares.[4]

Veritas, on the other hand, was an independent company which did nothing but equity research, giving Khmelnitsky more freedom. In July 2014, he was the first analyst to counter the prevailing enthusiasm for Valeant, putting a sell recommendation on the company.

More than a year later, struck by its similar focus on acquiring the rights to old medicines, he began looking at Concordia Healthcare. 'Those were two darling stocks,' he says, with their share prices rising 'astronomically' every year. Hedge funds had already poured money into the two companies and now more conservative asset managers running mutual funds were facing questions from investors about why they hadn't bought the stocks. 'If you're missing out on those returns that created pressure,' Khmelnitsky says, 'you don't want to miss out on the party.'[5] But, like Cohodes, when Khmelnitsky looked at Concordia's business model he had more questions than answers.

Khmelnitsky began poring over financial documents and other public filings. He wanted to assess whether the $3.5 billion valuation Concordia had put on the British company AMCo was a good deal. As far as he could see, Concordia's existing approach in the American market had been straightforward. 'They were buying old drugs where you don't need to invest much at all, and you can just jack up the price and that will generate returns,' he says.

It was easy to do in the US, where there were no price controls. But in the UK, with a large single payer in the form of the National Health Service (NHS), surely it would be very different. With an annual drug bill in 2015/16 of more than £13 billion, the NHS could wield enormous purchasing power when buying medicines, particularly older medicines like those owned by AMCo which were no longer protected by patent and so were open to generic competition.[6] Despite this, on the day the deal was announced Concordia was bullish about the growth prospects for the newly acquired business, and the potential to increase prices. It suggested the revenues from AMCo alone would rise to as much as $560 million in 2015, up from $454 million the previous year.[7]

On a phone call with analysts to discuss the deal, Mark Thompson, Concordia's founder and chief executive, was buoyant, describing the new business as a 'very, very powerful cash machine'.[8] It was, he insisted, a transformational deal which meant Concordia could now 'provide a one-stop shop for Big Pharma' looking to divest products sold around the world. Thompson was joined on the call by John Beighton, the chief executive of AMCo, who described how they acquired drugs from large pharmaceutical companies and 'breathe[d] new life back into them'.

'We like to describe these products as little jewels that we acquire and we polish up and turn into real shining stars,' he said. They were jewels because 'the majority of our products are either exclusive or semi-exclusive, and this is despite the fact that the products have been around, in some cases, for over eighty years'.

Asked if there was room for further revenue growth from the existing products, Beighton said, 'We haven't finished polishing. In fact . . . there are a number that have not been exploited yet. And we look at that both from a promotion and a price perspective.'

But the pair wouldn't be drawn on the secret sauce behind AMCo's success.

Thompson referred obliquely to AMCo being a branded medicines business with 'a very unique model, which I don't want to get into at this point in time. But you can look at it as a very similar model to Concordia.'[9]

What was really going on here? Khmelnitsky and others wondered. What are they doing that we don't know about?

The trick had emerged years earlier in the suburbs around London. At its core, it came down to the different way in which the UK seeks to control the prices of medicines sold under a brand name and those sold under their generic, scientific name.

Drugs sold under a brand name are usually introduced to the market as a new medicine which is still covered by a patent. As patents grant the supplier a monopoly for their duration, the prices for branded drugs in the UK are set by manufacturers before first entering the market. Once a drug is being sold, price regulation limits the ability of a manufacturer to change the price. If a company subsequently wants to increase the price it can petition the government for permission to do so. Alternatively, until 2019, it could agree to lower the price of one branded drug to match the extra cost of a price increase for another drug in its portfolio.[10] This set-up allows the NHS to retain control over its total spending on branded medicines. By contrast, cheaper generic drugs have much lighter regulation, with competition instead expected to act as the main driver in keeping prices down.

To move between the two categories, a drug could be 'debranded' and relaunched under a generic name, taking it outside the price restrictions and profit cap applied to branded medicines. The practice was not a new one, but by using it on medicines for which they were the sole or dominant supplier and combining it with dramatic price increases, a small group of companies were to discover it could produce lucrative results. Among them was Auden Mckenzie, then a small British company with a registered office on a dilapidated industrial estate next to railway tracks in Wembley, north London.

Auden Mckenzie was a family business launched at the turn of the millennium by Amit Patel and his sister Meeta, then both still in their twenties, with their father, Hasmukh. The elder Patel owned a pharmacy in Kensington in west London and had identified a gap in the market for a company making generic versions of specialised medicines.[11] He invested in the fledgling firm and the company set up a small manufacturing plant. Its first products included Synastone, an injectable version of the opioid methadone which is used as a pain-relief treatment and as a substitute for heroin in treating addicts.

Over the next few years, the company carved out a lucrative niche, reviving old drugs bought from large pharmaceutical companies and launching new formulations of generic drugs including several inject-able products. In 2008 they reached a deal with a large US company to buy the rights to Hydrocortone, a brand name for the drug hydrocortisone, a life-saving hormone replacement taken by patients with Addison's disease which had been around since the Second World War.

In order to sell a generic version of a drug in the UK, companies must obtain a marketing authorisation from the regulator. Auden Mckenzie had already applied for licences to make and sell generic versions of the two strengths of hydrocortisone tablets sold by the US drug giant Merck & Co. (MSD) in 2005, and in 2007, after success-fully demonstrating bioequivalence between the proposed generic versions and MSD's existing products, the applications were approved.

Several months later, in April 2008, the Patels struck a deal with MSD for the rights to the branded version. This version was easier to break into quarters – useful for those patients who needed only a partial dose – but it also meant that Auden Mckenzie would now be the only licensed manufacturer in the UK, giving it, at least for a period, significant control over pricing.

Without patent protection, anyone else could apply for a licence to sell their own generic version but this would be an expensive process which could take a year or two and the market had only limited value. There was also, in theory at least, a risk that health officials might notice if a drug rose dramatically in price and take steps to intervene. The government had some powers to step in if it deemed a price excessive but these had never been formally used, with official policy to instead let market forces control generic prices.[12]

After reaching the deal with MSD, Auden Mckenzie dropped the existing brand name and informed health officials they would instead be selling the drug under its generic name, hydrocortisone. At the same time, the drug's price changed.

The NHS publishes a monthly drug tariff, listing the price it pays to pharmacists for the different drugs they dispense, in addition to a fee for handling the prescription. The prices for generics set out in the tariff are calculated from data collected from manufacturers and wholesalers. Of course, if a drug has only one supplier, this price is closely linked with that manufacturer's ex-factory price, although it also reflects the margin received by others in the supply chain including wholesalers. For years, a packet of thirty hydrocortisone 10mg tablets, by far the most common strength, had been priced at 70 pence in the drug tariff. But in December 2008, the drug, now sold under a generic name, had a new reimbursement rate of £30.50. Nine months later, it rose again to £40. The cost to the NHS in England for community prescriptions alone increased from £400,000 in 2007 to nearly £32 million in 2009.

Boosted in part by hydrocortisone's soaring revenues, Auden Mckenzie rapidly grew in size. In 2007, its turnover had been just over £5 million a year, with post-tax profits of around £3 million. By 2009, turnover had risen to nearly £26 million and annual profits soared to £11 million.[13] The price rise was sufficiently dramatic to catch the attention of a journalist at the *Mail on Sunday* and in July 2010 he questioned Amit Patel at the businessman's house, where an Aston Martin and Mercedes were parked on the drive. Patel said the company had made a multi-million-pound investment in the manufacturing of the drug but had now recouped the costs. He promised that the price would 'creep back down because the company has recouped what it needed to . . . It was not simple and it was a very expensive process,' he added.[14]

However, the price paid by the NHS did not fall and from 2013 it began to rise again. By early 2015, when the Patels reached a deal to sell the company, the cost to the British health service of a pack of 10mg tablets had topped £66. It rose again under new ownership, peaking in January 2016 at nearly £88, an increase of more than 12,000 per cent since 2008.[15] Doctors, blissfully unaware of the price rise, continued to prescribe it. One, an endocrinologist and professor in London called Karim Meeran, later described how he had eventually discovered the price rise. He had a private patient brought in as an emergency case for whom he prescribed hydrocortisone. She came back from the hospital's pharmacy to tell him it was £100 a month and she couldn't afford it. 'I was really shocked,' he said. 'I said, "There's an error down there in the pharmacy," but, no, it was £100 for a month's supply, rather than £1.'[16]

Hydrocortisone and drugs like liothyronine, a treatment for patients with an underactive thyroid gland which was debranded at around the same time, showed that significant increases in the price of long-established medicines were possible even within the UK's supposedly closely regulated market. There were no signs of any push back from the British health service even as the companies involved notified officials of their new prices. Consequently, word of these successes, and the government's apparent willingness to tolerate it, soon spread and several companies began to hike the price of old medicines.

During Concordia's call with analysts in early September 2015, Mark Thompson was reticent to reveal the details of AMCo's business model. But the subsidiary's chief executive, John Beighton, had been far less discreet at a private industry event a few years earlier.

On a cloudy morning in November 2012, Beighton, then chief executive of the recently rebranded Mercury Pharma, and Guy Clark, the company's head of business development, gave a presentation at the Waldorf Hotel, a five-star establishment in the heart of central London. They were there to address movers and shakers from the pharmaceutical industry at an annual healthcare conference organised by the investment bank Jefferies.

Beighton, a slim but greying executive then in his early fifties, had joined Mercury just two years earlier after many years at Teva, the Israeli generics giant. He was recruited to lead a turnaround spearheaded by the private equity company Hg Capital, which had backed a management buyout in late 2009. At the time the company was still known as Goldshield, a name tainted by its involvement in a long-running price-fixing case which had cost the firm £4 million to settle and seen the business and its founders face criminal charges which had only recently been thrown out.[17] Under new ownership and leadership, the company embarked on a round of cost-cutting, closing loss-making parts of the business and shuttering a call centre of 550 people. The turnaround was rapid, with profits rising from £3 million to £13 million, as executives planned a new course focused solely on niche, off-patent drugs.

By early 2012, after paying out a £10 million dividend, the company was ready to be rebranded as Mercury Pharma and sold on by Hg Capital. The buyer, in a deal completed that summer, was another London private equity house, Cinven. Now Cinven planned to merge Mercury Pharma with another recently-acquired pharmaceutical company called Amdipharm to create AMCo.

Beighton and his colleague laid out the new company's planned business strategy to an audience of pharmaceutical executives. The talk was also something of a sales pitch, with Beighton well aware that Cinven would be looking to sell the combined business on to someone else within a few years.[18]

The slides from the presentation reveal that Beighton explained how Mercury Pharma focused on niche drugs which were off patent but had 'limited competition from originators or generics manufacturers or licence holders'.[19] It didn't carry out research into new medicines but worked on 'low risk' reformulations, launching new versions of existing drugs such as a tablet form of a medicine previously sold as a liquid or different strengths, and on taking generic products to new markets overseas.

In theory, generics companies face the constant risk of a rival company obtaining a marketing authorisation and entering the market, but Mercury and Amdipharm's most important drugs were protected by 'strong barriers to entry', one slide explained. Many of the existing authorisations dated back many years and were 'approved under "easier" regulatory regimes'. Some of the drugs were complicated to manufacture and many had a limited value, with total global sales of less than £10 million, giving little economic incentive for a rival to enter the market, particularly when seeking a new licence for a drug typically costs several hundred thousand pounds.

This limited competition and the British government's hands-off approach to regulating generics meant that prices could be increased, investors were told. The slides described the UK as 'an attractive market owing to unrestricted pricing on unbranded products'. The health service was paying limited attention to drug prices, which made up around 10 per cent of its budget, with pressure for savings focusing on other areas of spending. All told, the situation meant that there were 'significant volume / price optimization opportunities'. Beighton and Clark boasted of their 'proven track record' in carrying out this strategy at Mercury; now they planned to turn their focus to Amdipharm's 'underexploited' portfolio.

In some ways, Beighton, a mild-mannered, guitar-playing father-of-two, was an unlikely figure to oversee such a red-blooded capitalist strategy. He told friends he'd been a card-carrying socialist in his youth and remained a vocal supporter of the Labour Party when the hard-left backbench MP Jeremy Corbyn took over the leadership in 2015. Born in Sheffield, Beighton had once considered a career in politics, standing as Labour's candidate in the traditionally Tory stronghold of Ryedale, a rural constituency stretching into the North York Moors, in the 1987 general election. The seat was being defended by a Liberal Party candidate who had won a surprise by-election victory a year earlier and Beighton, who had little hope of winning, finished a distant third. Instead, the biochemistry graduate became a pharmaceutical industry lifer, starting out as a sales rep and, over the course of three decades, working his way up into senior management.[20]

Cinven's approaches to Mercury Pharma and Amdipharm were led by Supraj Rajagopalan, a partner at the private equity firm specialising in healthcare. Like Beighton, Rajagopalan had flirted with another career option in his youth. Educated at the fee-paying Abingdon School in Oxfordshire, he won a place at Cambridge University to study medical sciences and stayed on to complete a postgraduate degree in the same subject. A career in medicine beckoned but after two years as a doctor working for the NHS, he left the profession and ended up working in private equity.

Internal documents circulated within Cinven making the case for the investment allegedly pushed for a 'debranding' strategy and laid out the opportunity to increase prices and generate quick returns, according to a source who has seen the documents. Liothyronine, which had been rebranded by Mercury Pharma several years earlier, was highlighted as a key drug.

What was being suggested didn't break any laws; indeed, many in the generics market believed the British health department had no objection to the occasional price rise because it provided an incentive for rival generics to enter and force prices back down. In advocating this approach Cinven, like Concordia, was simply acting in the way the markets rewarded them: with a laser focus on maximising returns.[21]

The plan was given the green light and in March 2013 Cinven completed the merger of Mercury Pharma and Amdipharm, calling the new company Amdipharm Mercury, or AMCo, and installing Beighton as the chief executive. The new business wasted no time in getting to work to increase the value of its assets. The price of some of Amdipharm's bestselling drugs underwent regular increases after Cinven's takeover and by the end of 2013 an antiemetic had tripled in price while a thyroid drug had risen eight-fold.[22] Several aggressive price rises were also implemented on Mercury Pharma's portfolio. Meanwhile, the company went shopping for new assets. The first purchase, announced at the same time as the Cinven-initiated merger, was the rights to the Fucithalmic brand of eye drops used to treat bacterial conjunctivitis. The brand name was dropped the following year and the price paid by the NHS for the relaunched generic, for which AMCo was the only supplier, would be ten times higher than it had been before.

By 2015, as Thompson and other Concordia executives criss-crossed the Atlantic in an effort to land the AMCo deal, the debranding trick was being used by several drug companies on dozens of medicines. That year, large price increases for around seventy old medicines would cost the NHS an extra £262 million a year.[23] The technique was contagious. After selling Amdipharm to Cinven in late 2012, the two brothers who had founded the company began a new firm with drugs which they debranded and which then doubled in price every eight months. There seemed little need for caution. Beighton, the AMCo boss, told a US hedge fund at the time of Concordia's purchase that British government officials were well aware of what was happening and just waved the price rises through.

In the wake of Hillary Clinton's tweet in September 2015 promising to tackle price gouging in parts of the drug market, Concordia's share price, like those of many other drug companies, fell dramatically. By the time it was ready to sell eight million shares to help fund the AMCo deal, the sale price was $65 a share, significantly below the highs of nearly $90 which had been reached barely two weeks earlier.

While that offering, led by Goldman Sachs, was in progress, there was further bad news. The larger Canadian drug company Valeant found itself in the sights of Democrats in Congress who threatened to issue a subpoena if its chief executive refused to testify over the price increases of two heart drugs. Skittish investors took it as further indication that a crackdown on drug prices could be imminent and Concordia's stock took another hit. With the share offering still open, it meant that the financial institutions which had pledged to buy shares at $65 during the first twenty-four hours were now looking at a paper loss before they'd even received them.[24] The company was ultimately able to raise $520 million from share sales, down from the $700 million it had originally hoped for. It paid for the rest of the acquisition from $2.8 billion in debt financing, including a last-minute $180 million bridge loan from Goldman Sachs and the other banks which had underwritten the share offering.

Concordia looked to have weathered the storm. But in the following days, its larger peer, Valeant, would begin to unravel, raising considerable concern about the viability of both companies. In October, a study by Deutsche Bank revealed the scale of the price rises which had helped power Valeant's rapid growth. Politicians had singled out two heart medications but the practice extended to more than fifty drugs, with prices up by two-thirds on average in 2015 alone. Later that month, it faced further pressure over its close ties with a specialty pharmacy, Philidor, amid claims Philidor had been directing patients with prescriptions for cheap generics towards Valeant's expensive alternatives. Valeant's share price would fall to around $75, down from more than $250 a few months earlier.

In the wake of Valeant's sudden decline, Thompson and other Concordia executives who had previously welcomed the comparisons began to distance themselves. 'I think we're getting tarred with the same brush,' Thompson told a reporter in late October. 'We do have a very different model than they do. We buy products. We don't buy companies.'[25]

In November, during a conference call with analysts to discuss the business's latest financial results, Thompson insisted his company was 'not about price gouging or taking huge price increases'. He said that AMCo had raised the price of some of its products in the months before the sale but implied they were modest increases. 'The way they operate their business is very similar to ours,' he said. 'They are prudent and they take price where they think it's appropriate . . . What was a relatively small US business in 2014 is today a billion-dollar international pharmaceutical company,' he went on. 'The past two months has been an exceptionally challenging period for the entire specialty pharma industry and I recognise how difficult this period has been for many of our shareholders.'[26] He blamed much of the turmoil on 'misinformation that was communicated about Concordia that was patently false' but reiterated his faith in 'our business model strategy' and promised he would be buying more stock. The price increases implemented by Concordia in which their products doubled or tripled in price were not as eye-catching as Valeant's ten- or twenty-fold prices rises, but this belied the fact that they had typically already had their prices hiked shortly before Concordia acquired them.

Two months later, in January 2016, Thompson was interviewed at an investment conference by Prakash Gowd, an analyst at a Canadian bank. He gave an impassioned defence of Concordia's pricing strategy, saying 'we have always felt it was better to be conservative with price' and that patients have therapeutic alternatives so they didn't 'hold anybody hostage'.[27] He used the IBS drug Donnatal as an example, comparing Concordia's price of around $800 with a Valeant drug which cost $5,500. The comparisons weren't questioned in the room, but in reality the drug Thompson mentioned was rarely prescribed. Those that were cost one-third of the price of Donnatal, which was reliant on the loyalty of patients who had used it for years.

Inside Concordia, the acquisition of AMCo was seen as a 'pipeline play', attractive because of the reformulations and new versions of generic drugs which the company was developing and its potential for international expansion as much as the cash its current drugs were generating. Thompson's characterisation of AMCo's approach, with only modest price increases and a focus on growing through increased prescriptions rather than price, was at odds with what was occurring behind the scenes. While the deal was being agreed, AMCo had quietly implemented a host of large price increases on its medicines, as emails between the company and health service administrators reveal.[28] On September 7, the day before Concordia's deal to purchase the company had been publicly announced, an AMCo employee was asked by an administrator in the British health system to confirm price changes submitted for thirteen drugs, including several of the company's biggest earners. The drugs all increased in price by at least 50 per cent, with one, phenindione tablets, more than doubling from £237 to just under £520. The anticoagulant, which had cost just £18 a packet in 2010, had already trebled in price earlier that year. Over the rest of the month, before the deal had been formally completed, the prices of another fourteen drugs were increased.

Many of the same drugs would have their prices increased again under Concordia's ownership just a few months later. A liquid version of nitrofurantoin, which cost less than £100 a few years earlier, had already gone from £260 to more than £372 while the deal was being completed. In January, Concordia upped the price by another 20 per cent to £447. On the same day, liothyronine, which had gone up by around £50 a packet four months earlier, was bumped up by another 30 per cent to £258.[29]

These price rises didn't just carry a financial cost, draining millions from the taxpayer-funded British health system, they also had consequences for patient care. Liothyronine is used as a second-line treatment for patients with thyroid problems and has a small but passionate cohort who credit it with changing their lives. Patients with an underactive thyroid can experience weight gain, symptoms of depression and tiredness which is so extreme they cannot leave their beds. For those for whom the main treatment, levothyroxine, doesn't work, liothyronine can represent a lifeline.

In the late 2000s, the drug sold for 16 pence per tablet but it was debranded by Mercury Pharma in 2007 and the price began a steady rise which accelerated during Cinven and then Concordia's ownership of AMCo, reaching a peak of £9.22 for each pill. The cost to the NHS rose from under £4m a year to £31m in 2016.[30] In response, doctors in some parts of the country were told to take patients off the drug. Prescriptions dropped significantly and those who wanted to keep taking it had to resort to making trips to mainland Europe, where a packet of the tablets, made by a different manufacturer, sold for a few euros.[31] Others turned to online pharmacies with dubious credentials to source low-cost versions. In 2018, Melanie Woodcock, then a forty-seven-year-old woman living in Banbury in Oxfordshire, began using a 'website that is aimed at bodybuilders bulking up' to buy liothyronine after her doctors stopped prescribing it. She'd previously had her thyroid removed and has relied on liothyronine for more than a decade because the alternative medication left her with a litany of side effects: 'Feeling sluggish, constant headaches, dizziness, nausea feeling all day, it even affected my vision, just a constant brain fog . . . I wasn't going out anywhere. I wasn't going on holiday, I wasn't doing anything because I didn't have the energy . . . [Liothyronine] changed my whole outlook on life . . . I'm not happy about having to source it like this,' she says,[32] but she can't contemplate not being able to get the drug.

Meanwhile, the fight between management and Concordia's critics became increasingly public. Cohodes had finally placed his bet against the company after a shortfall in the equity fundraising round forced Goldman Sachs to step in with a bridge loan. A bellicose character, he began unleashing a barrage of disparaging tweets, describing Concordia as the 'poor man's Valeant' and questioning the track record of the company's chief executive, Mark Thompson. He was joined in his short position by other prominent short-sellers including Fahmi Quadir, a young analyst who had risen to prominence by betting against Valeant.[33]

Khmelnitsky had also gone public, becoming, in early March 2016, the first analyst to advise clients to sell Concordia's stock. The Russian-born accountant wasn't just facing the risk of embarrassment by going out on a limb. A decade earlier, an analyst at Bank of America named David Maris had been sued by Biovail, the predecessor of Valeant, after putting a sell rating on the company and questioning its account of missing earnings estimates because a truck transporting a large quantity of an antidepressant drug had crashed. He was ultimately vindicated when the lawsuit was dropped, but not before losing his job and having to endure private eyes hired by Biovail following his family around for months.[34] Maris is in no doubt about how hard it can be for an analyst to stick their neck out in criticising a company. 'People follow the crowd,' he says. When a company is doing well, 'everyone gets paid for supporting it and very few people get paid for calling it out as negative'.[35] Being on the other side can be a lonely game. 'I tell the business school class, I have seven brothers and sisters so I don't need friends,' Maris adds. 'You have to realise you are fighting for something much more important: you're fighting for the truth. You're trying to save people's retirement money.'

Nevertheless, Khmelnitsky didn't pull his punches. His report warned that despite 'aggressively pursuing' a strategy of 'buying developed drugs, hiking prices and skimping on R&D', Concordia was struggling to grow revenues. It also raised concerns about the sustainability of the drug company's low-tax structure, apparent reliance on price hikes and the amount of debt it had taken on, limiting its chance of making further acquisitions.[36]

A few weeks later another research firm run by former investigative reporter Herb Greenberg raised further questions about the future of the company's US business. 'While many investors were fixated on Valeant Pharmaceuticals, lesser-known Concordia Healthcare was pumped up on steroids,' he wrote. Greenberg pointed to the heart drug Lanoxin to dispute the company's claim that price rises on the drugs acquired from Covis hadn't led to a drop in the number of prescriptions.[37]

He also questioned whether Concordia had been aggressively selling into the channel during 2015, placing excessive amount of stock with wholesalers in order to boost revenue figures. The company booked such sales as revenue even though they hadn't yet been sold and the wholesalers were entitled to return unsold stock for a refund.

The pressure on Thompson was beginning to tell. Internally, there was a clamour to reduce the burden of long-term debt taken on to pay for the spate of acquisitions. It was now well north of $3 billion and interest costs alone were eating up $10 million a month.[38] In late March, the company's latest financial results showed revenues from its North American business were below expectations, but they were bailed out by growth from AMCo. Thompson issued a statement claiming that 'Concordia has been the subject of an unrelenting and malicious attack by a group of short-sellers for several months'.[39] A month later, he would single out Cohodes with a jibe delivered at the end of the company's AGM, defiantly proclaiming: 'If you are a chicken farmer, your chickens will come home to roost.'

Much of the short-sellers' case against Concordia was that it had overpaid for its acquisitions, loaded up on debt and would struggle to grow its existing business and find and pay for more acquisitions to maintain the growth which had powered its rise. But even these critics were unaware of the full extent of the price rises that had already been carried out by AMCo before it was bought by Concordia.

In the spring of 2016, one of Cohodes's friends, a thirty-three-year-old Dallas hedge funder called Chris Crum, began to analyse data released by UK health officials.

'I downloaded thirty-six months of data from the NHS saying how many prescriptions and how many pills, and at what cost. And it's all in Excel, and I wrote some codes to look up for some of these drugs. There are like ten thousand rows in some of these spreadsheets but I found it all and I aggregated it and I said, "Let's take a look at what's going on here."'

'And you can see, like nitrofurantoin, which was 7 per cent of AMCo revenue. The cost of [a] 100mg capsule which was manufactured exclusively by AMCo was 172 per cent more than 100mg tablets manufactured by Dr Reddy's. Fusidic acid, which is an eye drop, since 2013 they raised the price over 1,300 per cent. This is 8 per cent of AMCo revenue. So I figured out like, holy crap, they found a nice little loophole here. And is it legal? Yeah, it was legal. But is it right? It's not right.'[40]

He passed his analysis on to Cohodes.

'It was just great, you know, to be able to go after these guys and say, "Look, this is bullshit, right?" These drugs have been on the market for decades, in some instances, and you're jacking up the price now, because there's no, or almost no competition at all. And it's like free money for these guys. And that was the game.'

Crum thought the pricing behaviour revealed in his spreadsheets left Concordia vulnerable to regulators taking a close look at the company.

'You could see that these guys were jacking up the price. In the US people tolerated it a little bit . . . because there's not a lot of goodwill towards private insurers. In the NHS, you're ripping off the government and you're ripping off the taxpayers directly,' he says. 'You can be a profiteer, but once you get found out the game is over.' He was also struck by the fact that these weren't one-time price rises but a strategy repeated a number of times over several years.

By now, the mood in the United States and Canada, and among investors on Wall Street and Bay Street, was beginning to turn against the upstart drug companies they'd previously enthusiastically backed. In the same month Crum worked his way through dozens of spread-sheets, Valeant's chief executive Mike Pearson was summoned for a dressing down before a US Senate committee investigating excessive drug prices and Concordia's own share price was continuing a steady decline. Thompson had an added reason to fixate on the share price because he had used his shares as collateral to obtain loans. If it fell too far, a margin call would be issued and he'd be forced to liquidate part of his shareholding.[41] Then, suddenly, came an opportunity to rewrite the narrative.

On April 22, Bloomberg News reported that Blackstone Group,

one of the world's biggest private equity groups, was eyeing a take-over of Concordia.[42] Two other firms, Apollo Global Management and the Carlyle Group, were subsequently reported to have shown interest in bidding for the company.

Some analysts close to the company had long believed the plan had always been to grow it rapidly and then sell up to a larger pharmaceutical company or a private equity firm. 'They wanted to make a lot of money, make it really quickly and get out,' one says. Now, with private equity circulating, this opportunity was within their grasp. If they could seal a takeover deal and cash out, Thompson and other Concordia executives could count themselves among some of the biggest winners of a private-equity-fuelled transformation in how older medicines were treated by the drug industry.

In the UK, the trick was necessary as a way of getting around regulations governing the price of old drugs. In the US there was no need for similar gymnastics. In the absence of competition, companies enjoyed the same pricing freedom with old drugs as they did with new treatments. Concordia and Valeant were not alone in their willingness to embrace this, and in their wider business model which envisioned a new kind of pharmaceutical company. By 2015, at least two dozen companies were following a similar playbook. They had a simple pitch to investors: all the advantages Big Pharma enjoys, with almost none of the same risks.

What Thompson and other executives were doing was not unlawful; their actions were a product of the system, emblematic of an industry wholly focused on financial returns. These companies were the culmination of broader changes: the logical conclusion of investors' dissatisfaction with the high cost of R&D and a financialised business model which prioritised the short-term success of showing earnings growth every quarter.

But they emerged more specifically from a gap in the market created by large pharmaceutical companies' headlong rush into the blockbuster era. The myopic focus on products with the potential for billion-dollar revenues left behind many drugs which were profitable but would never reach those heights. This created an opening for a new sector within the industry: specialty pharma.

In the late 1980s and early 1990s, specialty pharmaceutical companies including Roberts Pharmaceuticals, King Pharmaceuticals and Jones Pharma sought to build a business without needing to fund the discovery of new drugs. Instead, they looked to pick up the underperforming assets developed by the big drug companies. Some were still under patent but had been overtaken by better, more lucrative treatments; others had been on the market many years, with steady but underwhelming sales from a small cohort of patients with residual loyalty to the brand. 'Back then a drug would go off patent and about 20 per cent of patients would stay on the brand,' says the former analyst David Maris.[43] 'Their doctors will say "I trust the brand, I don't trust these generics"', and write a prescription with a 'dispense as written' designation which meant pharmacists couldn't substitute in a cheaper generic version.

Larger drug companies were gradually persuaded to sell or license the rights to these assets to these new specialty pharma firms because, by their standards, the revenues were insubstantial. For the acquirers, on the other hand, a drug with sales in the low tens of millions was lucrative enough, and they hoped to revive these largely abandoned products into something even more substantial with a little care and attention.

In the early days, efforts were focused on boosting revenues by better marketing these unloved Big Pharma outcasts, some of which hadn't had any sales reps behind them for years. Specialty pharma companies also invested in some development work, seeking to find new uses for the drugs they acquired or perhaps finding new ways of formulating them, so that, for example, a two-times-a-day drug could become a more patient-friendly single pill. Doing so would provide a few years of exclusivity.

The price rises that followed these early acquisitions were generally modest and aimed at bringing the drug closer to the prices for other treatments in the same therapeutic area. 'There was no outcry back then because most of these were really small products and while some of the price increases were a lot, they weren't hundreds of per cent,' Maris says. 'They were just 20 per cent, 30 per cent. And they were a one-time price increase to get back to where the market is.'

In time, however, price rises became more central to the strategy. The number of off-patent drugs sold under a brand name which had more than doubled in price in a single price increase began to take off in the mid-2000s, with two or three a year becoming thirteen or fourteen from 2006 onwards.[44]

By finding drugs which had little competition, specialty pharma companies took the same price elasticity that the biotech industry had shown existed when there was only one supplier for a treatment and used it to demand higher and higher prices, even though the medicines they were hawking were old and previously cheap treatments. The prices demanded grew higher, in part, because of what had happened to the launch prices of new treatments across the industry. When early specialty pharmaceutical companies raised the price to something closer to rival products treating the same ailment, this would typically be a price rise of no more than one-third. By the early 2010s, a similar change to an old drug could mean a price increase amounting to thousands of per cent.

As specialty pharmaceutical companies pushed prices up, they found that insurers and health systems were either too focused on the cost of the highest-grossing drugs to notice what was happening or too afraid of being criticised for denying patients access if they did anything. Either way, the push back was minimal. 'The next generation of pharma guys (or the smart ones) understand the inelasticity of certain products,' the chief executive of one such company wrote in an email to an investor in May 2014. 'They just pass it through and focus on managing care for physician payments and blockbusters.'[45]

The threat of a patient outcry was dealt with using the industry's familiar methods – co-pay coupons were offered and patient assistance programmes set up to limit how much anyone would have to pay out of their own wallet. The result was a route to quick and seemingly easy profits. You didn't need to invest in drug discovery and patiently wait years. You didn't even need to build a factory; the original supplier would keep making it or else it could be outsourced to contract manufacturers. You could set up a company in your own living room. All it took was an ability to find a drug which, for whatever reason – commercial disinterest, manufacturing difficulties, regulatory quirks – had no significant competition, and a willingness to keep raising the price.

One of the first to demonstrate just how much the price of an old medicine could be increased in the US market was a Californian company called Questcor Pharmaceuticals. The company had bought the rights to the anti-inflammatory HP Acthar Gel from Sanofi in 2001 for $100,000 and a small royalty on future profits. The drug, an injectable hormone dating back to the 1950s, was prescribed by a small number of doctors for multiple sclerosis patients who suffered a relapse and was also the first-line treatment for a rare seizure disorder in babies, although it couldn't be directly marketed for this purpose because it had only been approved for other indications.

It sold for just $40 a vial when Questcor acquired it and, with a small patient population and a complicated manufacturing process, was still loss-making even when six years of price rises had taken it to $1,650 a vial.[46] Then, in 2007, with the company facing bankruptcy, a new chief executive, a veteran of the defence industry called Don Bailey, oversaw a change in strategy. The price of Acthar Gel was increased to more than $23,000 for a single vial.

Four months later, Danielle Foltz's seven-and-a-half-month-old son Trevor began suffering increasingly violent seizures and was diagnosed with infantile spasms. Neurologists warned that without urgently administering several injections of Questcor's drug Acthar, he would likely suffer irreversible brain damage. Each day that went by amounted to playing 'Russian roulette', Foltz told a 2008 congressional hearing, but their insurance initially baulked at paying for the medication and Questcor's patient assistance helpline said it would take several days to respond, with no guarantee it would provide the medication.[47]

'Just getting that kind of diagnosis shatters you, but then to add the guilt of realising that you may not be able to rescue your son because you can't afford to, it's unimaginable, and in my mind, unacceptable,' Foltz said.[48] Fortunately, her case had a happy ending. After five days, the insurer relented and agreed to pay and Trevor was successfully treated. She was at the hearing, she said, to plead for other families whose children would be diagnosed in the future: 'My heart cannot help but be consumed for those families devastated by infantile spasms. Will they have access to this drug, or will they be priced out?'[49]

For Questcor, the increased revenues from the price rise helped the company pull together sufficient data to secure approval to market the drug as a treatment for infantile spasms, something which doctors had been doing 'off-label' for decades.[50] It also funded studies into other uses of the medicine and boosted efforts to market the drug to patients with rheumatic diseases. The number of vials being sold ballooned and by 2013 Acthar was bringing in revenues of more than $750 million, up from less than $50 million when Bailey took over. A company which had been close to going out of business now had a drug which was well on its way to becoming a blockbuster.[51] It was so successful, in fact, that the British company Mallinckrodt Pharmaceuticals agreed to buy Questcor for $5.6 billion in March 2014, with Acthar Gel the sole meaningful source of revenue. Further price hikes followed under new ownership, with the list price of Acthar Gel approaching $39,000 in 2019, an increase of more than 97,000 per cent since 2001.[52] In 2013, Questcor acquired the rights to develop Synacthen Depot, a potential rival treatment which was being developed by Novartis.[53] It was promptly shelved. Four years later, Mallinckrodt paid a $100 million fine to settle charges that this had broken antitrust laws.

Another early proponent of large price increases was Ovation Pharmaceuticals, set up in Illinois in 2000 by Jeff Aronin, then a thirty-two-year-old business graduate with a plan to pick up the 'low-risk pharmaceutical products' from Big Pharma which were under-marketed or were in the late stages of development.[54] The company bought the rights to treatments for rare diseases and implemented sharp price rises. One former Abbott Laboratories medication went from $230 a dose to $1,900 after being acquired in 2003, while four drugs bought from MSD in 2005 underwent overnight price increases of up to 3,400 per cent.[55] A decades-old cancer drug went from costing $2,000 for a year's supply to $14,000.[56] Aronin sold the business for $900 million in 2009 and promptly set up a new firm, Marathon Pharmaceuticals, which later ran into trouble by proposing to sell an old muscular dystrophy drug for $89,000 a year, despite it being available cheaply in Europe.[57]

The scale of the price rises implemented by Ovation and Questcor on off-patent drugs with a single supplier drew a smattering of criticism, but it was Valeant, under Mike Pearson's leadership, which took the business strategy to a new level.

Pearson ruthlessly pared back costs, slashing the workforce of each newly acquired company and cutting R&D down to as little as 3 per cent of sales. This was typically accompanied by mammoth price increases. In 2013, Marathon had bought the rights to two heart drugs, Nitropress and Isuprel, and increased the prices from around $45 a vial to more than $200.[58] They were sold on to Valeant two years later and the Canadian company immediately implemented even more aggressive price rises, taking the drugs up to $880 and $1,760 respectively.[59]

By the time Thompson set up Concordia, specialty pharma's original focus on marketing niche drugs had morphed into a predatory, price-driven model. At least thirty American companies were buying old drugs and implementing sometimes enormous price rises. The frenzied hunt for acquisitions that resulted – Valeant alone made more than one hundred – meant some companies flipped already price-hiked drugs on to other upstart specialty pharma firms who then increased prices further.[60]

Valeant and others were acting, as a critical US Senate report later put it, 'more like hedge funds than traditional pharmaceutical companies'.[61] They were exploiting – in many cases ruthlessly – a market failure and were aided and abetted in this endeavour by financiers who rushed to give the businesses early-stage funding and major consultancy firms who helped to find suitable drugs. Private equity and venture capital firms, particularly a cluster based in the Chicago area, funded and set up several of the companies responsible for some of the largest price increases. Ovation Pharmaceuticals was able to acquire its first drugs after receiving $150 million in private equity financing.[62] Horizon Pharma, which put up the list price of a painkiller medication from $138 to nearly $3,000 per bottle, raised more than $50 million in venture capital funding before being listed on the Nasdaq in 2010.[63]

For those companies which were publicly traded, like Concordia and Valeant, their growing share price was crucial to the ability to fund each new drug acquisition. Hedge funds poured money into both companies. Bill Ackman's Pershing Square and another activist hedge fund investor, Jeff Ubben of ValueAct, were among the largest shareholders in Valeant during its rise, while the now-defunct hedge fund Visium Asset Management was among significant early shareholders in Concordia.

Alongside this, investment banks helped grease the wheels by orchestrating funding rounds and providing financing for new acquisitions, in exchange, of course, for lucrative fees; Valeant alone generated more than $400 million in investment banking fees.[64] Large consultancy firms were involved, too. Mike Pearson's views on the pharmaceutical industry had been shaped by his work as a consultant at McKinsey, where he spent two decades before making the leap to helming Valeant and applying his price-hiking, asset-stripping playbook there. Several other former McKinsey executives joined him at Valeant and the consultancy firm was also hired to provide advice to the drugmaker, including on pricing.[65] In late December 2014, a senior McKinsey consultant described several drugs Valeant was eyeing up, including two heart medications, as not being on insurers' radar and having 'material pricing potential'. A document attached to the email said that the 'products have been in the system for so long that reviews are practically rubber stamped'.[66]

During the same period, McKinsey was being paid to advise four companies who were seeking to boost sales of opioids. The company's consultants advised Johnson & Johnson on sales of a fentanyl patch, issuing recommendations on influencing doctors to prescribe stronger formulations, the *New York Times* reported.[67] They also spent years advising Purdue Pharma on how to 'turbocharge' sales of OxyContin, suggesting ideas like increasing visits from sales representatives to doctors writing large numbers of prescriptions and urging the company 'to consider mail orders as a way to bypass pharmacies that had been tightening oversight of opioid prescriptions'.[68] In 2017, with the devastatingly addictive effects of the drug well established, McKinsey proposed a plan to pay pharmacies a rebate of nearly $15,000 every time a customer overdosed or developed an opioid use disorder.[69] The company subsequently agreed to pay $573 million to US states to settle claims it faced over its role in the opioid epidemic, although it did not admit wrongdoing and maintained that its past work had been lawful.[70]

As old drugs became increasingly valuable to rival companies pursuing the same price-hiking strategy, novel ways of preventing competition were developed. One specialty pharma company, Amedra Pharmaceuticals, acquired the rights to an old GSK drug called albendazole, raised the price so an average prescription rose from $36 to $241, and subsequently acquired the rights to the only 'therapeutically interchangeable anti-parasitic agent'.[71]

Other companies were able to take advantage of a scheme run by the FDA to crack down on the sale of old and potentially ineffective drugs. Until 1962, drugmakers needed only to demonstrate that their product was safe in order to get it on the US market. There was no requirement to prove it actually worked as a treatment. A 2006 FDA initiative tried to clean up this historical relic by requiring manufacturers of unapproved drugs which were still being sold to go through the modern regulatory process. The first one to do so would be rewarded with several years of exclusivity, with unapproved rivals forced to withdraw their drugs.

The success of Donnatal, one of the first drugs Concordia bought, was based on what the company believed was a monopoly created by this Drug Efficacy Study Implementation scheme. Another drug-maker, URL Pharma, had benefited from the same programme a few years earlier when it was awarded exclusive rights to a gout treatment called Colcrys after funding clinical trials to show its effi-cacy. It then sued rivals to kick them off the market and put the price of the drug up to fifty times the previous level.[72]

Another approach was to limit the ability of generic companies to seek a licence for their own version of an original drug by tightly controlling who could obtain the product. By using a 'closed distri-bution' system which allows the manufacturer to choose who it sells to, generic companies could be denied access to the original product, something that was required by the regulator in order to demonstrate bioequivalence and get a competing version on the market. Turing Pharmaceuticals deployed this approach after acquiring a treatment for life-threatening parasitic infections in 2015. The drug being bought had already had its price increased several times since the rights were first divested by GSK in 2010. Back then, Daraprim cost $1 per tablet. Over five years the new owner, Amedra Pharmaceuticals, a subsidiary of CorePharma, pushed it up to $13.50. CorePharma was itself acquired in the spring of 2015 and the price rose again, to $17.50, before the US rights were sold on in August 2015.[73] The latest acquirer was a pale-skinned thirty-something who would subsequently find himself splashed across the pages of the *New York Times*.

Although Turing was only ever a minor player, Martin Shkreli would come to embody the ruthlessness of the drugs-as-financial-assets business model – a pantomime villain enthusiastic to embrace that role. He had previously founded a small pharmaceutical company called Retrophin, which had used the same 'closed distribution' approach for at least two drugs.[74] Shkreli fell out with the Retrophin board and was pushed out in late 2014, but not before the company had put up the price of Thiola, which it had just acquired, from $1.50 to $30 per pill, with patients requiring up to fifteen a day. Shkreli had reportedly pushed for a price increase of four times that amount but had been overruled by colleagues.[75]

Undeterred, he set up Turing Pharmaceuticals and acquired three of his former company's assets. Daraprim was secured in a $55 million deal a few months later. It was Shkreli who had written the email to an investor claiming that drug executives hadn't grasped just how far they could push prices without resistance from insurers and with Daraprim he intended to prove the point. In a presentation to investors about the drug, he boasted that it was 'the Gold Standard of care for toxoplasmosis' and so doctors, wanting the best for their patents, would continue to use the drug regardless of its price.[76]

In September 2015, the enormous overnight increase in the price of Daraprim became headline news.[77] Amid the torrent of opprobrium that followed, Shkreli was branded 'the most hated man in America'. The moniker left him unrepentant. At a Forbes healthcare conference less than three months later, Shkreli, dressed in a black-and-grey hoodie and jeans, was asked by a PR executive whether he wished he had handled anything differently.

'I probably would have raised the price higher, is probably what I would have done,' he said, slouching in his chair like a sullen teenager. 'I think healthcare prices are inelastic. I could have raised it higher and made more profits for our shareholders, which is my primary duty.'

It was a capitalist system and these were the rules, he said. 'My investors expect me to maximise profits. Not to minimise them or go half or go 70 per cent but to go to 100 per cent of the profit curve that we're all taught in MBA class.'[78]

The predatory model Valeant, Shkreli and others pursued reduced drugs to financial instruments from which value was to be extracted for as long as possible. As each well ran dry – as higher prices eventually scared off prescribers or belatedly drew competition to a newly-valuable market – the companies went on to the next one, a bigger and better acquisition to keep the whole enterprise growing.

As the model spread, hundreds of drugs were affected. In the United States, one in five generic drugs at least doubled in price between early 2010 and mid-2015, according to the government's own analysis of its spending on prescription drugs.[79] Over a similar period, more than four hundred products rose in price by at least 1,000 per cent.[80]

The rewards for those involved could be immense. One private-equity-backed company bought a former Genentech drug called Actimmune for $55 million, increased the price and sold it on for $660 million little more than two years later, Bloomberg News reported.[81] The Danish company Lundbeck paid $900 million for Jeffrey Aronin's nine-year-old business Ovation Pharmaceuticals in 2009. Questcor paid $100,000 for the rights to Acthar, the single product which saw the company sell for $5.6 billion thirteen years later. For those companies who didn't sell up, investors cashing out at the right moment could see huge profits on their initial investment. Valeant's stock had a sixteen-fold gain over five years, at one point becoming Canada's largest company by market value.[82]

The consequences were borne by patients and payers. In the US, increased costs meant higher out-of-pocket expenses for those who needed the drugs and patients had their treatment interrupted or decided to forgo it altogether because of cost pressures. In other cases, doctors stopped prescribing useful drugs after realising how expensive they had become. When Valeant dramatically increased the prices of two heart drugs, the number of patients treated with them fell by between one-third and one-half.[83]

The financial cost of this model, ultimately meted out to taxpayers and employers paying insurance premiums, was also enormous. In the United States, the more than 20 per cent of generic drugs which saw what the Government Accountability Office deemed 'extraordinary price increases' of 100 per cent or more, cost billions a year.[84] The cost to British taxpayers of price rises for seventy drugs was £368 million in 2016 alone.[85] Old medicines in other European countries have been subject to similarly dramatic price increases. Cancer drugs in Italy rose in price by up to 1,500 per cent after being acquired from GSK by the South African company Aspen Pharmacare.[86] In Denmark, the price of an injectable solution used to induce labour was increased by around 2,000 per cent, from the equivalent of €6 to more than €127 per vial.[87] Most dramatically of all, an old drug used to treat patients with a rare disease rose in price from 28 cents to €140 per capsule, increasing the cost of treatment from €300 to more than €150,000 per year in the Netherlands, Belgium, Spain and other countries. The price rises occurred after an Italian company bought the rights to rival suppliers of the drug, called CDCA, and withdrew them from the market.[88]

The Mississippi consulting firm set up by the drug-pricing guru Mick Kolassa, Medical Marketing Economics (MME), advised Valeant on the two heart drugs it bought from Marathon Pharmaceuticals, although he wasn't personally involved. The consultancy's 'Pricing Flexibility Review' concluded that the drugs, then costing around $200 a vial, could be priced much higher. 'MME believes pricing flexibility may still exist for the product up to the perceptual price point of $1,000 per vial,' the company wrote in 2015. It recommended a price of $700 for a single vial of one of the drugs, Isuprel.[89] Valeant duly increased the price but went even further – going to more than $1,700 per vial.

Back then, Kolassa was prepared to justify Valeant's decision to double the price of another drug, Seconal, immediately after acquiring it. The medication is used in assisted dying cases and Valeant increased the price of the required dose from $1,500 to $3,000. It had been sold for just $200 by a different manufacturer a few years earlier. 'Here's a company that said, well, we can raise the price, keep it on the market and make some money with it. Or we can walk away and the product goes away,' Kolassa told National Public Radio in 2016.[90]

But Kolassa now says it was these price hikes for old drugs which led him to walk away from the industry. In recent years, he says, he'd be called by companies who would tell him: 'We just bought this drug, it's off patent, but there's no generics. [It's selling] for $3 a day, can I get $50 a day for it?'

'And the answer at first was the market will let you do that, yes. But I just hated it over and over. They weren't bringing anything of value to the market, they were taking advantage of the fundamental problems in the market, and I couldn't be part of that any more,'

Kolassa says. 'At first I would advise these companies and after a while I'd just say, "You can leave me alone, what you're doing . . . I hate this. I'm not going to help you steal money from the system."'[91]

When the debranding trick later came to light, the main drug industry trade body in the UK was quick to condemn the price hikes for old medicines it facilitated as 'cynical and exploitative'.[92] But its use wasn't restricted to small upstart companies looking to grow rapidly – Big Pharma also got in on the act.

In 2009, Pfizer, one of the world's largest drug companies, was wrestling with a dilemma. One of the company's UK products, a treatment for epilepsy sold under the brand name Epanutin, had become loss-making. The drug, which had first been synthesised a century earlier, had now been superseded by other treatments and was only rarely prescribed for new patients. Nevertheless, there remained tens of thousands of patients, around 10 per cent of epileptic patients in the UK, who still relied on the drug.[93] The price, set many years earlier, was £2.83 for a packet of eighty-four Epanutin capsules – just 3p per capsule. By contrast, the much less popular tablet version of the drug cost more than £1 per pill after having its price hiked by the generics firm Teva.

Under the rules Pfizer had signed up to, in order to raise the price of the medicine it would have to drop the price of another of its branded products or potentially hand back the extra profits. The alternative was to make a request to the Department of Health and hope to persuade officials that a major price rise was justified. Neither option was particularly attractive. Fortunately, earlier that year, another proposal had emerged. Alison Stevenson, a veteran of the generic drug industry who had founded a small Somerset-based company called Tor Generics, contacted the pharmaceutical giant in May saying she had ideas about how the company could obtain a higher price for a number of drugs.[94] Several weeks later, she came in for a meeting and presented her idea to Jason Perfitt and Jenny Shaw, two Pfizer executives with responsibilities for mature medicines.

Stevenson suggested that Pfizer should license Epanutin capsules to her business, which would then debrand the product and sell it under its generic name as phenytoin sodium hard capsules. Pfizer would continue to supply the medicine but the new generic version, freed from the price restrictions on branded medicines, could then be sold at a higher price. It was a legal, if morally questionable, strategy. She believed it would be 'extremely challenging' for others to obtain a share of the market with a rival generic version and predicted a window of at least three to five years where the Pfizer-manufactured drug remained the only available version.

Phenytoin, the active ingredient in Epanutin, has what is known as a narrow therapeutic index, meaning patients are very sensitive to the exact level of the drug in the blood necessary to control seizures and avoid adverse side effects. Clinical guidance therefore recommended that once a patient was stable on the drug, they shouldn't be switched to a different medicine or even a version of the same drug from a different manufacturer, including, in this case, a more expensive tablet version made by the Israeli generics business Teva. As a result, it would need to be made clear to doctors and patients that the medicine wasn't being changed in any way beyond its new packaging. Stevenson's plan, she said, would increase revenues by £19 million a year, with profits to be split between Pfizer and Tor Generics.[95]

Internal emails later obtained by regulators show Pfizer officials wrestling with the ethics and viability of the proposal. After the meeting with Stevenson, Shaw emailed Perfitt and another colleague in late July to outline the idea. By doing it with Tor Generics, Pfizer would 'distance ourselves from the price increase', she wrote, explaining some of the mechanics of the proposed deal. She concluded by saying: 'My other concern is just an ethical one – the top line looks great, however this would increase the price of phenytoin capsules to the NHS drastically and to be frank, doesn't feel right.' Couldn't they instead approach the Department of Health, explain that it was loss-making and reach an agreement for a more modest price increase, she asked. 'Or on the other hand, maybe I'm just being to[o] nice!!' she signed off.

Others raised safety concerns. Dr Berkeley Phillips, Pfizer's recently appointed UK medical director, was unequivocal when he was informed of the prospect a few months later. 'I do not believe it is medically safe to switch between branded and generic AEDs [anti-epileptic drugs] and particularly with phenytoin as it has such a narrow therapeutic window,' he wrote in an email on September 18, 2009. 'Loss of seizure control would have a major impact clinically and also in terms of losing a driving licence which may have been regained after a long period free of seizures.'[96] Another senior employee replied, summing it up as an 'Interesting dilemma'. 'Agree that we have an obligation to do the right thing for patients, but equally we have obligation to do right thing for business,' they wrote.

Despite the concerns raised, discussions with Tor Generics continued. In late January 2010, Steve Poulton, head of Pfizer's Established Products Business Unit, circulated a summary of where things had got to, explaining that Pfizer needed to explore it because the 'potential upside is huge'. He later said he feared the drug would ultimately be discontinued by Pfizer if they didn't find a way to make it profitable. However, there were unresolved issues. One was listed under the heading 'Trust'. 'We need to work out how we can position this as "no change" with patients & physicians; and at the same time "change" with [the Department of Health] and payers without being accused of hypocrisy by pursuing a trust agenda, yet taking the opportunity to fleece the NHS in [a] time of funding crisis,' he wrote.[97]

Pfizer ultimately decided to reject a deal with Tor Generics. But a few months later, the company initiated contact with another small drug company, Flynn Pharma, and discussed a similar proposal.

In a slideshow presentation to Pfizer executives in 2010, Flynn outlined the potential for price hikes to cause reputational damage but proposed that 'Pfizer uses Flynn Pharma as the MA [marketing authorisation] holder to avoid pharmacopolitical damage'. A note of a phone call in June 2011 between Paul Wilson, a Pfizer commercial account director, and Flynn Pharma made it clear that, whilst Pfizer could debrand the drug themselves, Flynn was there to shield the larger company's reputation. 'It's ALL about reputation' the note read, with Flynn questioning whether 'Pfizer execs want the *Daily Mail* camped on their doorstep', a reference to the article that had appeared about Auden Mckenzie's price increases for hydrocortisone the previous year.[98]

Under the deal, Pfizer would continue to manufacture the drug with Flynn buying the stock at a price which was higher than Epanutin's current selling price. Flynn was then free to debrand and significantly increase the price of the product. They hoped to avoid patient safety concerns by making doctors and other healthcare professionals aware of what was planned.

The deal was finally signed in January 2012. The only real difference to Tor's proposal was that Pfizer would transfer the marketing authorisations to Flynn Pharma, something which required permission from the Medicines & Healthcare products Regulatory Agency (MHRA). When Alison Stevenson got wind of what had happened, she took legal action, ultimately reaching a settlement in which Pfizer paid Tor Generics a seven-figure sum.

In early March, the marketing authorisations were successfully transferred to Flynn but when the company then sought approval to change the name, MHRA officials were reluctant because of the risk it could lead to 'undue alarm and confusion for patients'. Flynn responded by warning that supplies of the branded version would run out within weeks and that 'a discontinuity of supplies may lead to fatalities'. Following a 'very difficult' phone call with Flynn in late June 2012, an MHRA official reported back to the Department of Health. 'Flynn effectively threatened to stop the product if they do not get the generic name approved,' they wrote. 'Whilst this is completely irresponsible of Flynn, we do not see an easy way out of this.'[99] Eventually, Flynn submitted a new plan with a detailed communication strategy and it was approved. Flynn has denied ever threatening to stop supplying the drug.

The renamed drug was launched by Flynn in late September 2012.[100] The price increase meant that a pack of eighty-four 100mg capsules, the most common strength, now cost the NHS £67.50 compared with

£2.83 when it was called Epanutin, an overnight increase of 2,285 per cent.[101] Even when another generic manufacturer unexpectedly launched their own version a few months later, the price only fell by 20 per cent. All told, the drug cost the British health service around £50 million in 2013, compared to just £2 million the previous year.

The debranding trick and other attempts by small drug companies to profit from hiking the price of old generic drugs often benefited from a lack of competition. But in recent years, patients have also seen the cost of old drugs rise even when there are many companies making the drug.

In July 2014, a lawyer working for George Jepsen, the elected attorney general for the state of Connecticut, was flicking through a newspaper when one particular article caught his eye. It detailed how the price of a handful of old generic drugs had more than doubled in price in recent years, much to patients' and doctors' chagrin. In one case, a drug was made by three different manufacturers and yet all had raised their prices at around the same time. The lawyer, Mike Cole, thought it looked 'a bit squirrely', Jepsen recalls, and the antitrust team he worked for got permission to issue subpoenas and see what they could find. Joe Nielsen, the antitrust lawyer asked to take the lead on the investigation, didn't get very far on those particular drugs, but 'in the course of getting information in response to the subpoenas they saw other opportunities of possible price fixing,' Jepsen says. The sprawling conspiracy they would eventually uncover was described by one Justice Department official to a member of Jepsen's team as 'probably the largest US-based cartel in history'.[102]

Jepsen, a broad-faced, down-to-earth lawyer, stepped down as state attorney-general in 2019, deciding not to run again after two four-year terms. He is now back in private practice but retains a keen interest in the lawsuit as it works its way through the American legal system. More than forty US states have joined the case and the Department of Justice has also opened a criminal investigation. Jepsen says his team realised early on that they were on to something.

The generic drug industry in the US was extremely 'tight-knit', with companies clustered around New Jersey and eastern Pennsylvania and regularly socialising together. 'There are several hundred executives . . . [and] these folks all know each other,' he says. 'They do golf outings, girls' nights out, they see each other all the time at trade shows, and so we started a peek into that world.'[103]

Their gut feeling was bolstered as they began to fire off what would become hundreds of subpoenas requesting documents from telephone companies and generic manufacturers. 'We noticed very quickly when the subpoenas started that the prices didn't come down, but the frequency of price increases diminished quickly,' Jepsen adds.

In a functioning competitive market, the presence of multiple generics manufacturers should help to drive down the cost of these gradually ageing medicines. But if drug companies agreed not to compete, they could all be assured of higher profits, even if these came from a smaller market share than they might otherwise be able to obtain. Social events offered ample opportunity to discuss prices and markets for different drugs without leaving a paper trail. 'The incentives were all there and the means to do it were all there,' Jepsen says.

Meanwhile, the records of phone calls and text messages from hundreds of drug executives were now in the lawyers' possession and software allowed them to analyse patterns behind the communications. 'We can track phone calls that took place between two telephone numbers and the date and the time of each call, and the duration of each call. These are nominal competitors, they're supposed to be at each other's throats to gain an advantage. What we found was that they were talking to one another dozens, even hundreds, and even more than 1,000 times over the course of a year-and-a-half period,' he says. 'We found collusion to be pervasive throughout the industry.'

Jepsen initially went after a smaller generic company, Heritage Pharmaceuticals, which had been caught 'red-handed'. In December 2016 he published a complaint naming Heritage and five other companies, focusing on just two drugs. In the months that followed, several drug executives came forward as cooperating witnesses, helping the lawyers to build their case alleging a much wider conspiracy.[104] As Jepsen sees it, a huge number, perhaps even a majority of generic drugs, were affected by a seemingly industry-wide agreement to divide up the market and give each company a 'fair share'. That phrase kept coming up in communications between drug executives at different drug companies discussing a wide range of drugs. Another term that was used was 'playing nice in the sandbox'. If one company was playing by the rules and not competing on price, others wouldn't compete for their customers.

The alleged conspiracy was laid out in full in a 500-page legal filing which was made public in May 2019. It pointed the finger at twenty companies and more than 100 drugs. Teva, the Israeli generics giant, was central to the charges, and companies owned by large drugmakers including Pfizer's Greenstone and Novartis's Sandoz were also among the accused.[105]

The complaint claimed that generic companies would carve up the market for different generic drugs, sharing out the available distribution and retail customers. Markets would normally be split equally between those making the drug unless one company had been the first to launch a generic, in which case it could expect a larger share. By dividing up customers, generic manufacturers avoided undercutting one another on price. The legal filings laid out occasions when customers had gone to a generics manufacturer and asked it to bid for a contract, only for that company to decline to do so, apparently because that customer was assigned to a different manufacturer. Information was shared, it was alleged, at cocktail parties, industry dinners and golf outings, with executives meeting at a steakhouse in New Jersey and at 'Women in the Industry' events in Minnesota, among other places.

The cosy arrangements between supposed rivals kept prices higher than they would otherwise be and had existed for several years when Teva and other companies 'sought to leverage the collusive nature of the industry to not only maintain their "fair share" of each generic drug market, but also to significantly raise prices on as many drugs as possible', legal papers claimed.[106] From 2012, Teva allegedly developed an understanding which meant that when it raised prices, it could be assured that competing companies would follow suit and raise their own prices rather than seizing on the opportunity to gain new customers with a cheaper generic product. One of the examples cited came in 2012 when Teva raised the price of a beta blocker called nadolol and was followed by Sandoz, which did the same thing a month later. By 2013, the third manufacturer of the drug, Mylan, had also increased its prices.[107] The three companies had matched one another's price hikes and different formulations of the drug now cost as much as 2,700 per cent more than it had previously.[108] In the days leading up to the increases, executives from the three companies were in frequent phone contact.

Jepsen believes the alleged collusion has cost American consumers tens of billions of dollars, but he is all too aware of the ways in which high drug prices can have other costs. 'These are drugs that people need for their health and even for their life and so the high cost of these drugs are forcing people to make choices they shouldn't have to make – between paying their mortgage or paying their rent or . . . their family's health,' he says. 'It's a terrible human cost.'

CHAPTER SEVEN

The acquisition game

The blockbuster era left research-led companies reliant on a small number of drugs for the bulk of their profits. Patent thickets, evergreening and other tricks could help extend the length of time during which these billion-dollar drugs enjoyed a monopoly, but they couldn't keep generic competition away for ever. One large 'patent cliff' came in the early 2010s, as a series of bestselling drugs launched in the late 1990s lost their patent protection and became exposed to generic competition. Among them were Eli Lilly's antipsychotic drug Zyprexa, Sanofi and Bristol-Myers Squibb's jointly-marketed blood thinner Plavix, and Pfizer's cholesterol-lowering drug Lipitor. The impact of losing their legally enforced monopoly was often dramatic. Within a year of Lipitor going off patent in 2012, Pfizer had seen 60 per cent of the drug's $9.6 billion annual sales revenues disappear.

To make matters worse for an industry looking to fill a series of blockbuster-sized holes, by 2010 the number of new products coming through drug development pipelines had been in a decade-long slump, with fewer than twenty-five new drugs, on average, each year.[1] The blockbuster model was pursued on the basis that funding R&D would produce a regular supply of new mass-market drugs, but drug discovery was getting more expensive and less productive.

Amidst these challenges, the pressures of being a listed company didn't let up. Drug executives weren't simply expected to replace lost sales but to continue to grow revenues beyond where they had been before. The initial response of many was to fall back on the business-school toolkit: mergers, budget cuts and layoffs.

The turn of the millennium was marked by a series of mega-mergers which remodelled the industry, creating GlaxoSmithKline, AstraZeneca and other twenty-first-century titans of Big Pharma. In this frenzy of dealmaking, it became a case of finding a rival to take over or risk being taken over yourself. A new round of mergers and acquisitions arrived a decade later, often accompanied during the global economic downturn of that period by large-scale cuts to head counts and existing research projects. Between 2009 and 2012, more than thirty Big Pharma research sites were shuttered.[2] Pfizer cut more than 50,000 jobs over a seven-year period while its annual R&D budget was reduced from $9.4 billion in 2010 to $6.7 billion in 2013.[3] Between 2000 and 2010, the number of people working at research-led drug companies fell by 300,000.[4]

Although mergers were thought to be popular with shareholders, they were ultimately self-defeating, providing a short-term boost at the expense of longer-term damage. John LaMattina served as a research chief at Pfizer before leaving the company in 2007. A few years later, he examined the impact of mergers on R&D, publishing his findings in a medical journal. LaMattina concluded that large mergers had a 'devastating' effect on research. 'Not only are R&D cuts made, but entire research sites are eliminated,' he wrote.[5]

This had happened when Pfizer bought three drug companies, Warner–Lambert, Pharmacia and Searle, and shut down several research centres. But the merger also disrupted the speed with which new compounds were brought through the development pipeline, LaMattina found. He blamed the slow process of integrating R&D divisions and assessing their projects. 'During this period – which can take at least 9 months – generally no new programmes are started and hiring will be frozen.'

One former Big Pharma chief executive paints a similar picture. 'In a big merger of companies, one that is spending $6 billion [on research] and one that is spending $4 billion, you don't end up spending $10 [billion], you probably end up spending $7 billion,' he says. 'Research spending is being driven out by the industry.'[6]

The appetite for mergers has already consumed many of the mid-sized players in the industry and shows no sign of slowing. In mid-2019, with the US patent for Humira due to expire and generic competition preparing to enter the market, AbbVie struck a $63 billion deal to buy Allergan, a drug company best known for selling the cosmetic treatment Botox. It said it eventually expected to save $2 billion a year as a result of the acquisition.[7] In the same year, Bristol-Myers Squibb paid $74 billion to take over Celgene, while in late 2020 AstraZeneca announced plans for a $39 billion acquisition of Alexion Pharmaceuticals.

Across the industry, the proportion of revenue devoted to research and development had consistently risen since the 1980s but after 2000 it began to fall. This slide was finally halted in 2011 and there have been modest annual increases since 2015, although R&D expenditure as a share of sales is projected to fall again in the first half of the 2020s.[8]

Within this, the amount of money spent by large pharmaceutical companies on the kind of in-house early-stage research which is essential to producing genuinely new treatments has fallen significantly. The cost of running clinical trials to test potential drugs on patients has ballooned in recent years, taking up a bigger and bigger proportion of the money drug companies dedicate to research. The changes become clear from data buried at the back of an annual membership survey conducted by the industry's main US trade body, Pharmaceutical Research and Manufacturers of America. In 2008, R&D spending on preclinical work – research before the first clinical trial including into furthering our understanding of diseases and identifying new drug targets and potential compounds – amounted to 28.8 per cent.[9] By 2019, this had fallen to 15.7 per cent.[10]

Part of the problem for the lumbering giants of Big Pharma was a brain drain as scientists in industry and academia succumbed to the allure of setting up or joining a fledgling biotech. If they had a good idea and it could be demonstrated to have clinical uses, the rewards on offer far exceeded anything a salaried research scientist could expect. Alongside this, as we shall see, was a slump in R&D productivity which led many executives to conclude that increased investment in drug discovery would just result in losses. The rational alternative was to hand more and more money back to investors in the form of dividends and share buybacks.

Buybacks, a once obscure financial manoeuvre, became particularly popular because of their additional benefits. By using earnings to purchase shares back from investors, the number of shares in a company is reduced. This in turn improves a metric known as earnings per share, which can serve to boost a company's share price. The economist Lazonick believes share buybacks are among the worst manifestations of a financialised industry because they extract value from a company, depleting resources which could otherwise be used to increase investment in innovation and reward workers for their prior contributions to value-creation. The effect on the share price can be short-lived, but there are often significant personal incentives for executives to follow that course of action. Research has shown that companies are more likely to make use of share buybacks if they place a heavy emphasis on stock options when compensating executives.[11]

Over a ten-year period from 2007 to 2016, nineteen large drug companies spent a combined $297 billion buying back their own shares and $267 billion paying out cash dividends. This was equivalent to all but $2 billion of the companies' net profits over the same period and $75 billion more than was invested in R&D.[12] These buybacks came on top of revenue-boosting financial shenanigans such as moving intellectual property offshore or lining up a 'tax inversion' deal in order to slash tax bills. Tax inversions, which analysts thought Concordia, with its Barbados subsidiary, might become a target for, involve a large company buying a smaller one in order to move its corporate headquarters to a country with a lower tax rate. Several drug companies including Mylan and Allergan did this and

Pfizer was proposing to make the same move before President Obama changed the rules in 2018, killing that deal.[13]

This financial engineering was accompanied by the continued increase in how much was being charged for drugs around the world. The days in which new products in an existing drug class tried to grab a share of the market by launching with a much lower price were long gone. One study by researchers at Oregon State University found that when a new multiple sclerosis drug came onto the market, the manufacturers of older treatments actually increased their prices to match. With no generic versions of these old drugs on sale, their manufacturers saw more profit in relying on brand loyalty and marketing efforts to persuade doctors to prescribe their treatments.[14]

Drug executives had also picked up a lucrative new habit: price rises for existing drugs. They weren't on the same scale as the thousands of per cent increases pushed through by some specialty pharma companies, but when the drugs involved have annual revenues in the billions, a 10 or 20 per cent yearly increase meant huge sums for those footing the bills.

Many countries impose price or spending controls which severely hamper the ability of manufacturers to change the price of a patent-protected drug once it's on the market. In the UK, for example, drugmakers must hand back extra revenue above an allowed increase of 2 per cent in expenditure across branded drugs.[15] The US has never had such measures but for a long time drug executives were nevertheless wary of a backlash if they imposed above-inflation price rises on existing drugs. The chief executive of one of the largest research-led drug companies, speaking anonymously, says that in the early 2000s he would limit annual price rises to the rate of inflation, which was typically no higher than 3 per cent. 'Historically I would never want my average prices going up more than the rate of inflation,' the former executive says. 'I just felt that would bring enough scrutiny, enough political pressure, legislation, that that was just a risk I wasn't willing to take.'[16]

By the latter part of the 2000s that hesitation began to disappear.

After all, if drugs were viewed by their manufacturers as nothing more than financial assets, why not increase prices as much as the market allows? There has been a 'sea change [with a] shift to counting on more revenue growth from price', the executive argues, adding that this 'probably accounts for a lot of the criticism of the industry today'. Large annual price increases in the United States became commonplace. By 2008, a drug pricing expert in the US was telling a congressional hearing that 'a 10 to 20 per cent increase, from month to month or from year to year . . . [is] just viewed as normal now'.[17]

'Companies were losing revenue from patent expirations and they did not have follow-on compounds and the only avenue they had was to raise price,' the former Big Pharma chief executive says. 'I suspect they were made out of desperation that "Look, we're losing volume from patent expiration, we're not launching new drugs fast enough to make up the difference, our licensing compounds aren't being as successful. The only way we can continue to show revenue is to raise price." That is what shareholders pay CEOs to do.'[18]

Regular price increases meant Viagra's list price doubled in the decade after its launch. Pfizer continued to increase the cost even when two similar so-called 'me-too' products, Cialis and Levitra, entered the market and took a significant share of patients.[19] A recent study looking at a sample of thirty-six top-selling brand-name drugs in the United States found that since 2012 costs to insurers or un-insured patients have increased by more than half for 80 per cent of drugs, and have doubled for 44 per cent.[20]

The increases weren't limited to the period when a drug had patent protection, with the hikes also enabling manufacturers to draw more revenue from the small number of doctors and patients who remain loyal to a brand name even when there are generics available. Others, particularly biological medicines which are much harder to make, had no competition even after losing patent protection and were happy to continue exploiting their pricing power. More than two decades after its launch, Avonex, which treats multiple sclerosis, had averaged annual price rises of 36 per cent.[21] The actions of Valeant, Concordia and others in the specialty pharma sector demonstrated to mainstream drug companies just how much their pricing power over drugs which were already on the market can be exploited before payers, whether that be insurers or governments, take action.

When prices went up overnight by thousands of per cent in a way that was clearly unfair there might an outcry. But if only one company is supplying the drug a patient needs, they only have two choices: pay up or go without. Economists call this 'pricing elasticity', a measure of how much of an impact a price increase will have on demand. Medicines are very inelastic because of the lack of alternatives.

Price increases became an important way of delivering sales growth from big blockbuster drugs, making up for the damage that increasing generics prescriptions was doing to revenues from those that had slipped off patent, and they remain so. Internal emails and other documents obtained from drugmakers by a congressional investigation in 2020 found evidence that price rises for several bestselling drugs were implemented when a company feared it might miss revenue targets.[22]

Despite commitments to limit the size of price rises, they are still regular occurrences in the US market. Many companies increase list prices at the start of each year and 2021 was no different. One company, GoodRx, tracked more than 800 price rises as the calendar ticked over into a new decade. They increased by an average of 4.5 per cent, more than three percentage points above the rate of inflation, and included, for the second year in a row, a 7.4 per cent hike for Humira, the drug with the largest annual sales revenue.[23] A report by an analyst at the investment bank Leerink found that price rises were responsible for more than 60 per cent of sales growth for the top forty-five largest-selling drugs in the US between 2014 and 2017.[24]

Although these regular price hikes for existing drugs while they were still under patent were largely a US phenomenon, they had global significance because of the way in which they help to push up the launch price of the next generation of treatments in that therapy area. If the existing drug has become more expensive, this sets a higher benchmark for the next drug aimed at the same patients.

The same inflationary effect holds true for other markets, even if companies expect to obtain reimbursement for their products at prices which are lower than those charged in the US.

When in-house efforts failed to produce the new products needed, drug companies started to scour other, smaller firms for promising drug candidates. This had the added advantage of allowing executives to be much more strategic in the products they went after. Large companies had traditionally maintained a research and commercial infrastructure capable of handling a diverse range of therapeutic areas but the switch towards buying in assets made this expense less necessary. Promising drug candidates might be of interest because they were in a similar area to the company's existing drugs, taking advantage of institutional knowledge and a ready-made sales force and enabling the company to develop new two- or three-drug cocktails which could extend the revenue-earning life of an existing product. Or maybe companies saw a weakness in their portfolio, perhaps a lucrative new field they didn't have a drug in, and wanted to skip the decade or more of research and development required if they started from scratch.

If a key drug was running out of patent life, a well-timed acquisition allowed executives to replace the impending revenue shortfall and keep markets happy. The price paid for a company, or to license a drug, could be reduced to a calculation: how much risk was there in the next stage of development; how big was the market likely to be; what was the anticipated competition; and, above all, what sort of reimbursement price could be expected. The approach didn't remove risk, but it made it much more quantifiable than the hopeful leap of in-house scientists embarking on new basic research or early-stage development.

Little wonder then that financiers ushered the industry down this path with enthusiasm. In 2010, the American investment bank Morgan Stanley laid out the case for Big Pharma cutting their in-house research efforts and using the money to buy later-stage assets from smaller firms or divest into non-pharma assets.[25] The bank's analysis found that in-licensing had three times the likely return on investment compared with in-house research. Of course, this approach can still go wrong for companies, as AbbVie found when it bought a San Francisco biotech called Stemcentrx in a deal worth $5.8 billion in 2016. The company was developing a lung cancer treatment but it subsequently faced setbacks in clinical trials, prompting AbbVie to record a $4 billion impairment charge. But when a company makes a good assessment of the chance of success of a drug candidate and then takes an aggressive approach to pricing, the potential rewards are enormous.

As we shall see, much of the basic scientific advances which take place occur in university laboratories or the offices of publicly funded researchers. This new approach of relying on acquisitions, however, allowed the industry's giants to outsource another large chunk of the drug discovery process. Now, new drugs are more likely to have emerged from a venture capital-funded start-up set up by researchers who worked on the basic science – hence why clusters of biotechs are found around university towns in Britain and America. Investors put in enough money to get through the initial clinical trials and then the firm looks to sell out to large drug companies. They, in turn, can leverage their expertise to bring it through late-stage testing and regulatory approval before deploying their legal and marketing muscle to launch it around the world.

The acquisition model which proved so lucrative to specialty pharmaceutical companies buying the rights to old drugs has become the norm for new drugs, too. Nearly three-quarters of new drugs sold in the United States were acquired by the manufacturer from another company.[26] More than half of the drug projects in Big Pharma pipelines originated at other companies.[27] Pfizer, one of the world's largest drug companies, hasn't launched a drug with significant sales which originated and was developed internally since 2005.[28]

Large pharmaceutical companies have moved their R&D operations close to universities to 'operate like head-hunters, identifying local academics . . . working on promising new biological medicines which [the] pharmaceutical company could use in their own innovative drug-discovery programmes'.[29] Publicly-funded research has always played a huge role in advancing scientific understanding and identifying plausible targets for pharmaceutical intervention, but as in-house R&D has been stripped back, it has taken on an even greater importance in applying that basic research to drug development. A recent study found that public research had played a 'major role' in the late-stage development of one in four new drugs over the last decade.[30]

For Bernard Munos, the veteran of Eli Lilly, the triumph of the acquisition model marks the completion of a transformation in the industry's culture which began when the first biotech companies helped to drive through a more aggressive attitude to pricing. 'In the early days, you basically had a club of well-behaved companies,' he says. 'Most of them had a history long dominated by the founding families and they really were in this thing for themselves of course and their investors, but also for the public good.'[31]

He says there was an understanding that patents were 'in a way, a licence to print money but there's an implied covenant there – society basically has granted their intellectual property rights, and in turn society is expecting for the industry not to abuse those rights.'

'This culture changed when most of the new drugs are brought in by small companies funded by venture capitalists or financial people,' he says. 'The only reason why they do that is basically to make money and this old covenant about behaving well and not abusing your freedom of pricing, that pretty much went out the window.' The new culture stems from 'financiers who put some money in this game and expect to get as much back as they possibly can – and damn the consequences'.

The acquisition model has created huge windfalls for a select few. Many biotechs fail, but when one does get snapped up by a larger firm for billions, the founders and early-stage investors often stand to make a fortune. Two brothers who founded a biotech-focused hedge fund, Baker Bros. Advisors, are now worth a reported $4 billion, while Dr Patrick Soon-Shiong, a doctor who developed a

cancer drug, became a billionaire when he sold the company for
nearly $3 billion in 2001.[32]

Neither the hedge fund nor Soon-Shiong are accused of wrongdoing; they are operating within the system as it has evolved. But
for the public at large, it is far less advantageous. Although significant
risk now lies elsewhere, large pharmaceutical companies continue to
enjoy the patents, and ensuing pricing power, granted in exchange
for this endeavour. There is also evidence to suggest that the acquisition model has contributed to increasing prices. The global
consultancy firm Deloitte produces an annual report examining the
industry's research and development efforts. It has found that drugs
acquired from other companies have 'historically launched at higher
rates than the industry benchmark'.[33]

As Big Pharma becomes increasingly reliant on smaller companies,
usually biotech start-ups, to carry out early-stage research and development, competition for those with viable and potentially lucrative
drug candidates has only grown more intense. This pushes up the
acquisition cost. The sum paid for a drug sets a floor for the amount
the company is hoping to recoup. More importantly, it ensures that
the company which believes it can charge the highest price for the
drug is likely to bid the highest sum for the assets.

Drug companies have always subjected new compounds to regular
assessments through the research and development process, disre-
garding those which were thought not to have sufficient commercial
potential. But within that they were willing to make some allowances,
to draw the lines differently for projects of genuine clinical importance. It was the mindset that meant Burroughs Wellcome sold
treatments for tropical diseases that barely paid for themselves and
Merck & Co. developed a drug for river blindness which it ended
up giving away.

When Sanofi-Aventis closed nearly half of its research facilities
in 2009, a senior R&D executive admitted that it heralded a change
in approach. 'Just because a project is innovative does not mean it
will be funded,' he said, suggesting the company had previously not
exposed truly novel therapies to the same commercial considerations

as other drugs. Now they would have to 'go through the same selection procedure for investment as any product in the company'.[34]

Large companies have historically tolerated a portfolio with mixed profitability. In the switch to an acquisition model, this is no longer feasible. Shareholders scrutinise the numbers and deliver an instant verdict when a deal is announced in the form of a red or green arrow showing a slumping or soaring stock price. The only way to justify a multi-billion-dollar acquisition is to point not simply to their clinical importance, but to the commercial promise of the pipeline drugs being acquired.

One company which illustrates how drugmakers have changed in the pharmaceutical industry's new era was set up by a brilliant and idealistic young scientist who was convinced he could change the world; it ended up, thirty years later, as a lightning rod for criticism over drug pricing, with its executives hauled before Congress to face accusations from US senators of shameless profiteering and greed.

Founded in June 1987, Gilead Sciences was one of scores of start-ups looking to take advantage of the promised biotech revolution. The company was established by Michael Riordan, a charismatic twenty-nine-year-old medical researcher turned venture capitalist from Kansas who saw huge possibilities in the new field of nucleic acid chemistry. Like many of the scientists flocking to the nascent industry, Riordan, who had obtained an MBA from Harvard after completing his medical degree, wasn't content to stay in the laboratory, watching the rewards of any successes eventually flow to some distant behemoth. He wanted to be at the coalface of the revolution.

At the Johns Hopkins School of Medicine, Riordan had become interested in what he called 'gene targeting'. It involved creating an 'anti-sense' compound which could penetrate a cell and bind to mRNA, the chemical messenger molecule which conveys information from DNA in order to create a protein, thereby blocking the production of specific disease-causing proteins. This targeted approach promised to avoid the toxic side effects of traditional small molecule drugs.

The young scientist and entrepreneur planned to develop this technology for commercial use, believing it would, within a decade, allow the creation of a new class of drugs which 'could be used to treat 70 per cent of human diseases'.[35] Riordan named his new company after a play he had read as a student, *Balm in Gilead*, which referred to the extract of an ancient willow tree with healing powers found in the Middle East and which was seen as 'one of mankind's first genuine therapeutics'.[36]

Shortly after launching the business, Riordan tapped up his former employer, the venture capital firm Menlo Ventures, for a $2 million investment and in 1988 moved Gilead to laboratories in an industrial park in Silicon Valley. The co-founder of Intel joined to offer business advice and within months Riordan was also able to persuade Donald Rumsfeld, a former – and future – US defence secretary, to join the board of directors.[37]

Gilead's growing cadre of scientists soon expanded their approach, working on a range of ways in which nucleotides, the building blocks of the nucleic acids DNA and RNA, could be chemically modified and used to disrupt the replication of genetic or viral diseases. As well as using an anti-sense compound which can interfere with mRNA, they explored 'triple helix' compounds which would bind to the DNA double helix and block selective genes from replicating. Gilead also began looking at compounds which targeted specific proteins inside and outside the cell. In 1989, John Martin, the head of Bristol-Myers' HIV drug programme, jumped ship from Bristol-Myers after being wined and dined by Riordan in a Manhattan steakhouse.[38]

By 1992, despite never having launched a new drug or posted a profit, Gilead went public. The IPO raised more than $85 million, with Wall Street happy to bet on the promise of future riches. The company told investors that its genetic code blocker programme had projects underway which it hoped would result in treatments for cancer, malaria and dengue fever.[39] But it was its antiviral programme, collaborating with research scientists in Prague on compounds with uses against the herpes virus, hepatitis B and HIV, which would hold the most promise.

Several years later, an antiviral, an injectable treatment for AIDS-related blindness called Vistide, became Gilead's first drug. By this point Martin had taken over as chief executive and, just a few months later, the founder was out, stepping down as chairman, with Rumsfeld taking his place. Riordan cut his ties with the company altogether in 1998.

The promise of blocking genetic code and transforming healthcare which had led the young scientist to create Gilead had proved elusive. Instead, under the new leadership of Martin, Gilead became focused exclusively on developing AIDS drugs and other antivirals. A series of setbacks followed. Vistide was found to cause significant kidney damage, preventing its use in more lucrative indications beyond AIDS-related blindness, and another AIDS treatment, adefovir, had significant toxicity and was rejected by the FDA when Gilead sought approval in the late 1990s, although it was later sold in lower doses as a hepatitis B treatment.[40]

Meanwhile, the company was developing tenofovir, a compound first synthesised and developed in the 1980s by two men working on either side of the Iron Curtain: the Czech scientist Antonín Holý in Prague and Erik De Clercq, a biologist in Leuven, Belgium. After they discovered its antiviral properties, they teamed up with John Martin, who brought the project across when he moved from Bristol-Myers.[41] The drug was launched on the market by Gilead in late 2001 as an anti-HIV treatment and quickly became a key driver of the company's growth.

Gilead was not the only biotech company on the hunt for AIDS drugs.

David Barry, the Burroughs Wellcome research scientist who had been integral to the development of AZT, the first AIDS drug, had left that firm in 1995. He took the core of his HIV research team and, in keeping with the entrepreneurial spirit of the age, established a new start-up called Triangle Pharmaceuticals.

The company's star asset was an HIV drug called emtricitabine, or FTC, which had been discovered by scientists at Emory University in Atlanta, Georgia, in 1990. Barry had originally worked on developing the drug at Burroughs, which licensed it from Emory, but the project was halted after the company was taken over by Glaxo PLC in 1995. Glaxo was developing a competing nucleoside analogue called 3TC and the Emory scientists who discovered FTC believed this was no coincidence, concluding that it was 'hard to ignore the possibility that the merger also provided an attractive opportunity to block the development of the [competing] product'.[42]

With the merged Glaxo Wellcome having dropped the project, a new licensing agreement for development and commercialisation rights allowed Barry's new team at Triangle to continue their work. Glaxo Wellcome, however, kept hold of crucial clinical data and patent rights for several years, which resulted in lengthy legal proceedings.

In early 2002, Barry died suddenly at the age of fifty-eight and in the wake of his passing Triangle Pharmaceuticals was sold to Gilead for around $500 million. FTC was already close to hitting the market at the time of the acquisition and it was duly approved as a once-a-day pill with the brand name Emtriva in July 2003.[43]

But the real value, Gilead executives had always believed, would come from creating a single-pill combination drug for the treatment of HIV, replacing the scores of pills a day that some patients were taking. A year later, they launched Truvada, a new drug which combined FTC with tenofovir, the reverse transcriptase inhibitor which the company had been selling since 2001. On its own, FTC had sales of barely more than $50 million a year in the US. When combined with tenofovir into Truvada, however, it became a blockbuster drug, reaching sales of $1.2 billion in 2006.[44] Nor did Gilead's deal-making end there. It struck an agreement with another company, Bristol-Myers Squibb, to combine its drug Sustiva with Truvada to create a triple-combination pill which also became a blockbuster, with sales of $1.5 billion in 2008.

All told, Gilead's acquisition of Triangle Pharmaceuticals was, by 2008, responsible for 80 per cent of its $5 billion revenues. The journal *Nature Biotechnology* describe it as 'Gilead's deal of a lifetime' and yet, just three years later, Gilead made an even more lucrative acquisition.

The three Emory University researchers who had discovered the HIV drug FTC were Dennis Liotta, Raymond Schinazi and Woo-Baeg Choi. In 1998, Liotta and Schinazi founded a new biotech company to develop antiviral drugs. The company was called Pharmasset, reflecting the intention not to bring drugs all the way through development to market, but to 'create assets that would be sold to companies'.[45]

More than a decade later, in the summer of 2011, Gilead was on the hunt for a new acquisition. All its revenues were coming from one area, HIV treatments, and its lacklustre share price reflected shareholders who were anxious to see what it would do next. 'They were bringing in billions of dollars in revenue around their chronic treatments for HIV patients but there wasn't any other growth stream' of the kind Wall Street demanded, says Victor Roy, who wrote a PhD on Gilead at the University of Cambridge and is now doing a medical residency at Boston Medical Center in the United States.[46]

The company wanted to use its expertise in antivirals to enter the market for hepatitis C drugs and, at the urging of their head of liver disease research, John McHutchison, had zeroed in on a highly promising candidate being developed by Pharmasset called PSI-7977. McHutchison, a hepatitis C expert, had been hired from Duke University where he had worked on clinical trials for several experimental compounds, including Pharmasset's. 'He spent a good year persuading the board and the company that the compounds [being developed internally were no match for Pharmasset's effort and] that's going to be the one that we really want,' Roy says.

A task force was assembled within Gilead to complete the acquisition, dubbed 'Project Harry'. Gilead was concerned that if they didn't move quickly to buy Pharmasset, other companies would sweep in. These concerns only grew with the release of Phase II clinical trial results for PSI-7977 which proved spectacular: 'Show-stopping amazing,' Roy says. With no time to waste, Gilead offered $8 billion for Pharmasset. It twice increased its bid in the face of competition before an eventual sale price was agreed: $11.2 billion for a business with just eighty-two employees and a track record of losing money every year.

The deal represented a particularly lucrative outcome for Schinazi. He had been the one to lobby Emory to file patents for 3TC and FTC, a decision which made the university, and the drug's inventors, a fortune. In 2005, the university sold the future royalties of FTC for $525 million. Schinazi, Liotta and Choi split a $210 million share of the windfall.[47] 'He's got natural entrepreneurial talents that most people have to teach themselves,' Liotta said of Schinazi at the time of the deal. 'I think he can smell money.'[48] The sale of Pharmasset brought further riches. Although he was no longer a company director, Schinazi retained shares which were worth $400 million when the business was sold.

At the core of Gilead's valuation of Pharmasset was how much money could be made from PSI-7977, a compound subsequently given the generic name sofosbuvir. Pricing decisions are often shrouded in mystery but in this case Gilead's approach is revealed in documents obtained by a later congressional investigation. Before buying Pharmasset, the 'Project Harry' team at Gilead had assumed a price of around $65,000 per patient, a US Senate committee report concluded.[49] This figure, which emerged from pricing modelling carried out by Barclays bank, nearly matched the cost of the existing standard-of-care treatment for hepatitis C, a three-pronged approach involving Vertex's Incivek alongside interferon and ribavirin. A year after the sale, as Phase III clinical trials for sofosbuvir were underway, an internal presentation shows Gilead was still contemplating a price of around $65,000 per patient, with an expected discount of 25 per cent for sales in Europe.

However, in the run-up to launch, the company's expectations shifted. Armed with the results of a survey of ninety payers asking the perceived value of the treatment, executives now believed that 'price sensitivity begins at $90,000'. By Gilead's estimate, the average cost of existing three-part treatments had also risen because of annual price rises and was now pegged at $83,000, with Incivek, the pill sofosbuvir would be replacing, costing $55,000.[50] Executives started to contemplate a higher price.

Crucial to Gilead's decision was the fact it was planning a two-stage strategy. Sofosbuvir, sold under the brand name Sovaldi, was to be followed onto the market by a new combination called Harvoni which would eliminate the need for interferon injections. The company didn't want to undermine the price it could command for Harvoni, particularly if a rival company managed to launch a competing interferon-free product before this second Gilead treatment hit the market. If they set the price of Sovaldi at $60,000 'achieving more than an $80K Wave 2 price will be unlikely, eroding shareholding value', the company concluded.[51]

A price of between $80,000 and $85,000 was ultimately settled on, under the belief (which would later prove mistaken) that this price would 'allow Gilead to capture value for the product without going to a price [which] . . . could hinder patient access to uncomfortable levels'. Gilead planned to offer discounts of a little under one-fifth of its list price, but, as it transpired, the offers would rarely be accepted because they were 'tied to loosening access restrictions', requiring payers to cover the cost of the drug for a wider pool of patients and wiping out the budget savings from the discount in the process.[52]

The launch would be accompanied by all the familiar bells and whistles. An extensive advertising and sales force effort was planned to increase awareness of the disease and expand the number of patients seeking treatment. Millions would be paid to doctors to speak about the drugs, while a company-funded 'HepCHope' campaign would direct callers towards Gilead's products.

Later on, with two years of discussions resulting in a price of $81,000, equating to $27,000 for a twenty-eight-pill bottle, senior executives suggested rounding it up to a neat $28,000 per bottle. Martin, the chief executive, noted in an email that this price would 'be easy [for] the press release, from twenty-eight days and $28,000' – a round figure of $1,000 a day. Patients would still need to take interferon or ribavirin, or, for some genotypes, both, alongside

Sovaldi, so the price represented a significant hike on existing treatments. The declared price of Sovaldi was also based on a twelve-week
treatment course but for some patients a twenty-four-week course
would be required, doubling the cost. Gilead considered lowering
the price for this patient group, who, research indicated, would also
have a lower cure rate, but ultimately decided to have only one price.[53]

In a report on Gilead based on access to thousands of internal
company documents, the US Senate Finance Committee concluded
that Gilead had been focused on 'maximising revenue – even as the
company's analysis showed a lower price would allow more people
to be treated'.[54] A 'key consideration', the report said, was to prepare
the market for its next hepatitis C treatment, Harvoni, to have a
higher price. That part of the strategy worked. Sovaldi was approved
in December 2013, and generated sales of more than $10 billion in
its first year on the market, effectively doubling the company's revenues.[55] Gilead's next hepatitis C offering, Harvoni, a combination of
sofosbuvir and ledipasvir, a drug developed in-house, launched less
than a year later with a price tag of $94,500 for a twelve-week course.
Sales topped $14 billion in the first full financial year after its launch.[56]

The hepatitis C drugs brought to the market by Gilead reflect the
best of the pharmaceutical industry – an extraordinary clinical advance
from the previous highly toxic treatment options. They are also,
however, an embodiment of what market forces have done to drug
prices. Pharmasset had spent just $62.4 million researching PSI-7977
and had budgeted a further $120 million to take it through Phase III
clinical trials. Gilead told the US Senate Finance Committee that it
had spent $880.3 million on developing sofosbuvir and three other
compounds used in combination with the drug but did not provide
figures for sofosbuvir alone. The biggest cost, the $11.2 billion paid
to acquire Pharmasset, was nearly matched by the $10.3 billion in
sales of Sovaldi in 2014 alone. Even with an allowance for the risk
taken in placing such a big bet on Pharmasset's fledgling assets, the
returns were enormous. The prices, on a par with orphan drugs but
set for a treatment with a huge market, were so high that even Schinazi,
one of the co-founders of Pharmasset, branded them 'obscene'.[57]

Sovaldi and Harvoni highlight how higher and higher prices have become an intrinsic part of an industry that increasingly relies on being able to acquire promising drugs rather than developing them in-house. The expectation that a new drug will be at least as expensive as the existing standard of care, with a premium added on at the drugmaker's discretion based on the value they believe it adds by being more clinically useful, allows biotechs to win backing from venture capital. In turn, those high prices drive up the acquisition costs of smaller drug companies. When the drug goes on sale and the rewards are reaped, they are frequently used to build a war chest for the next acquisition, perhaps with a sizeable spend on stock buybacks or dividends along the way. 'That entire flow of capital relies on almost an assumption that the launch price of any new treatment is going to be higher than the current price of the existing standard of care in that disease area,' Roy says.

In the aftermath of its hepatitis C treatments hitting the market, Gilead spent nearly $26 billion on stock buybacks in a three-year span.[58] In the same period, Gilead executives were among the best paid in the industry. Martin, the company's chief executive, had always been one of the industry's better-paid bosses, with annual remuneration of between $30 million and $60 million in the years leading up to the Pharmasset deal. Almost all of his compensation was linked to Gilead's soaring stock price, meaning the success of the hepatitis C treatments generated huge personal wealth. His compensation was worth $170 million in 2013 and had touched $232 million by 2015. He wasn't alone. The company's president, John Milligan, had a pay package worth $100 million in 2015 while Norbert Bischofberger, who was in charge of clinical research, was close behind with $96 million.[59] Two years later, Gilead used the revenues from Sovaldi and Harvoni to buy another drug company, Kite Pharma, for $11.9 billion. The key product was a cellular therapy called Yescarta which launched with a US price tag of $373,000 and a list price of nearly £300,000 in the UK.[60] And so the cycle began again.

Faced with a backlash, Gilead turned to the language of the 'value-based' approach Kolassa and others had pushed to justify the price of its new hepatitis C treatments. 'We stand behind the pricing of our therapies because of the benefit they bring to patients and the significant value they represent to payers, providers and our entire healthcare system,' a senior Gilead executive wrote to a medical journal.[61] He argued that the price would ultimately save money for health systems because they would no longer have to pay for liver transplants or other treatment costs as the disease progressed. This argument is regularly wheeled out by other drugmakers as a selling point for their latest product. It plays on the fact that the cost of healthcare in the US is hugely expensive across the board, for everything from doctors' fees to diagnostic tests and inpatient stays.

In Gilead's case, an independent analysis by a US non-profit found that the argument didn't stack up. Even over a twenty-year timeframe, the upfront cost of the new hepatitis C treatments would remain one-third higher than the later savings.[62] This was before including the costs of treating other ailments which would inevitably arise from the fact that patients cured of hepatitis C could then be expected to live longer. The non-profit concluded that money would only be saved if the new treatment was restricted to the most unwell patients, those with advanced liver damage. Trying to help a wider group would simply be too expensive at the price Gilead was charging.

At the turn of the millennium, the industry's business model seemed under threat. The slump in new drugs, and particularly in mass-market blockbusters which could be sold to huge numbers of patients, threatened to reduce revenues from on-patent drugs and was coupled with research-led companies losing a growing proportion of sales once their products went off patent. Generics accounted for only 50 per cent of drugs prescribed in the United States in 2000 and around 45 per cent in the UK. By 2020, they made up 90 per cent in both countries.[63]

The industry's efforts to meet these challenges had mixed success. Mergers and layoffs designed to placate shareholders failed to prevent the first ten years of the twenty-first century becoming known as a lost decade for Big Pharma's stock prices.[64] But things improved markedly in the 2010s as acquisitions and swelling prices allowed the industry to maintain its spectacular profitability even as a growing proportion of these profits came from treating smaller and smaller patient groups. For patients, however, the picture was a little different.

Before Solvadi launched, Gilead had steeled itself internally against any backlash over the price. 'Let's hold our position whatever competitors do or whatever the headlines,' one senior employee had instructed others.[65] The company had observed the opprobrium that had been poured on the manufacturers of AIDS medicines a generation earlier over the cost of the drug in the developing world and planned to offer far lower prices or strike deals with generic manufacturers to avoid the same criticism. A deal was subsequently reached with the government of Egypt, which had a high number of hepatitis C patients, to sell a twelve-week drug regimen for $900. Several Indian manufacturers were granted licences to make the drug providing they paid a royalty and only sold it to less well-off countries.

But Gilead hadn't counted on the level of outcry that its $1,000-a-day price would provoke in the richest nations. Such was Sovaldi's promise that, for years, doctors had been 'warehousing' hepatitis C patients, telling them to wait until a new generation of interferon-free cures hit the market. Now the price tag, and the huge number of patients waiting for the treatment to hit the market, meant that the drug single-handedly threatened to bankrupt health budgets across the United States.

In the UK it was priced at nearly £35,000 for a twelve-week course – around $57,000 at the exchange rates of the time.[66] Curing the country's 200,000 hepatitis C sufferers was now clinically possible, but it would consume one-third of the yearly drugs budget. In Spain, Italy, Portugal and Poland, the cost would exceed their entire annual budgets.[67]

Rationing care was the only answer. Even with a discount which brought the price down, the UK government determined that it could only afford to treat 10,000 patients a year.[68] In the US, only a small proportion of hepatitis C patients who qualified for Medicaid received the drug. Even small numbers placed a huge financial strain on the programmes. In 2014 alone, state Medicaid spent around $1.3 billion on Sovaldi (excluding rebates) to treat just 16,281 patients, less than 2.5 per cent of those with the disease.[69]

Gilead responded to criticism of its pricing decision by publicising its licensing agreements with Indian manufacturers to sell a cheap version to poorer countries as well as its patient assistance programme for those in the US. But both had significant limitations. The assistance programme offered to cover almost all of the money insured patients were required to personally pay but was of no benefit to anyone on a government-funded scheme like Medicare as they weren't eligible. A separate programme offered the drug free of charge to patients without adequate insurance, helping 4,000 patients in the first eight months after launch. Meanwhile, the agreements with Indian manufacturers resulted in much cheaper versions of Harvoni and Sovaldi becoming available. Under the terms of the licence, however, the generic companies could only sell to a specific list of countries. Among those excluded were many middle-income countries including eastern European nations where hepatitis C is prevalent. The health systems in these countries fell between two stools, unable to afford anything close to the prices charged in the US and major European markets and barred from importing cheap Indian generics.

Sovaldi and Harvoni, which can be made for $10 a bottle, raised the prospect of curing tens of millions of people diagnosed with hepatitis C and ridding countries of the life-threatening disease within a generation.[70] Instead, the high prices set by Gilead – and resulting restrictions imposed by health systems on which patients would receive the new drugs – meant that initial progress was painfully slow. In 2015, two years after launch, more people died from hepatitis C than received Gilead's new treatments.[71] Even with a reduction in prices which, as we shall see, came when earlier-than-expected competition arrived on the market, by 2020 wealthy European countries had still treated only around half of those diagnosed as carrying the virus.[72]

CHAPTER EIGHT

A one-sided tug of war

In late May 2015, Dr Leonard Saltz, a pensive man in round, thin-rimmed glasses, took to the stage before an audience of his peers in a room the size of an aircraft hangar.

It was the annual meeting of the American Society of Clinical Oncology, a prestigious gathering of tens of thousands of medical professionals, government officials, biotech investors and pharmaceutical reps in an enormous Chicago conference centre on the banks of Lake Michigan. Saltz, an oncologist at Memorial Sloan Kettering Cancer Center in New York, had been invited to speak during the plenary session, the conference's most high-profile platform, which is typically devoted to presentations on the most significant new scientific research. But he wasn't there to talk about clinical breakthroughs. He planned to use his keynote speech to raise what for many doctors was a taboo subject – the cost of drugs.

The fifty-eight-year-old began by talking about new data presented at the conference which showed promising evidence of the benefits for skin cancer patients of an experimental combination of two Bristol-Myers Squibb drugs.

'As a researcher, I am deeply gratified to see how basic science has been elegantly translated into useful drugs that are benefiting patients today,' he told the audience. 'As a clinician . . . I want these drugs, and drugs like them, available for my patients.'[1]

'As one who worries about how we will make them available and minimise disparities, I have a major problem – and that is that these drugs cost too much.'

Together, the price per milligram of the two drugs is 'approximately 4,000 times the cost of gold', Saltz said.[2] At $300,000 for a year's treatment, a typical US patient required by their insurance plan to pay 20 per cent of their costs would need to find $60,000. The price of these drugs and other cancer treatments was not based on their therapeutic value, the soft-spoken oncologist argued, but simply 'what has come before and what the seller believes the market will bear'.

He put up a new slide, showing what had happened to the launch price of cancer drugs in the United States going all the way back to the mid-1970s. Back then, they cost an average of $129 a month. By the late 1980s, this had reached $1,000 a month with no sign of slowing down. From the early 2000s, the chart jags violently upwards, passing $2,000, $5,000 and reaching almost $10,000 a month.[3] The point was clear: the Bristol-Myers drugs were not outliers. This was a systemic problem.

Traditionally, doctors aren't meant to concern themselves with drug prices, let alone complain about them to an audience of several thousand physicians.

'It is drilled into doctors in their training and in their existence that it's not your job to worry about price,' Saltz says, speaking by phone from his office in New York. 'But I started to ask, "Well, then whose job is it?" because we started to hear an awful lot of people worrying about healthcare costs.'[4] He'd first broached the topic at a much smaller event during the same annual conference in 2004 but, although his fellow physicians had been surprised by the prices he revealed, he'd made little headway in bringing the issue to the fore.

This time, things seemed different. For many in the audience, Saltz's admonishments were 'uncomfortable', Dr Alan Venook, a professor of medicine at the University of California San Francisco and the man who had invited Saltz to speak, told a reporter.[5] The conference is sponsored by pharmaceutical companies, making criticism of the drug industry from this platform unusual. Saltz, though, was greeted by rousing applause when he finished his talk. The speech made headlines and, for months afterwards, other doctors and academics would get in touch, asking to replicate his slides. Speaking out had been an easy decision, Saltz says. He saw the impact of soaring prices every week in the consulting rooms and hospital wards where he worked as patients grappled with the financial consequences of their illness.

In the US, even those with health insurance are often required to make a substantial contribution to the cost of their medications. In oncology, this can easily amount to a four-figure sum each month. Saltz says he's seen patients 'trimming the doses' they'd been prescribed in order to save money, or having to choose between a new treatment and giving up their house or life savings. In other wealthy countries, health systems have rationed the availability of cancer therapies because of their high cost. It seems particularly cruel, Saltz says, for those with a type of cancer where the only drugs available offer small, incremental benefits, measured in weeks or a few months rather than years.

From cancer drugs to insulin, the prices of prescription drugs have soared across a wide range of therapy areas since the late 1990s. Multiple sclerosis treatments, for example, cost between $8,000 and $11,000 in the mid-1990s. By 2015, they averaged $60,000 a year.[6] Again and again, companies have found markets willing to bear prices that had previously seemed inconceivable. AZT once caused an outcry with a proposed price of $10,000 a year; now there are scores of drugs costing more than $10,000 per month. Breakthrough drugs which could help tens of millions of people have launched with six-figure price tags and there are treatments for rare diseases on the market costing more than $1 million a head.

As prices have risen, so have the number of prescriptions, compounding the problem. The amount spent on prescription drugs in the US tripled between 1997 and 2007 and has increased by another 60 per cent since then.[7] Large European countries are spending 40 or 50 per cent more on drugs than they did a decade ago. All told, global pharmaceutical spending after discounts and rebates reached $1 trillion in 2019, up from less than $800 billion just five years earlier.[8] Western populations are getting older and more medicated, but a significant chunk – estimates suggest around one-third of the growth in spending in the United States – is down purely to price rises and more expensive new medicines.[9] It reflects drug companies' willingness to push things further, but also the failure of markets, regulators and governments to push back with enough force. The result is that even in rich, industrialised countries, beneficial medicines are increasingly out of reach for many patients because they or their health system simply can't afford them. When those medicines treat a potentially fatal condition, the cost can be measured in lives.

Insulin was discovered by four Canadian scientists in the early 1920s. Two of those involved, Frederick Banting and John Macleod, took the view that any involvement in patenting the discovery was at odds with the Hippocratic oath they had sworn to uphold and kept their names off the patent. The other two, a medical student and PhD researcher, transferred the patent to the University of Toronto for a single dollar because they believed 'that insulin should be made as widely available as possible, without any barriers such as cost'.[10] By harvesting animal insulin from the pancreatic ducts of pigs and purifying it into a form which was injectable into humans, the scientists created an effective treatment for diabetic patients who had previously faced the prospect of a heavily restricted diet and near-certain death within a couple of years.

When the University of Toronto partnered with Eli Lilly to begin mass-production of insulin soon after its discovery, the low life expectancy meant there were relatively few diabetics. A century later, the number of people with diabetes is approaching 500 million, a fast-growing health crisis which has pushed the value of the global insulin market above $20 billion.[11] Most have type 2 diabetes, in which the insulin produced by the body is insufficient or not working properly. A minority of around 10 per cent have type 1 diabetes, in which the body's own immune system attacks insulin-producing cells in the pancreas.[12] Type 1 diabetics cannot produce any insulin of their own and so are completely reliant on daily injections of lab-grown or animal insulin.

By 2018, Meaghan Patterson, a forty-seven-year-old nurse in Dayton, Ohio, had been living with type 1 diabetes for the best part of twenty years. When she was diagnosed, a vial of insulin, which would last her about ten days, cost $30. By 2018, the same medicine had risen to nearly $300.

Because of the cost, Meaghan, a larger woman with short-cropped hair and a loud laugh, had been stretching her diabetes supplies for some time. 'I don't know any type 1 [diabetic] that hasn't, at some point, tried to stretch what they have,' her sister-in-law Mindi Patterson says.[13] She was well aware of the dangers of not managing her blood sugar levels, having twice gone into diabetic ketoacidosis (DKA), a life-threatening complication brought on by a lack of insulin in the body, but had little choice.

Meaghan needed three or four vials a month, costing up to $1,200, in addition to other supplies including testing strips. 'She was making $30,000 to $40,000 a year and she was single so she was able to cover most of what she needed,' Mindi says. But in mid-June Meaghan lost her job. Uninsured, and only able to get short-term work, she quickly struggled financially.

The jobs she found paid OK, 'but the problem at that point is you're behind on your rent, you're behind on your phone, you're behind on your car payment, you can't really afford groceries. How are you going to handle purchasing not just one vial . . . but three or four?' Mindi explains. As Christmas approached, Meaghan had been rationing her insulin injections for some time, but, with a new job lined up for the start of January, she had nearly made it through.

On Christmas Eve, Mindi later learned, Meaghan had started throwing up. She had continued periodically vomiting throughout the night and the next morning her roommate, Cookie, urged her to go to hospital. Meaghan insisted she was fine and her roommate left her sleeping on the sofa as she went to work.

Meaghan was still asleep when Cookie returned at around 11 p.m. that evening. Pleased she was getting some rest, she didn't want to disturb her. But when Cookie got up the next morning, Meaghan still hadn't moved. She had passed away.

In the aftermath, Mindi and her husband, Rockwell, were able to piece together what they thought had happened. While cleaning out Meaghan's apartment, they found an empty sample vial of Humalog, the insulin she typically took, an empty vial of another type of insulin and a receipt for a cheaper, older version of the hormone sold by Walmart. The scrunched up paper showed it had been purchased on December 20th. 'It was partially used, so we know she used that for the last five days of her life.'

Mindi had previously discussed Walmart's intermediate-acting insulin with her sister-in-law to discourage her from using it without being monitored by a doctor. 'It's more unpredictable [meaning] your blood sugars will go higher and drop down more,' Mindi explains, which can be dangerous for a type 1 diabetic. But she understands why her sister-in-law took it.

'She was desperate,' Mindi says. When Meaghan died, she had just $25 left in her wallet but received the final payment of $2,000 from her previous short-term job on Boxing Day and was due to start a new nursing job, which offered health insurance, the following week.

'Knowing Meaghan I'm sure she was like, "I just have to wait a day, I get my money tomorrow. I can get what I need then",' Mindi says. She is convinced that Meaghan died of diabetic ketoacidosis, although no autopsy was ever performed. The cause of death was listed on her death certificate as a cardiac arrest, which can be caused by DKA.

For forty-nine-year-old Mindi, the price of insulin is still a constant concern. Her two teenage sons, Pierce and Martin, have both been diagnosed with type 1 diabetes, as has her husband, who is disabled and cannot work. She currently gets medical insurance through her job at Costco, but, as the sole breadwinner, worries what would happen if her situation changed or if the insurance cover or co-pay requirement is altered.

'In a family like ours, every penny counts. I run out of money about a week and a half after I get paid, and that's because I'm paying for the food, and the diabetes supply. My husband's social security disability pays for our electricity, our gas and then |his| parents pay our mortgage. My in-laws are in their seventies and they're still working because they have to help us.'

Insulin has been deemed an essential medicine by the World Health Organization because of the threat to life for type 1 diabetics who cannot access it. If blood sugar levels slip out of control, the consequences for patients can include kidney failure, blindness or death.

Just three companies, Sanofi, Novo Nordisk and Eli Lilly, produce almost all of the world's insulin. In a well-functioning market, competition might be expected to drive prices down, but for years the three firms followed similar pricing strategies: when one increased prices, the others typically moved to match them.[14] Companies aren't allowed to discuss prices and doing so would amount to price-fixing but if one manufacturer simply follows the lead of another this perfectly legal behaviour can achieve the same result.

Banting and his colleagues had found a way to extract animal insulin, which was purified and then injected into humans. Since the late 1970s, however, scientists have been able to produce genetically-engineered versions of human insulin which have fewer side effects. This synthetic 'human' insulin has become the standard treatment for diabetics and has allowed companies to obtain fresh patents by rolling out a series of incrementally improved versions called insulin analogues. Sanofi alone had filed more than seventy additional patents for Lantus, their version of the drug, since launching it in 2000 before losing a legal challenge from a generic drug manufacturer in 2018.[15]

The lack of competition globally has long hindered access to insulin. 'We have estimated that half of those who need insulin are having access problems,' says Margaret Ewen of the Dutch non-profit Health Action International. 'This medicine that's been around for

100 years still has very limited competition,' she says.[16] A number of factors have contributed to diabetics facing difficulties obtaining insulin including shortages, the cost of test strips and glucose monitors, and the differing policies of health systems as to whether they cover the cost of insulin. At its heart, though, is the pricing of the drug and how affordable that is for patients.

Nowhere is the problem caused by pricing more acute for diabetic patients than in the United States. Between 2002 and 2013, the published prices of insulin in the US tripled, and they have risen further still.[17] The most commonly-prescribed form of insulin, Lantus, cost two federal healthcare programmes in the US $5.7 billion in 2015, the second highest expenditure of any medicine over those twelve months and an increase of 15 per cent on the previous year.[18] In 2019 researchers at Yale found that one in four Americans had rationed their insulin because of the high cost of the medicine.[19] Campaigners have documented more than a dozen deaths among patients who tried to eke out their supplies or ran out altogether.

There is no intrinsic reason why insulin must be so expensive. It is relatively cheap to make. While American prices have soared from $20 to $275 per vial, those in Canada and many European countries held steady at around $20 to $30. Even at this price, manufacturers could enjoy a healthy profit, with one study estimating a fairer price would be less than $6 a vial for analogue insulin and cheaper for the human version.[20] That would mean a year's supply would cost around $100, rather than the average out-of-pocket cost of $6,000 in the US.[21]

In some ways the pricing of insulin is unusual, a uniquely American problem and a direct consequence of the country's uniquely flawed healthcare system. But in other ways, it is no different than the problems afflicting scores of drugs around the world. The social contract hands drugmakers enormous pricing power. If there is little or no commercial pressure on a price from manufacturers of rival treatments, and no generic manufacturers selling the same product, the only remaining brake is the willingness of those paying the bills to use their purchasing power or pricing regulations to push back.

The ultimate counterbalance in any negotiation with a monopoly supplier is the buyer's ability to walk away if they are not prepared to meet the asking price. Drugs, of course, are different. Someone with type 1 diabetes cannot produce their own insulin. Without medication, they are likely to die within days. When Gilead's pills were launched, a hepatitis C patient faced the unenviable alternative of a year-long treatment regimen with severe side effects and only a 50 per cent chance of working if they could not access the new drugs.[22] Pharmaceuticals are also unusual as products because of the distance between the buyer and the beneficiary since they are rarely paid for by the person who will directly benefit from them. In these circumstances, it is vital that those paying use their purchasing power to negotiate reasonable prices.

But the most important market for pharmaceuticals in the world, the United States, is failing to offer any meaningful resistance to price growth in a way that benefits the insurance policy-holders and taxpayers who ultimately foot the bills. In fact, the system is so riddled with absurdities that powerful market players are incentivised to increase drug prices further.

The United States spends at least $350 billion a year on pharmaceuticals, an annual budget that has risen by $100 billion in a decade.[23] The sheer scale of American spending on drugs dwarfs every other country in the world, with US sales worth more than the next nine largest markets combined. Annual spending on pharmaceuticals per person in the US is 25 per cent higher than any other major economic power.[24] The drug industry relies on American profits. Yet, instead of leveraging this bargaining power, American patients face the highest drug prices in the world.

At the centre of the American system is a complicated and opaque series of discounts, rebates and fees which mean the price of medicines often varies hugely between different buyers. Insurance companies, large employers and the US government's health programmes, Medicare and Medicaid, typically don't negotiate directly with drug companies but instead use middlemen known as pharmacy benefit managers (PBMs).

PBMs first proliferated in the 1970s, initially operating as claims administrators handling paperwork for health insurance companies. Over time they grew in size and influence, masterminding innovations like prescription benefit cards and mail order services that made it easier for insurance customers to obtain their medicines.[25] By the 1990s these entities played a key role in negotiating prices, reimbursing pharmacies and deciding which drugs were given preferred status. Their success in inserting themselves into the pharmaceutical ecosystem prompted a string of large drugmakers to acquire PBMs themselves, although they were subsequently forced to sell them off because of concerns they could be used to push their owner's drugs. Changes to Medicare signed into law by President Bush which came into effect in 2006 enhanced the growth of PBMs further as they were handed responsibility for administering prescription plans for millions of elderly patients. Since then, a series of mergers and acquisitions have left three large PBMs with a dominant market share in the US.

The idea of PBMs is that by representing large numbers of patients, they will have significant bargaining power. By maintaining lists of which drugs are covered, they can use their buying power to seek rebates from manufacturers to reduce the list price of medicines – payments which reached $90 billion in 2016.[26] In theory, these savings are passed on to the insurer who, in turn, passes the benefit to patients in the form of lower premiums. However, discounts and rebates take place in secret. Even the insurers often don't know the extent of a discount or rebate secured by PBMs, and so there are no guarantees the benefits are being passed on in full. Critics say the system encourages drug companies to push up list prices in order to facilitate larger discounts and rebates with which to tempt PBMs and insurers into favouring their drugs. After all, if a drug is more expensive than a rival but offers a larger rebate, the PBM stands to gain more from putting the higher-priced drug on its formulary. Recent years have been marked by a spate of lawsuits accusing PBMs of overcharging their clients by enormous amounts. One, filed by America's second-largest health insurer, alleged it had been paying an extra $3 billion a year.[27]

PBMs capture an estimated 14 per cent of total spending on pharmaceuticals in the United States and the sums involved have made the three largest PBMs enormously profitable.[28] They have also been blamed for the growing gap between list prices and the amount actually received by drug manufacturers.[29] In recent years, this gap has grown significantly as PBMs became very adept at leveraging deep discounts when drugs are therapeutically interchangeable.

Between 2007 and 2018, list prices in the US rose by 9.1 per cent a year, but net prices only grew by 4.5 per cent.[30] While the average discount secured in the early 1990s stood at 16 per cent, some companies now claim to be giving discounts of 45 per cent or more on the list prices for their branded drugs.[31] This gap between list prices and the sums drugmakers receive is particularly pronounced in the insulin market. Between 2007 and 2013, the list price of Lantus went up by 252 per cent, but the actual price the manufacturer received increased by the significant but substantially lower sum of 57 per cent.[32] It is no surprise that patients with diabetes are among those who have filed lawsuits attacking PBMs, accusing them of conspiring with manufacturers to inflate insulin prices.

In February 2019, when senior executives at three insulin manufacturers were among those summoned before Congress for a dressing down on drug prices, they were quick to point fingers at PBMs. Olivier Brandicourt, the chief executive of Sanofi, told the assembled politicians that the net price of Lantus, meaning the amount the manufacturer actually receives, had gone down over the past two years. He said this had been intended to improve the affordability of the medicine for patients, adding: 'Unfortunately, under the current system, savings from rebates are not consistently passed through to patients in the form of lower deductibles, co-payments or co-insurance amounts.'[33]

'All players – wholesalers like McKesson and Cardinal, pharmacies like CVS and Walgreens, pharmacy benefit managers like Express Scripts and CVS Caremark, and drug companies – make more money when list prices increase,' Alex Azar, a former senior Eli Lilly executive, told an industry conference in 2017, months before he was named US health and human services secretary. 'The unfortunate victims of these trends are patients.'[34] If PBMs use their power to favour those drugs with the largest rebates, plumping up their own profits even as they drive patients towards more expensive drugs, the cost is ultimately borne by health insurance policy holders in the form of higher premiums.

Higher list prices also have a direct impact on many patients' ability to access medicines even if insurers and government programmes are getting sizeable discounts. Changes in the US health insurance market mean that large numbers of patients are no longer cushioned from list prices in the way they once were. The average size of the deductible which an insured patient must pay out of their own pocket before insurance steps in has gone up steeply in recent years and can often reach several thousand dollars. Even after paying this, patients remain exposed to high list prices because many schemes also impose a co-pay requirement. These used to be fixed sums, perhaps $10 or $20 per medication, but are now more likely to be based on a percentage of the drug's price. Meanwhile for those like Meaghan Patterson who lose their jobs and become uninsured, the list price of a drug is the amount of money, in full, they must pay to obtain the medicines they need.

While handing the private, for-profit PBMs a huge but secretive role in determining drug prices, the American system also handicaps the government's own ability to drive down prices. Under the law as it currently stands, government officials are legally prohibited from negotiating lower drug prices on behalf of Medicare Part D, the programme which pays for prescription drugs for elderly Americans. What's more, for six classes of drugs, which includes cancer drugs taken by patients at home, antidepressants, AIDS treatments and insulin, Part D plans are required to cover 'all or substantially all drugs' on the market, regardless of the cost. Although the private health plans that provide Medicare coverage can negotiate, these restrictions severely hamper their efforts.

Insurers theoretically have more freedom in deciding what to cover but the commercial reality is that health plans are expected to cover most drugs. If they don't, customers will take their business elsewhere. On top of those expectations, three-quarters of Americans with health insurance live in states which have passed laws requiring insurers to cover cancer drugs for on- and off-label uses.[35] For other high-priced drugs, insurers are more likely to impose restrictions to try and limit their use rather than refusing to pay for them altogether. This can be achieved by requiring prior authorisation before it is prescribed, or placing it in a tier which commands a higher co-pay.

Oncology treatments are among several therapeutic areas where the US system has inadvertently pushed manufacturers to set higher prices. A scheme passed by Congress in 1992 known as 340B requires the industry to grant discounts of at least 23.1 per cent to some public health clinics and other government-funded institutions. Since it was introduced, rule changes have seen a huge expansion in the number of providers eligible. In an effort to offset the discounts they must offer, drug companies responded by setting higher launch prices.[36]

For those cancer treatments which require infusion under medical supervision, and all other biological medicines, there are financial incentives for doctors to prescribe more expensive treatments. Such medicines come under Medicare Part B and are reimbursed on the basis of the average sales price of the drug, plus a set profit margin of 4.3 per cent.[37] The fixed profit margin calculated on the basis of the drug's price means that, perversely, hospitals make more money from administering a more expensive drug. Oncologists, and the hospitals they work for, can also benefit from the difference between wholesale and retail prices. Irinotecan, a cancer drug sold under the brand name Camptosar, became subject to generic competition in 2008, bringing the price down by 80 per cent. Despite the price fall, oncologists' use of the drug actually fell, with one explanation pointing towards a reduction in the money made on the difference between how much hospitals were reimbursed for the drug and how much they paid for it.[38]

Far from controlling costs, the US system is so badly flawed, so punctured with skewed incentives and shrouded in mystery as to

who is paying what for different drugs, that products can succeed
which appear to defy basic logic. Duexis is a pain relief drug for
patients with rheumatoid arthritis. It is a simple combination of two
medicines: ibuprofen, the common anti-inflammatory, and famotidine, an antacid which reduces the risk of ibuprofen causing an ulcer.
Both of the medicines are long off patent and are sold generically
as over-the-counter medicines available without a prescription for a
few cents a pill. Taking generic versions of ibuprofen and famotidine
instead of the branded Duexis would cost just $15 to $30 a month.
However, the combination drug, which is taken three times a day,
costs $27 a pill at full price, or around $2,500 for a month's supply,
with its manufacturer receiving around $400 of that because of heavy
discounting.[39] Despite this astronomical mark-up on drugs easily
available in pharmacies, Duexis generated net sales of more than
$500 million in the space of five years.[40]

The drug was launched by Horizon Pharma in 2011 and met the
US regulator's requirements by demonstrating safety and efficacy,
leaving the manufacturer free to launch it on the market at any price
they wished. In turn, the body responsible for Medicare is not allowed
to negotiate with manufacturers over pricing. So when the drug
company persuades doctors to prescribe the medicine, US taxpayers
duly meet the cost. For commercially insured patients, any potential
worries about the cost are negated by patient assistance programmes
which limit out-of-pocket costs to no more than $25.

Sales eventually began to decline when doctors and insurers finally
cottoned on to the extremely high cost of the drug, but at that point
Horizon managed to get an addition made to the prescribing information leaflet. Since 2017, the package insert states: 'Do not
substitute Duexis with the single-ingredient products of ibuprofen
and famotidine'. The evidence it used to persuade the FDA to allow
this used several familiar tricks from the pharmaceutical industry's
toolkit.

First, Horizon Pharma found a specific new niche which hadn't
previously been covered as an approved indication for famotidine.
The generic could be marketed as a treatment for two common types

of ulcers but not specifically to 'decrease the risk of developing upper gastrointestinal ulcers in patients taking ibuprofen'. Duexis secured approval for this use by demonstrating efficacy in a clinical trial in which it compared patients who took the combination drug containing 800mg of ibuprofen and 26.6mg of famotidine with those taking only ibuprofen in the same dose. Finally, it argued that the 'unique combination of active ingredients in Duexis is not available OTC [over-the-counter]' because famotidine is only available generically in 10mg or 20mg doses. Duexis is taken three times a day, meaning a total dose of 79.8mg – for all intents and purposes the same as four 20mg tablets. Nevertheless, it secured the labelling change and continues to bring in more than $100 million a year.[41]

There are scores of similar drugs. A 2018 study found that twenty-nine combination medicines, sold under brand names, cost Medicare, and therefore US taxpayers, an extra $925 million in 2016 compared with the cost of generic versions of the constituent parts.[42] Yosprala, which combines aspirin and the stomach drug omeprazole, drugs costing just a few dollars, has been listed for pharmacists with a price tag of more than $1,100 for thirty tablets.

These drugs take advantage of the market and the lack of effective regulation or push back from payers, but also of the ignorance or indifference of many doctors towards pricing which Saltz looked to challenge. The distance between prescribing doctors and the insurers or health systems who ultimately pay the bill helps to reduce price sensitivity. Doctors who have prescribed the same drug for decades are all too easily oblivious to the regular price increases the manufacturer has been implementing which now mean it is several times the price of a similar medicine. Others remain wedded to brand name products even when generics are available and many countries prohibit so-called 'generic substitution', where chemists can substitute the cheaper product even when the brand name version has been prescribed. For newly-launched drugs, even if time-pressed doctors were to study the clinical evidence behind the treatment in depth, they face an uphill struggle to ascertain whether a higher price is merited by the relative benefit over another treatment because drug companies work strenuously to avoid straightforward head-to-head comparison with rival products unless they know it is going to show a clear benefit.

Almost every aspect of the system plays to drugmakers' strengths. The fierce secrecy that surrounds prices, discounts and rebates leaves unsuspecting insurers unaware that another company is paying 20 per cent less for the same cancer treatment or arthritis drug. In the US, the industry also benefits from a different attitude to healthcare and pharmaceutical intervention than is found in Canada, Europe, Australia and New Zealand. Fuelled by drug industry lobbying, US patient groups stand primed to oppose the faintest whiff of anything that looks like rationing or withholding treatment.

American patients who have a serious illness and are covered by insurance want and expect every medicine going, regardless of the cost to the insurer or the relative benefit. Anything less is seen as an attack on fundamental individual freedoms. While Europeans, perhaps used to seeing national health systems with strained budgets visibly having to struggle with the demands of huge numbers of patients, are accustomed to some degree of cost–benefit analysis and rationing, American individualism demands the best no matter the cost. As a result, any talk of price or budgetary controls in the United States quickly descends into heated partisan rhetoric, as epitomised by Sarah Palin's accusation that President Obama's health reforms were an attempt to bring in 'death panels' – faceless bureaucrats who would deny care to the elderly or disabled because they were not worthy of treatment.

As well as having the highest prices, the US makes greater use of drugs at the more expensive end of the scale than other rich countries.[43] Those with insurance provided by their employers typically have a maximum amount set on the costs they can be required to pay. Once they have passed this threshold, there is little reason for patients not to push their doctor to prescribe any drug that could conceivably help, even if it offers only minimal gains at a very large price. Meanwhile, the underinsured and more than one in twelve Americans without health insurance are left behind.[44]

To call the US system broken is to do it an injustice. Broken might imply that what was once a functioning system has simply fallen into disrepair and needs fixing. It doesn't capture the extent to which the mass of misaligned financial incentives and opaque prices actively make things worse. Of course, the problems with US healthcare extend far beyond pharmaceuticals; American patients face far higher prices for everything from routine operations to diagnostic tests, ambulance call outs and overnight hospital stays. Despite having the highest spending per person, the US healthcare system routinely ranks well below those of other economically developed countries.[45]

These costs mean that the poor in America simply can't afford to get sick. For others, becoming seriously unwell can push them into poverty. These are problems that generations of US politicians, to their shame, have failed to address. But while the high cost of hospital care is essentially a domestic issue, the huge growth in pharmaceutical prices in the US has ramifications all over the globe.

Chantelle Lindsay never wanted her diagnosis to define her. When she played lacrosse, she played as hard as any of the other girls in the small Canadian town of Truro, sprinting across the concrete floor even as she then spluttered and coughed her way through the rest breaks. 'This new girl started playing and she didn't realise Chantelle had CF,' Chantelle's father, Mark, recalls. 'And she made a joke: "I'm going to have to get you some cough drops."'

'Chantelle kind of laughed [along] and said, "Yeah, maybe you should," and never even told her,' he says. 'She went through the whole year, didn't even know that Chantelle had CF. It's not some-thing that she dwelled on or wanted any pity for, she just worked through it.'[46]

Chantelle had been diagnosed with CF – cystic fibrosis – when she was three months old. As she grew up, she didn't complain about the regular physiotherapy sessions or taking her aerosols; nor did she let these things hold her back. As well as lacrosse, she played football and ice hockey, refusing to let the disease stop her from joining in the same activities as her friends. 'She was Chantelle,' her father says. 'Not Chantelle with CF.'

Patients with cystic fibrosis, which is inherited, suffer a gradual deterioration as their lungs and digestive systems become clogged and around half do not live past the age of forty. In early 2012, Vertex Pharmaceuticals, a Boston-based biotech company, launched Kalydeco, the first of a series of revolutionary new drugs which targeted the underlying cause of cystic fibrosis, halting the progression of the disease. For a while, Chantelle took another of Vertex's new drugs, Orkambi, but in January 2019 she turned twenty-two and was no longer covered by the health insurance offered through her father's job as a car mechanic. It didn't seem a significant issue at first. Her lung function hadn't really improved while on Orkambi but it also hadn't declined further, staying 'at about 60 to 70 per cent lung function, which was quite manageable', Mark says.

It was around six months later when Chantelle's health began to decline. She started getting more lung infections, each one requiring a course of antibiotics to treat. By December, one particularly belligerent infection left her in hospital, where doctors cycled through different combinations of antibiotics trying to find one that worked. She was discharged but returned less than two weeks later. As the new year dawned, Chantelle's lung function was down to 37 per cent. Her doctors were running out of options.

Orkambi, the drug Chantelle had been taking until early 2019, was one of several recently launched combination drugs. Now, fresh off the pipeline, was Vertex's latest offering, a triple-combination pill called Trikafta. While Orkambi could slow decline in lung function and help patients avoid being hospitalised, Trikafta was far more impressive, with studies showing it could actively improve lung function for up to 90 per cent of cystic fibrosis patients.[47]

Trikafta had received regulatory approval in the US in October 2019 but the manufacturer, concerned about the Canadian government's proposed changes to how much it is willing to pay for new drugs, was yet to submit it for approval in Canada. In the meantime, Vertex, like many drug companies, had an 'expanded access' programme which offered the drug free of charge to patients with an urgent need. Chantelle's new readings dropped her inside the threshold required to be eligible for Vertex's compassionate use programme and so her doctors wrote to the company to make the case on her behalf. And then they waited, and waited.

'That's when our real fight started,' Mark says. The family got in touch with another cystic fibrosis patient, Stephanie Stavros, who had just become the first Canadian to receive the drug under Vertex's compassionate use programme. Stavros had peppered Vertex with letters and pleas. 'She didn't really know what particular thing helped her get it but she went as far as having her little four-year-old write to Vertex in crayon trying to get them to understand the importance of her getting this drug,' Mark adds. Stavros had seen a rapid improvement after taking the drug. 'You keep fighting, you'll do fine,' she told them.

Hundreds of letters, maybe even thousands, were sent. 'Our friends were writing letters to Vertex and the government officials. We were on the news. We were just doing everything we could to try and pressure someone,' Mark says. 'We figured someone somewhere will have a connection with somebody to try and help us get this drug that we need.'

The family appealed to the Canadian government too but officials said their hands were tied; it was down to Vertex to take the first step before they could approve the drug under a special access scheme. Fundraising efforts were organised. A dance and silent auction in Chantelle's hometown raised $17,000 (around £10,000). Doctors helped get her back on Mark's insurance by declaring her long-term disabled, allowing her to try another of Vertex's older drugs. It wasn't successful.

Mark and his wife contemplated seeking a lung transplant in Toronto if Chantelle got sufficiently well, or driving across the US border to get hold of Trikafta there. At one point, he received a call from a wealthy would-be Good Samaritan. 'He said, "How can we get this drug for Chantelle? How can we get her down there and get treated?",' Mark says. 'The trouble with it is, you go down, get treated,

but you can't bring the drug back across. We would have had to
move to the States. And then he asked about getting the drug and
having it brought up here.'

Two others offered to send Trikafta from the US. 'The trouble
with that is you're sending an illegal drug across the border. It
would be confiscated and we'd probably be charged for trying to
import it so we couldn't even do that,' Mark says. Even if they
somehow got it to Canada, Chantelle's doctors wouldn't be allowed
to administer it unless it came through the government's special
access programme, something that wasn't possible without Vertex's
help.

Eventually, Chantelle's doctors got a response from the drugmaker.
'It was probably five or six weeks after we had applied,' Mark says.
'They came back and told us no.'[48] She died a few days later.

Vertex was in no rush to launch the drug in Canada because 'they
were afraid of the impact that the new regulations in Canada would
have on their price around the globe', says John Wallenburg, chief
scientific officer at the non-profit Cystic Fibrosis Canada.[49] When a
new drug makes it through clinical trials, it is not launched everywhere
at the same time. Each new market has different regulatory requirements and fees to obtain market approval as well as requiring
investment in safety monitoring and a sales force to push the drug.
Some drugs, particularly complex biological medicines, may also
initially be in short supply as the drugmaker ramps up its manufacturing capabilities, so it makes commercial sense to prioritise the
most valuable and accessible markets.

The United States is usually at the top of the list but other countries are dependent on their market size and how favourably their
regulatory or health system's approach to new drugs is viewed. If a
country is seen as having particularly onerous or difficult regulators,
it can expect a longer wait than one that will wave a drug through
rapidly. Similarly, if a country is seen as having particularly harsh
price controls or a reputation for tough negotiating, it can expect to
fall further back in the queue.

While the US largely leaves drug reimbursement decisions to the free market, many other countries take a more proactive approach in trying to drive down costs. As well as seeking to use their buying power to negotiate better prices, several have set up agencies or panels as gatekeepers to determine the maximum price they are prepared to pay.

In Canada's case, a body called the Patented Medicine Prices Review Board sets limits on the price of a new drug based on the cost of comparable treatments and prices in other countries. It is then up to individual provinces to negotiate with the manufacturer on possible discounts and to decide whether it will offer the drug. The price of new drugs in Canada, though lower than in the US, had long been amongst the highest in the world, but in 2019 the Canadian government announced that it was pushing ahead with changes which aimed to reduce the cost of patent-protected medicines by one-fifth.

Not only were other health systems likely to offer more favourable financial terms for Trikafta, there was also the danger that the drug could be rejected by the Patented Medicine Prices Review Board as excessively priced. Such a decision could have significant ramifications in how it was viewed in other markets. Even if Vertex did lower its price sufficiently to win acceptance, this would also come at a cost. This is because many countries use something called 'external reference pricing' which pegs what they are prepared to pay for a treatment to the average cost of the drug in a number of designated markets. Canada uses the United Kingdom, Germany and several other countries, including, until July 2020, the high-priced US and Swiss markets. It in turn serves as a reference market for prices in Brazil and South Africa.

External reference pricing is used in more than thirty countries, including Australia, Brazil, Japan and many European nations, either in conjunction with other judgements on cost-effectiveness or the therapeutic benefits of a new product or as a direct means of setting a reimbursement price.[50] The consequence is that prices in one country ripple across the globe. Large Western economies have a particularly outsized impact in this respect. One study by researchers at the Berlin University of Technology found that dropping the price of a drug by €1 in Germany would reduce the price paid for the same product by 36 cents in Italy and 28 cents in the Netherlands.[51] Prices obtained in the United Kingdom are also influential, both because it is used as a reference price by at least seventeen European countries as well as Canada and Australia but also because of the well-respected approach the British healthcare system takes when appraising the prices of new medicines.[52]

The British approach centres around a gatekeeper called the National Institute for Health and Care Excellence (NICE).[53] Set up in 1999, with offices in two monolithic towers in London and Manchester, NICE is an independent body tasked by the government with assessing new medicines and issuing guidance on whether they should be paid for. Initially only a proportion of new drugs were referred to NICE by the British government, but since 2019 all drugs are expected to be appraised by the cost-effectiveness body. The assessment process involves a measure called the Quality-Adjusted Life Year (QALY), which applies a cost–benefit analysis to a drug's effectiveness when compared with the best existing treatment. A QALY is a year of healthy life, meaning drugs get credit not simply for extending life but also for relieving pain or other symptoms for a period of time.

The use of a QALY is intended to force drugmakers to justify their prices with clear evidence of how their drugs can help different patient groups and NICE sets explicit thresholds for what it considers to be a fair price. A treatment which costs up to £30,000 per QALY gained from the intervention is generally considered cost-effective, while pressure from patients and drugmakers has led to higher thresholds for end-of-life treatments and drugs treating very rare diseases.

Drugs which fail NICE's assessment are not deemed cost-effective and are rejected unless drugmakers are prepared to discount the price to fall within the body's thresholds. Putting a price on someone's life may sound cold-hearted but it is something that already underpins a wide range of decisions from setting speed limits to environmental regulations. In any event, when a drug is so expensive it is out of reach, a price has already been placed on that person's life.

NICE requires companies to submit additional data beyond what is required to get marketing approval, including economic modelling demonstrating the drug's value. It is well regarded internationally for the scrutiny it applies. As a result, NICE's approval is a valuable prize which the manufacturer can use in negotiations in other markets to demonstrate that the product has been deemed cost-effective. On the other hand, if a drug is rejected, or if conditions are attached to its acceptance, it can have a damaging effect on the prospects of securing reimbursement in many other countries.

In theory, this approach sets a firm ceiling and should help in the global push back against excessively high drug prices but in reality almost all drugs approved by NICE only secure approval after agreeing to sizeable confidential discounts on their list price. These discounts aren't made public and so are limited in the impact they have on prices elsewhere.

Health technology assessments (HTAs) – the evaluation of the benefits, costs and wider impact of healthcare interventions such as pharmaceuticals or medical devices – like those carried out by NICE also have limitations as a means of pushing back on escalating prices. The approach is intrinsically inflationary, with each new drug which demonstrates a therapeutic benefit setting a pricing floor for the next one. In the UK, because HTAs haven't been carried out on all new drugs in the past, the modelling used to assess drugs will accept higher prices for different diseases depending purely on what has been paid for a treatment for that ailment before.

This can be seen when a medicine gains a new indication. The drug alemtuzumab was launched by Genzyme under the brand name Campath in 2001 as a treatment for leukaemia. While it was on the market, doctors realised it could also be used to treat some multiple sclerosis patients and began prescribing it on an unlicensed 'off-label' basis for this purpose. In 2012, a year after Genzyme had been bought by Sanofi, the drug was withdrawn from the market and relaunched with a licence to treat multiple sclerosis.

The relaunch, under the name Lemtrada, also carried a new price tag. Campath had cost around £2,500 for a full treatment course; Lemtrada cost around £56,000.[54] The new price reflected what Genzyme believed it could now sell the drug for when compared to other multiple sclerosis treatments and it was duly approved by NICE for use in Britain's health service. Because the value of a new drug is judged in relation to an existing treatment, the NICE approach creates an escalator effect which presumes that each new and better drug will inevitably have a higher price than the one that came before.[55]

Political pressure has also meant that the ceiling set by NICE's approach is not always a robust one. Andrew Stevens, now a professor of public health at the University of Birmingham, chaired one of NICE's appraisal committees for thirteen years. In 2005 the health secretary had intervened to push for patients with early-stage breast cancer to be given access to a Roche drug, Herceptin, even before it had been approved for use for that indication in the UK. As a result, NICE felt obliged to approve it, Stevens says. 'When there's a NICE appraisal there is always quite a lot of wriggle room in the economic models that are presented. So a committee if it's completely sort of unpressured will probably be very sceptical about the economic model which a company puts through,' he explains.[56] 'But where there's, as in the case of Herceptin . . . a strong perception pushed by the chairman of the committee that yes has got to be the answer, the least untidy way of doing it is by not picking apart the company's model.' As a result, it appears that the QALY threshold hasn't been breached 'whereas in fact it probably has been breached were the model to have been picked apart more assiduously'.

Overall, the UK pays prices which tend to be towards the cheaper end of the scale compared to other large European economies. The UK spends less on retail prescriptions – drugs sold by pharmacies – than Italy, France and Germany but more than the Netherlands, Portugal and Poland.[57] Gilead, when assessing the pricing landscape for its hepatitis C drugs, believed the British health system would drive a harder bargain than other large European markets. The UK was expected to 'set the European price floor and Germany to set the ceiling', the US Senate Finance Committee's report said, with an anticipated wholesale price in Germany of $63,198.70 compared to $57,100.20 in the UK.[58]

Nevertheless, the cost of drugs is contributing to significant financial strain for the British health system. Like other wealthy countries, it struggled to pay for Gilead's hepatitis C medicines. NICE was initially unpersuaded by the data Gilead presented to make its case for Sovaldi's £35,000 price tag for a twelve-week course. In the summer of 2014, the body said it was 'minded not to recommend' the drug but it eventually gave its approval the following year, and later deemed Harvoni to be cost-effective as well. Approval from NICE legally requires the NHS to offer the drug to patients, but on this occasion there were concerns that, with more than 200,000 people infected with hepatitis C across the UK, the expensive treatment could leave it unable to fund treatments for other patients, potentially causing thousands of unnecessary deaths.[59] The health service in England worked around these rules by imposing annual quotas on how many people could be treated. It was only years later that the introduction of competing hepatitis C treatments reduced the price to £10,000 per patient and meant English patients could be treated on a wider scale.[60]

The UK's efforts to reduce the price of drugs also suffers, like other healthcare systems, from the distorting effect of the US market. If a country is too successful at negotiating down prices, drugmakers can simply withhold their drug to protect American revenues. The US accounts for more than 40 per cent of global drug sales, far ahead of the second-largest market, China, which makes up 11 per cent. Even large European countries pale in comparison, with the combined sales figures for France and Germany amounting to less than one-fifth of those in the US.[61] The changes which have resulted in huge price inflation in the American market have pushed up drug executives' expectations of the prices they can command for their products elsewhere.

For some drugs, particularly those for extremely rare diseases with only very small numbers of patients, manufacturers often expect to sell the drug at a fairly uniform price around the world. For others, it is accepted that US prices will be higher, but manufacturers are nevertheless keen to push for the highest price possible in other markets. The British system, like many others, successfully limits price rises once a drug has gone on sale but NICE appraisals enable launch prices to continue to rise, even if they restrict the rate at which that can happen.

The problem is that the rewards on offer in the American market are so exaggerated the revenue from even large European countries is not enough to force drug companies to stay at the negotiating table. If the reimbursement prices on offer are considered too low, manufacturers have been prepared to walk away or withhold their drug for several years in order to protect revenues in the US and other countries. In Germany, where prices for new drugs are nego-tiated by a central organisation representing insurers, twenty-eight drugs, a little over 12 per cent of those submitted, have been with-drawn by their manufacturers since 2011 because they weren't happy with the price.[62] The US has also been willing to use its clout to apply pressure to countries who try and force drugmakers to sell their products at lower prices.

'In some cases, medicine that costs a few dollars in a foreign country costs hundreds of dollars in America for the same pill, with the same ingredients, in the same package, made in the same plant,' said then-President Donald Trump in a speech in May 2018 delivered from the White House lawn. 'And that is unacceptable.' He accused foreign countries of 'freeloading' on American research and develop-ment. Instead of seeking to reduce US prices directly, Trump pledged to use trade negotiations to force other countries to pay more for new drugs. He said he had directed officials to make fixing this a top priority and that they 'have great power over the trading partners; you're seeing that already . . . America will not be cheated any longer, and especially will not be cheated by foreign countries.'[63]

Small countries which are not used as reference markets can sometimes secure significant discounts on the prices paid for new drugs elsewhere, something New Zealand has largely managed to do. But for most countries, for all their efforts to control prices, drugmakers hold the upper hand. Patents offer the ultimate trump card, meaning no one else is permitted to supply a drug which may be the only treatment for a disease. Governments have powers to override patents in such situations but, as we shall see, very rarely use them.

Drug companies have used the power of being the only supplier of a medicine to play hardball with the price of drugs of all kinds. In 2009, the South African company Aspen Pharmacare struck a deal with GSK to buy the rights to six branded cancer drugs which had been off patent for many years but had attracted no generic competition. A few years later, Aspen decided it wanted to significantly increase their prices, which had gone unchanged for many years. It claimed they were loss-making, although the Italian competition watchdog, which later investigated, disputed this, saying it had seen internal financial documents which disproved the claim. Either way, Aspen was not prepared to take no for an answer as it sought to impose price changes in Europe. When several countries tried to resist, it threatened to stop making the drugs altogether. In Italy, the country's competition watchdog alleged, Aspen manipulated supplies so that there would be shortages of some of the essential medicines during price negotiations. The Italian health authorities agreed to price changes which forced up the cost of the drugs from less than €2 million a year to €7 million.[64] In Spain, where the authorities refused to acquiesce to a price rise from €2 a pack to €100 for one drug, it followed through on a threat to halt supply.[65] Emails show that, like Vertex, Aspen was willing to allow stock to expire rather than sell it at a lower price than the company wished.

Just as Canadians have struggled to access some of Vertex's cystic fibrosis treatments, so too have patients in Britain. The NHS agreed to pay for one of the earlier treatments, Kalydeco, which could help only about 5 per cent of those with the disease, even though it had not been assessed by NICE. The decision was quickly a cause of regret, with a senior official later telling a parliamentary committee the health service had spent more than £200 million 'above what we would see as a fair and reasonable price' over the course of that ill-judged five-year deal, benefiting just a few hundred patients.[66]

When the next drug, Orkambi, was ready for launch, NICE's verdict was unequivocal. The independent body agreed that the drug offered clear benefits for patients but judged it to be hugely over-priced. With a cost of around £350,000 per QALY, it was more than ten times more expensive than the maximum permitted for cystic fibrosis treatments.[67] An independent cost-effectiveness assessment in the US later took the same view, suggesting price cuts of more than 70 per cent were needed.[68] However, whereas US insurers covered the drug anyway, Vertex refused to sufficiently lower its UK asking price of £104,000 per patient per year and so the NHS refused to offer it to patients.

The standoff that followed lasted almost four years. During that time, Vertex destroyed nearly 8,000 packs of Orkambi which had passed their expiry date, while as many as 200 cystic fibrosis patients died waiting for the treatment, according to one campaign group.[69] Vertex also refused to submit data on its next cystic fibrosis drug, Symkevi, to NICE and wrote a letter to then British prime minister Theresa May suggesting it was rethinking its commitment to basing its international headquarters, employing 250 people, in the UK. A deal was finally agreed with the British health service in October 2019, shortly before a snap general election was announced.

If a country has baulked at the price of a manufacturer's previous treatment, it can expect to fall down the pecking order in future. The system reduces access to drugs and a willingness to pay for innovation to a binary choice. In fact, many countries don't get to make a choice at all. Under the tiered approach which the industry takes to the global market, some countries have long been accustomed to getting limited or no access to new drugs. Middle- and lower-income countries are rarely on the radar of large drug companies when they contemplate their launch strategy for a new product. In some cases, drugmakers won't bother to register their patents and seek regulatory approval at all because the market is too small and there is no prospect of the health system being able to pay a price that would generate sufficient revenues to be of interest.

In the poorest countries, it is left to corporate philanthropy, non-governmental organisations and humanitarian charities to deliver vaccines and other much-needed medicines. Cutting-edge drugs are only available to those wealthy enough to meet the full cost themselves, something the World Health Organization has acknowledged is the case with the majority of patent-protected cancer treatments.[70] As with richer countries, the US is willing to throw its weight around to protect drug companies when governments seek alternative means to access the medicines being offered at an unaffordable price.

In 2017, the Malaysian government, exasperated by the price of Gilead's hepatitis C treatments, struck an agreement with an Egyptian generics company to make cheaper alternative versions. The deal relied on compulsory licensing, a provision in a 1995 international agreement on intellectual property which allows governments to issue licences for patent-protected drugs without the consent of the patent-holder. Malaysia came under significant pressure to reverse its actions, with Gilead calling on high-level American officials including the US Trade Representative to help out.[71] The government held firm but the threat of diplomatic repercussions has contributed to how rarely compulsory licensing provisions have been used.

The result of the interconnectedness of global drug prices is that it is not just American patients who have reason to complain about the cost of medicines. Countries across the globe are battling with increasing drug bills, strained budgets and problems accessing new medicines. Pharmaceutical sales in Australia rose by 50 per cent over the last decade while the amount spent on medicines per person in Germany has increased by more than 40 per cent over the same timeframe.[72] In Britain, officials have negotiated an agreement with drug companies to cap the growth in medicine spending, but even with this in place the amount spent on branded drugs in England rose by one-sixth between 2014 and 2019.[73] In a sign of how the health system is struggling, policymakers were forced to introduce a budget impact test meaning that new drugs which pass NICE's cost-effectiveness test but are likely to cost more than £20 million a year can have their adoption by the NHS delayed.

These growing costs come even as health systems are having to turn down innovative new drugs because the prices being demanded are too high to fall within cost-effectiveness thresholds, or because the budgetary impact is too large. Single products can cripple entire health systems in even some of the wealthiest nations. In 2015 the Dutch government had to stop automatically paying for new medicines when it discovered that a lung cancer treatment would cost €200m a year, more than one-tenth of its annual budget.[74]

Health systems around the world have struggled with drug prices for years, and yet there is little sign of the problem easing. In fact, there is reason to believe new drugs will get exponentially more expensive.

CHAPTER NINE

The drugs we get

With hundreds of billions spent on pharmaceuticals each year, and tens of billions of that used to fund drug research, it is worth considering what we get for all that money. The new drugs which emerge are not necessarily those with the most clinical value, they are the ones which can command the highest prices and the largest profits. At the moment this means cancer patients and those suffering from some rare diseases are in luck. For schizophrenics reliant on outdated medicines with harsh side effects and patients with antibiotic-resistant infections, the message from the industry is tough luck; the financial rewards just don't look as good.

It hasn't always been this way. In the first decades of the industry, similar profits could be made across an array of therapeutic areas. Today, the industry spends more than £130 billion on research and development each year, funding thousands and thousands of clinical trials. From this, perhaps forty or fifty novel drugs will emerge onto the market each year. Each one is the product of countless choices made along the way. For the scientists these are often practical: selecting the biological target to go after, for example, and the type of assay to use. For those on the corporate side there are different considerations: what are the commercial prospects for this promising new compound? How does a particular disease or therapeutic area fit with the company's existing strengths?

Given such a vast spend, and the enormous number of diseases and conditions identified in humans, it might seem natural to assume that the drugs that emerge would treat a diverse range of therapeutic areas. Instead, the net result of all these choices is an astonishingly narrow range of new medications. If you were to randomly select a drug launched in the last five years, it would be more likely than not that it would fall into one of two categories: either a treatment for cancer or an orphan drug for patients with a rare disease. Many fall into both camps. In 2018, cancer and orphan drugs accounted for nearly two-thirds of new treatments.[1] It is no coincidence that drugs in these two fields dominate another list: they are among the highest priced in the world.

When the Orphan Drug Act was signed into law by US President Ronald Reagan in the first days of 1983, Abbey Meyers, the self-described 'housewife from Connecticut' instrumental in pushing for the legislation, shared the view of US health and human services secretary Margaret M. Heckler who had declared that orphan drugs 'will make nobody rich, but will help treat a small group of tragically handicapped people'.[2] When the legislation passed, these drugs cost the modern equivalent of $1,600 a year.[3] For those launched today, the average is around $150,000.[4]

In the decade before the US Orphan Drug Act came into force, there had been only a handful of treatments for rare diseases developed. This soon turned into a steady trickle of new treatments and Japan was persuaded to adopt its own incentives for rare diseases in 1993. At the end of the 1990s, the European Union followed suit, granting a longer marketing exclusivity period of ten years. Since the mid-2010s, around twenty new drugs with orphan status have hit the market each year.[5]

The incentives on offer to encourage these treatments were intended to ensure companies could make a profit in an area where the commercial prospects were otherwise poor. But the huge price tags which have become the norm for orphan drugs upended this, enabling pharmaceutical firms to enjoy blockbuster profits even when their drug can only be used by a small number of patients. With few if any alternative treatments for these patients with rare diseases, insurers and health systems have often struggled to negotiate the prices down, while cost-effectiveness bodies like NICE set much higher thresholds for high-cost, low-volume drugs.

The success of the expensively priced orphan drugs sold by some of the first biotechnology companies helped establish an expectation of high launch prices and the upward trajectory has continued. One study found that, over three decades, the average cost of a newly-launched orphan drug designed to be taken for years rather than on a short-term basis had doubled every five years.[6] At the end of the 1980s, the majority of orphan drugs had annual sales of less than $1 million and only three exceeded $100 million.[7] By 2008, there were forty-three blockbuster orphan drugs with annual global sales above $1 billion. They included Genzyme's Cerezyme and Amgen's Epogen, still going strong nearly two decades after their launch.[8]

While it used to be the case that patients with rare diseases couldn't receive treatment because of a lack of drugs, the pendulum has now swung the other way and orphan drugs exist which patients can't access on cost grounds. New Zealand's drug-pricing agency has refused to fund Soliris, which is administered by IV transfusion to patients with very rare blood disorders. Although it expected a maximum of twenty patients, it said paying the 'extreme' £300,000 price tag would 'mean potentially tens of thousands of New Zealanders missing out on new medicines which offer more health gain overall'.[9]

Soaring prices have encouraged companies to pour resources into developing more and more orphan drugs – and to find ways of seeking orphan status for as many medicines as possible. 'Originally orphan drugs were for treating unmet need,' says Donald Macarthur, a retired British pharmaceutical industry consultant who specialised in orphan drugs. 'There was no other treatment, there was nothing that the country could reference against when pricing that drug . . . so the company could charge almost what they liked. And this was fine when there were only a few orphan drugs and a few orphan drug companies. The payer was quite happy to pay this for the handful of patients. But now there's several hundred orphan drugs and the price is going through the roof and the costs are just growing exponentially.'[10]

The incentives offered for companies to manufacture medicines for rare diseases were designed to encourage the development of useful compounds which, for purely commercial reasons, might otherwise have been left gathering dust on a laboratory shelf. They were aimed, in short, at undeveloped drugs with small potential markets. But the rules didn't prevent drugs which were already on sale from obtaining an orphan designation for a new use – and with it, the opportunity for a sizeable price rise. Pentamidine, one of the early orphan drugs we met in a previous chapter, was sold as a treatment for tropical diseases before scientists discovered it could treat a type of pneumonia common in AIDS patients, enabling the manufacturer to quadruple the price.

In other cases, mainstream drugs which were already being used off-label to treat a small number of patients with rare diseases were formally registered for this purpose. The fact a medicine had already been used successfully by doctors helped the new manufacturer to secure regulatory approval, with a price rise invariably following. 'When it was an old drug, it was compounded by the hospital pharmacy at say 5p per tablet,' Macarthur explains. 'A company would take this chemical and produce it industrially and sell it for £500 per tablet. But to add insult to injury, they would use the data gained on the hospital-made product [and the] patient use for that to justify them getting marketing approval. So that was a real insult to the payer.'[11]

This practice has become more prevalent in recent years as the commercial prospects of orphan drugs grew. Dichlorphenamide is a white powder first sold in 1958 as a treatment for glaucoma. By the early 2000s, Daranide, as it was branded, had been overtaken by more modern alternatives and, with the patent long expired, was available with a list price of just $50 a bottle.[12] Seeing little commercial future, Merck & Co. pulled the drug from the US market in 2002. The news was a blow for a small group of patients with a rare neuromuscular disorder called periodic paralysis, which causes sudden and random episodes of muscle weakness which can leave sufferers bed-bound for days. These patients had found that Daranide helped relieve their condition and so, with MSD no longer manufacturing the drug, some began paying to import it from Europe or Asia.[13]

In 2007, researchers at the University of Rochester in New York obtained sponsorship from the US government-funded National Institutes of Health to put the drug's use as a rare disease treatment to the test. The Phase III trial they ran would prove to be a success, concluding that the drug was an effective treatment for patients with periodic paralysis.[14] At this point, a subsidiary of Sun Pharmaceutical Industries, an Indian drug company which had acquired the product from MSD, used the clinical trial data to re-launch the medicine on the American market with an orphan drug designation. The treatment, which was given the brand name Keveyis, was now priced at $13,650 for a box of 100 pills, the *Washington Post* later reported. US rights were subsequently sold on to another company, Strongbridge Biopharma, for $8.5 million and the price was increased further still, to $15,001.[15] Meanwhile, Sun Pharma sought to relaunch the drug at a higher price in Europe, with the British health service agreeing to pay £4,110 for 100 tablets for a drug which had previously cost £400 for a whole year's supply.[16]

This 'repurposing' of existing treatments can result in the bizarre situation where different forms of the same drug have hugely different prices. Generic versions of hydroxycarbamide capsules, which are prescribed for cancer patients, are widely available and cost around £12 for a box of 100 capsules in England, meaning two 500mg capsules would cost 24 pence. The same dose in tablet form costs £16.67, making it around seventy times more expensive, because a French company obtained an orphan designation to sell this version as a treatment for sickle-cell disease.[17] Prescribing a drug – in this case the capsule version – off-label is considered unethical by some doctors when there is a licensed version available, so the tablets continue to bring in a few hundred thousand pounds a year in Britain.

As well as obtaining orphan designations for drugs which were already on sale, companies have found workarounds to the intended limits on market size. To qualify for orphan status, a drug must treat a disease which is rare enough to be present in no more than between 1 in 1,500 or 1 in 2,500 people, depending on the country.[18] To get round this, companies have subdivided diseases into smaller groups of patients. Attempts to do this were already commonplace by the late 1980s, when the US regulator complained that the 'practice has got so absurd . . . that one company tried – and failed – to get orphan status for a drug to relieve knee pain. Left knee pain.'[19] Amgen's Epogen won orphan drug status as a treatment for anaemia associated specifically with end-stage renal disease. Although drugs can only be marketed for their approved use, doctors are free to prescribe the drug on an off-label basis if it is thought to work for other indications and off-label prescribing of Epogen soon ensured it 'became widely prescribed for a wide variety of patients with anaemia'.[20]

As an alternative technique, companies have taken drugs which their research teams suspected would have broad uses and started by seeking approval only for one narrow indication. This allowed the drug to be launched within the higher price ranges expected for orphan drugs, rather than on the lower scale for the broader therapy areas its manufacturer would subsequently seek marketing approval for. 'They sought orphan drug designations for their new drugs to treat a particular rare disease. And then once they get it on the market, they add other indications, some of which may be for treating common diseases, but they hold their price and absolutely rake it in,' Macarthur explains. 'There are many orphan drugs starting with one rare disease indication, they'll now have half a dozen or more indications, some for very, very common diseases.'[21]

It has also been exploited in the other direction, with well-established blockbusters already on the market securing orphan status for a new use in treating a rare disease. A recent investigation by Kaiser Health News identified seventy drugs which had obtained orphan status, and the attendant financial benefits, while already sold as a mass-market treatment. Among them were blockbusters like

Humira, the world's bestselling drug, and the cholesterol treatment Crestor. Humira, which is used by millions of patients with rheumatoid arthritis, received orphan status as a treatment for children with the condition and has since added four other rare diseases.[22] In 2017, half of the ten bestselling drugs had received orphan drug designations.[23] Orphan drugs are now so lucrative some companies have built their entire business around these products, with one, Alexion Pharmaceuticals, going for $39 billion when it was bought by AstraZeneca in a deal announced in late 2020.

Another big driver of growing healthcare costs has been the flurry of new cancer therapies, which, thanks to scientific advances, increasingly qualify for orphan status themselves. Cancers were once defined by broad categories based on where they occurred in the body but in recent years it has become apparent that different genetic mutations are responsible for the same disease.[24] Non-small-cell lung cancer, which makes up about 85 per cent of lung cancer cases, was previously split into three main types, but it can now be subdivided into much smaller patient groups. For example, three lung cancer drugs with orphan drug designations treat only those patients with non-small-cell lung cancer who have a particular gene mutation which is present in just 5 per cent of cases.[25] These advances in scientific understanding have allowed drugmakers to develop more targeted treatments which can qualify as orphan drugs, and deliver the higher level of prices such medications command.

Cancer, across all its forms, is the second leading cause of death globally, affecting, in some countries, as many as one in two people over their lifetime.[26] It, understandably, enjoys huge amounts of public research funding – the US National Institutes of Health alone devoted more than $6.5 billion to oncology in 2019[27] – while there is no shortage of interest from private companies attracted by the steady stream of new technologies and approaches and the high prices available for oncology drugs. All this spending has brought a raft of new cancer drugs – they now make up one in four of all new approvals – but for a lengthy period over the last decade, oncologists raised concerns that escalating prices were not necessarily matched by escalating benefits.[28]

In the United States, the launch price of cancer drugs has risen at a steady pace with little regard to how innovative a new drug is or the size of the benefits it offers. 'I can tell you the price of the next drug that's going to come out regardless of how good it is,' the cancer doctor Leonard Saltz says. 'Because it's going to be somewhere around 10 per cent over whatever the aggregate cost of the last three drugs that came out was.

'It's only based on what the market will bear, what came before, and not on any degree of how much good it does,' he adds.

Academic analysis has borne this out. A study which examined fifty-one cancer drugs launched in the United States between 2009 and 2013 found little difference between the list prices of novel drugs when compared to less innovative treatments. Launch prices had spiralled up even if the benefits they brought were small, 'typically measured in months, not years'.[29] A separate study by the economist Ernst Berndt pegged the 10 per cent annual increase in the average price of cancer treatments between 1995 and 2013 as amounting to $8,500 each year.[30] Companies were simply looking at what was already on the market for the same type of cancer and setting a slightly higher price rather than weighing up the benefits of their drug, Berndt concluded.

'The system is incentivising the development of incremental drugs,' Saltz says, 'because the price on an incremental drug is going to be just as much as the price on a transformative drug and it's much easier to make an incremental advance.'

Patients are also led to believe that drugs offer more benefits than they really do, Saltz argues. 'We were claiming bigger victories than we had,' he says.[31] 'The simplest was "significant survival advantage". I can say the word significant, but you hear substantial.' In reality, though, a statistically significant advantage can translate into a small improvement in real terms. 'We have drugs on the market with highly significant survival advantages of two weeks,' Saltz says, 'at many thousands of dollars per month.'

He believes the term 'progression-free survival' is even more problematic. 'Patients think progression-free survival means survival, and they think survival means cure.' He has urged fellow doctors to use the 'more precise, if less rosy, term "progression-free interval"',[32] because it simply denotes 'the amount of time from when you start using a drug until the drug is not working'. 'If we really discuss with patients what the data are for the drug that we're offering, they're often shocked at how little it is,' Saltz says.

In the US, television adverts help push patients to demand new drugs from their doctors, but even in countries where pharmaceutical advertising is banned, anyone turning to the internet to research their disease will quickly become aware of the latest treatments. The most recently released new drugs in Saltz's own specialty, colorectal cancer, are Lonsurf, a combination drug sold by Taiho Pharmaceutical and Servier, and Bayer's Stivarga. 'Each afford less than a [three-] month median survival benefit over a placebo in the best-case survival population, which doesn't exist very much. And each costs in the range of $17,000 to $20,000 a month,' Saltz explains. 'They didn't have to be very good. They just have to get on the market and then they can charge whatever they want.'

Because the US market shapes which products are developed, the problem of high-priced cancer drugs which offer only minimal improvements on existing treatments is a global one. As long ago as 2011, the British medical journal *The Lancet*'s Oncology Commission on Global Cancer Surgery recognised how limited many new drugs were in improving treatment options and laid out demands for a 'radical shift' in cancer policy. Oncologists and the drug industry, the commission argued, 'should take responsibility and not accept a substandard evidence base and an ethos of very small benefit at whatever cost'.[33]

The rocketing price of cancer drugs in the US and elsewhere has been possible because, like rare-disease treatments, health systems have given such products a special status with fewer restrictions than other areas. Even a few extra weeks have huge value to patients with a terminal diagnosis and, recognising this, health systems like the

UK's which rely on cost-effectiveness measures have introduced special rules for end-of-life care. These types of treatments, as for orphan drugs which hold the power to give a desperately ill child with a rare disease a normal life, also carry huge emotional weight which patient groups, often bolstered by pharmaceutical industry funding, have used to apply pressure on governments and insurers to pay for these drugs.

In contrast with Peter Staley's band of AIDS activists who at one point occupied Burroughs Wellcome's offices, oncology and rare-disease groups are more likely to work with drug companies than criticise their pricing practices. They know that the high prices the drugs command is what is incentivising more companies to develop treatments for that disease rather than a different one and don't want to kill the golden goose. In Canada, Chantelle Lindsay's father, Mark, continued to campaign for access to Trikafta in order that other cystic fibrosis patients don't have to follow his daughter's fate, with his ire largely focused on the Canadian government's proposed changes to pricing rules and their seeming unwillingness to pay.[34]

In the UK, articles about cancer patients being denied a drug which was available in other countries have been a media staple since the mid-2000s. The story of patients whose only hope lay in some new treatment which a faceless and presumably uncaring bureaucrat had blocked in order to save money regularly featured in mid-market newspapers and on television news shows. Because of this, in 2010, a newly elected British coalition government set up a special fund for cancer drugs, allowing manufacturers to bypass the usual cost-effectiveness assessments made by NICE.

The fund allowed patients to access exactly the kind of expensive and only modestly beneficial drugs which Dr Saltz had decried. It was only meant to be a temporary measure but the power of patient groups and drug company lobbying made it impossible to curtail even as it rapidly exceeded its budget. The eventual cost to taxpayers was £1.3 billion over six years, money which, a report later concluded, had 'not delivered meaningful value to patients and society'.[35] Many treatments covered by the programme did not extend life and the period of 'progression-free survival' they offered instead, during which the cancer's spread is halted, did not improve the quality of a patient's life because of the unpleasant side effects caused by the toxicity of the drugs.[36] Even with a higher threshold adopted for end-of-life treatments, NICE still periodically finds itself being criticised by patient groups, charities and the media for blocking or reducing the eligibility for cancer treatments whose high prices mean they struggle to pass cost-effectiveness assessments.

It is not just high prices that have made treatments for cancer and rare diseases attractive to drugmakers. Their profitability is also boosted by the way in which they are handled by regulators and by the smaller clinical trials required, meaning more patent-protected years are left when they go on sale. Cancer drugs typically have to clear a lower regulatory bar than other new medicines to prove that they work. Clinical trials testing the efficacy of new drugs generally involve giving half of the patients enrolled the new medicine and half the existing standard of care – or a placebo if there are no effective treatments. Researchers then measure how many members of each cohort remain alive over a number of years. It is an effective means of establishing the efficacy of a drug but it is also time-consuming.

During the AIDS crisis thousands of patients faced an effective death sentence without treatment while promising drugs worked their way through clinical trials. As a result, some drugs can now be approved on the basis of so-called surrogate endpoints. Instead of looking at overall survival rates, a faster indicator is used: something else testable and deemed relevant to the progression of the disease, such as the size of a tumour. The hope is that showing the drug's effect on the body will be a good indicator of the effectiveness of the drug at keeping a patient alive or improving their quality of life. Drug companies are usually required to carry out post-approval clinical trials which, it is hoped, will subsequently confirm that.

However, once a drug has hit the market, the manufacturer may feel there is little to be gained and much to be lost in funding the expensive business of finding out whether it actually works.

Researchers at the National Cancer Institute and the Knight Cancer Center in the US looked at what happened in the years after thirty-six cancer drugs were approved on the basis of surrogate endpoints. More than four years after approval, thirteen drugs were yet to report back on the results of testing. Of those that had, eighteen drugs had failed to show that they improved survival rates while just five had shown that they worked.[37]

The same problem exists in Europe. More than half of sixty-eight cancer medicines approved by the European Medicines Agency between 2009 and 2013 had not established that they could prolong survival or improve quality of life at the point when they were given the green light to be sold to patients, a study found. Three years after hitting the market, only six more of these drugs had been able to show their benefit to patients. Among those which had been able to show that they improved survival rates, half had gains that were so small – in some cases just a few weeks – that they were not held to be clinically meaningful.[38] 'Accelerated approval [means] we approve drugs with very limited data, and the companies charge maximum prices for them and when later data shows they have to be withdrawn they keep the money,' says Peter Bach, a colleague of Saltz's in New York, where he also studies health outcomes.[39]

Rare-disease drugs have also benefited from the use of surrogate endpoints and are, in general, cheaper and quicker to develop than drugs aimed at larger patient groups.[40] With fewer patients affected, there is no need for the enormous Phase III clinical trials which have become the norm for drugs aimed at diseases with large patient populations. Researchers in Canada found that, because of a higher probability of success, orphan drugs had development costs more than 40 per cent lower than non-orphan drugs.[41]

A final boon to drugmakers selling treatments for cancer and rare diseases is the lack of competition even once a patent-protected period ends because the vast majority are biological medicines rather than small molecule drugs. A recent survey found that only half of orphan drugs faced competition from rival versions.[42]

Generic versions of traditional pills and tablets play a central role in the social contract with the pharmaceutical industry. Once a drug is off patent, the launch of rival generic versions should bring a reduction in prices down towards commodity levels. In hotly contested markets for the most enduringly popular old medicines, this may be barely more than the cost of manufacturing. Drug companies are, in the words of biotech venture capitalist Bruce Booth, 'handing society an in-perpetuity gift', to be enjoyed long after the original inventor has received their reward.[43]

Making generic versions of traditional small molecule drugs is cheap and it is a relatively quick process to jump the regulatory hurdles required to get them on the market once the original drug's patent has expired. The injectable biological medicines made in living cells which were pioneered by the biotech industry are, however, an altogether different proposition for a generics manufacturer. Biological medicines, known as biologics, involve a much more expensive and complicated manufacturing process. Lipitor, a blockbuster small molecule drug, is made up of seventy-six atoms; by comparison, the biologic Humira contains more than 20,000.[44] This is a particularly significant problem because the prevalence of biologics is growing. More than 200 have made it to the market and they make up eight of the ten bestselling medicines, including Humira, the first drug to have sales of more than $20 billion in a single year.[45]

Biologics are made of proteins from living organisms, which creates a natural variability which means exact copies – true generics – are impossible. Instead, competing versions are called biosimilars and work in a similar way without being exact copies. For a time, there was no abbreviated route to market for a biosimilar, as there is for a generic drug. While generics simply have to show bioequivalence with an existing drug – meaning they act in the body in the same way – biosimilars were treated as an entirely new product, required to fund the full gamut of clinical trials to demonstrate safety and efficacy.

The European Union changed this in 2004, allowing generic drugmakers to use comparability studies to show their versions were clinically similar to an existing biologic and the first biosimilar was approved in 2006. Since then, take up has improved but overall numbers remain low. By the start of 2020, only fifty-eight biosimilars were approved for use in Europe.[46] In America, things have progressed at an even slower pace. Henry Waxman, the Democratic congressman who played a pivotal role in the passage of the Orphan Drug Act, introduced a bill in 2009 to follow Europe's lead in bringing in a regulatory pathway for biosimilars. In a concession to biotech companies, it proposed guaranteeing a minimum exclusivity window for the original biologic of at least five years regardless of its patent status, but extensive industry lobbying managed to increase this to twelve years. The US didn't get its first biosimilar until 2015, and only a dozen or so have been launched in the following five years.[47] With the biosimilar industry still in its infancy across the globe, the first biosimilars launched have offered only a fraction of the savings of the more competitive generic markets, typically setting their prices just 10 or 20 per cent below that of the biologics they are competing with. This represents a huge challenge to the social contract. Without this generic competition, drugmakers selling biologics effectively enjoy much longer exclusivity periods in which they can impose high prices, meaning much longer periods for healthcare systems to have to try and meet these costs.

The ever-rising prices of orphan drugs and cancer treatments have allowed drugmakers to continue to find blockbuster profits even as new mass-market treatments dried up. These kinds of drugs pose a challenge to some of the industry's established approaches to boosting revenues. With elevated blood pressure or high cholesterol, lobbying and marketing could expand the definition of ill health and sell pills to millions of healthy people. With a treatment for cancer or a specific rare disease, this simply doesn't apply. No matter how much is spent on celebrity TV adverts and free pens for doctors, there are only so many patients with Gaucher's disease or non-small-cell lung cancer. That leaves price as the only lever left to pull.

Fortunately for drugmakers, when prices get high enough, even small numbers of patients can generate billions of dollars in revenue. Orphan drugs cost, on average, five times as much as non-orphan medications. They already account for one-sixth of global spending on drugs despite representing less than 0.5 per cent of prescriptions and their sales are expected to increase by 50 per cent between 2020 and 2024.[48]

Oncology and rare diseases are valuable areas of clinical need where new drugs can be life-changing for patients. But having such a large proportion of new drugs in areas with some of the highest price tags puts huge pressure on limited healthcare budgets. High drug prices don't simply hit access to new medicines for patients, they also distort the market further up the pipeline, determining which areas attract the brightest minds and the lion's share of research funding. The high prices of orphan drugs and cancer treatments has created a self-perpetuating bubble which draws in new investors attracted by the potential rewards on offer. Each new launch pushes up the benchmarks further.

Disproportionately high prices in a select few areas has contributed to the trend of large drug companies narrowing the breadth of their research efforts. When Emma Walmsley took over GSK in 2017, she laid out plans to focus 80 per cent of research spending on four areas believed to have the best returns. She said they had been too 'thinly spread' and needed to 'make sure we are backing the assets that are winning'.[49] Sanofi, the large French company, halted thirty-eight pipeline projects in 2019 as it sought to prioritise oncology, immunology and rare blood disorders while saving €1.5 billion a year.[50] The projects which paid the price for this narrower focus included ALX-0171, a promising treatment for respiratory syncytial virus (RSV), which can cause pneumonia and bronchitis. Nearly 60,000 children under the age of five die each year from respiratory infections caused by RSV.[51]

The divestments which resulted from Big Pharma's strategic narrowing of focus provided the inventory for the predatory model which arose. Daraprim had been a GSK drug until it sold the marketing rights off to a company called CorePharma in 2010. Five years later, the drug was sold on twice more, ending up in the hands of Martin Shkreli and his company Turing Pharmaceuticals.

The biotech companies which increasingly carry out the bulk of the early-stage research on drug candidates are even more susceptible to clustering around the same therapy areas than Big Pharma. Part of this is the scale of returns the venture capitalists funding the nascent companies demand, but it is also because those behind the firms tend to live and work in the same circles. 'Anecdotally, it seems like moving to more and more VC-backed early innovation is leading to more herding not less herding,' says Josh Krieger, an assistant professor at Harvard Business School who has studied the problem. The same investors go to the same conferences and talk to the same scientists, clustering around 'what is the new hot thing'.[52]

Meanwhile, other areas of clinical need are not viewed as favourably and get far less research funding. 'Heart disease kills more people than cancer,' says Bach. 'I don't think we had a single drug approved in the US for cardiovascular disease [in 2018].' By comparison, there were fifteen approved in oncology. 'That's stunning,' Bach adds.[53] 'I think it's very hard to argue that heavy focus on extremely rare diseases and diseases associated with cancer that are going to be fatal but can be forestalled is the best use of biomedical innovation,' he says. 'But it's the most profitable one in our current system.'

The drug development work which gets funded is driven by economic incentives and, all too often, these incentives are at odds with society's most pressing clinical needs. While drug companies pour money into oncology and rare diseases – more than one-third of all drug discovery efforts are currently devoted to oncology and there are over 1,000 clinical trials underway for immunotherapies; so many that there aren't enough patients to fill all of them – other areas attract scant investment because the financial rewards are not sufficiently high.[54]

Diseases which afflict those in less economically developed countries have long been neglected, with campaigners accustomed to relying on global health donors and companies' willingness to fund work as part of corporate social responsibility efforts rather than commercial incentives. Given the relative wealth of the patients who would benefit, any successful product, while not necessarily loss-making, would have little hope of making money on the sort of scale that large drugmakers normally require to attract their interest. The Access to Medicine Foundation, a non-profit based in Amsterdam, produces an annual scorecard assessing how much different drug companies are doing to research the medicines and other medical advances most needed by those in middle- and low-income countries. Its most recent assessment found 149 of the 211 'identified priority gaps' were not being addressed.[55]

Aidan Hollis, an economics professor at the University of Calgary, has studied the link between drug discovery funding and the relative affluence of those who suffer from disease. The results were striking, if not unexpected.

'There's this enormous bias towards the diseases of high-income people and away from the diseases of low-income people,' he says. 'And it's not only true from clinical trials funded by pharmaceutical companies, it's also true for trials funded by governments. Because high-income country governments, not surprisingly, put their money into diseases which affect their own people.'[56]

Globally, diabetes and malaria account for roughly the same number of lost years of healthy life, 'but there are ten times as many trials on drugs for diabetes'. The trend holds true even within a therapeutic area, Hollis has found. Those cancers that are most prevalent in high-income populations get a disproportionate amount of the funding compared with those, like ovarian cancer, that are more common in poorer countries.

The discoveries of penicillin and sulphanilamide in the late 1920s and early 1930s paved the way for a new era of medicine. Over the next four decades, scores of new antibiotics were developed including ten distinct new classes of drugs. They helped to transform medical science, meaning bacterial illnesses like pneumonia, tuberculosis or typhoid fever could now be treated and making childbirth and routine surgeries significantly safer. However, the steady supply of new antibiotics has dried up. There have only been two new classes of antibiotics introduced since the late 1960s and neither treat Gram-negative bacteria, the cause of most antibiotic-resistant superbugs.[57]

In the meantime, the liberal use of existing antibiotics in animal feed and as treatments for everyday illnesses like colds, sore throats and ear infections has led to the growing prevalence of bacterial infections which are resistant to antibiotics. The warnings of this impending global crisis have been frequent and unequivocal.

Drug-resistant diseases already claim 700,000 lives a year and a review commissioned by the British government warned that this was on track to swell to 10 million by 2050, more than currently die from cancer. A UN report in April 2019 found that 'common diseases are becoming untreatable'. 'There is no time to wait,' it exclaimed. 'Unless the world acts urgently, antimicrobial resistance will have disastrous impact within a generation.'[58] Despite this, only a handful of large pharmaceutical companies are actively seeking to develop new antimicrobials.

The two-year independent 'Review on Antimicrobial Resistance' commissioned by the British government in 2014 was headed by Jim O'Neill. Born in Manchester in northwest England, O'Neill, a plain-speaking son of a postman, became chief economist at Goldman Sachs and a man talked about as a contender to become Governor of the Bank of England. He is a proud capitalist but can make no attempt to hide his contempt for the pharmaceutical industry's unwillingness to invest in new antibiotic drugs.

'The amount of talk that's gone around the topic makes virtually anything else I've experienced in around thirty-five years of a life involving business to be like a garden party,' he says. Since the dire warnings in his review, 'absolutely nothing's happened', he complains.[59] A succession of large drug companies have left the antibiotics field, often handing off their pipeline assets to smaller firms which have struggled to stay solvent.

The problem, from the industry's perspective, is that, although there is huge need for new antibiotics, the development of a new class is unlikely to bring a financial windfall to the company behind it. Existing antibiotics are cheap, easily available as generics and are only taken for a short time. Even in the hyper-charged US market they cost no more than a few thousand dollars per course. To make matters worse from a commercial perspective, there would be little scope to make up for an underwhelming price through volume. Given the inevitability of resistance eventually building up against any new drug, it would be in doctors' and society's interests to prescribe the new agent as little as possible to maintain its effectiveness for as long as possible. So after investing vast sums in research and development, a drug company proudly wielding a new antibiotic would be left with it serving as an agent of last resort, to be used only in the worst of cases. The estimated value of a new antibiotic would be just $50 million, a far cry from the billions brought in by blockbuster drugs.[60] Large drug companies backed a new $1 billion fund announced in the summer of 2020 to help biotechs developing promising novel antibiotics stay afloat but it will take billions more to conquer the current barriers to taking these drugs through latter-stage clinical trials and onto the market. In the meantime, the number of deaths from antibiotic-resistant infections continues to rise.

The risk of antibiotic resistance has long been highlighted by public health and national security experts. So too have warnings of another threat: an outbreak of a novel infectious disease with no available cures or treatments. Once a mainstay of large pharmaceutical companies who helped the world eradicate polio and smallpox, vaccines came to be seen as a backwater with little money to be made. Between 1967 and 2004, the number of vaccine manufacturers dropped from twenty-six to five.[61] By the early 2000s, there were shortages of vaccines for influenza and several vaccines recommended for young children including measles, mumps, rubella, tetanus and chickenpox.[62] Vaccines were unattractive in part because their main customers were governments, buying on a massive scale to inoculate whole populations, and 'governments have tended to be tough negotiators', Hollis says.[63] Vaccine production is also more expensive than the typical manufacturing process for drugs, with more complex regulatory hurdles and requirements for enormous clinical trials because, as Dr Paul Offit, who heads the Vaccine Education Center at a Philadelphia hospital, puts it, 'the current culture does not allow for any serious side effects from a vaccine' even if it will help more people than will be harmed.[64] The fortunes of vaccine divisions have been somewhat reversed over the last fifteen years, boosted by growing demand from developing countries – thanks in large part to the Bill Gates-funded Gavi Vaccine Alliance which underwrites the cost – and the launch of several vaccines for adults which became blockbusters. A vaccine for cervical cancer developed by publicly funded researchers in Australia and the United States was approved for sale by the American company Merck & Co. (MSD) in 2006. By 2018 it was bringing in $3 billion in annual sales, while Pfizer's pneumonia vaccine Prevnar had sales of nearly $6 billion in the same year.[65] Pfizer has even been able to impose post-launch price rises on its vaccine. The current version of Pfizer's Prevnar, called Prevnar 13, was launched at $108 a dose, already one-third higher than its predecessor, and has since risen to $188.[66] The introduction of high-dose flu vaccines for the elderly has also boosted profits and helped push up prices.

Nevertheless, until the coronavirus pandemic hit, vaccines remained a relatively under-resourced area. Vaccine sales made up around 2 or 3 per cent of global sales and just four large drug companies – Pfizer, GSK, MSD and Sanofi – have large vaccine divisions. For the well-established markets, like flu, there is little incentive to risk fortunes in pursuit of a more effective vaccine when small annual tweaks bring in reliable long-term profits. With most vaccination funded by governments, there can be little market left for any vaccine deemed inferior to a rival's version, as GSK found when the runaway success of MSD's HPV vaccine led to a commercial decision to pull its own effort, Cervarix, from the US market.[67]

While some vaccines have been developed for previously neglected diseases, such as Sanofi's transformative dengue fever vaccine, large drug companies have proven slow to commit resources to developing threats until it becomes clearer that they will be able to generate a return on investment. If they then rush to fund trials for experimental treatments and increase supplies of flu shots in the face of a pandemic, they can find themselves out of pocket when the product hits the market too late and remains unsold.[68]

The Ebola virus had first appeared in 1976, taking its name from a river in the Democratic Republic of Congo, then known as Zaire, where one of two simultaneous outbreaks occurred. Ebola is a deadly viral disease, killing as many as 90 per cent of those infected, and in the decades after its emergence there were a number of small-scale outbreaks. But as these occurred in poor African nations, there was little commercial interest in developing a vaccine. 'Ebola victims are among the poorest people in the world and they live in the poorest countries in the world and neither the countries nor the individuals were in a position to pay high prices for vaccines so this never became an attractive market,' Hollis says.

Some public funding had been made available for research into the virus as part of biosecurity measures and during the 2000s Canadian scientists developed and began testing a genetically engineered vaccine candidate. The animal testing showed promising results and in 2010 Canada's Public Health Agency licensed the vaccine to a small American company called NewLink Genetics for $200,000.[69] NewLink was expected to fund clinical testing in humans, the point in the process where costs leap into tens of millions of dollars, and to jump through the regulatory hoops so it could be sold. But with little prospect of a return on investment, the vaccine instead sat on a shelf for several years without any further testing, the *New York Times* later reported.[70]

It was only in 2014, after the emergence of a large new outbreak in West Africa which threatened to spread further afield, that Western governments and companies began to devote significant resources to the virus. Nearly a year after the outbreak had begun, NewLink finally launched Phase I clinical trials and then sub-licensed the vaccine to MSD for $50 million.[71] It would be another five years, long after the epidemic in West Africa had ended, before MSD was able to bring the vaccine to market.

In the wake of Ebola, the Zika virus and other outbreaks, several companies indicated they were not prepared to continue responding in the same way. 'We do not want to have these activities compete with in-house programmes,' Dr Rip Ballou, a research chief at GSK Global Vaccine, told reporters. 'And our learnings from Ebola, from pandemic flu, from SARS previously, is that it's very disruptive and that's not the way that we want to do business going forward.'[72]

The World Health Organization (WHO) keeps a list of 'priority diseases' which pose the gravest threat to public health and for which there are no adequate treatments. Among them is Disease X, which represents 'the knowledge that a serious international epidemic could be caused by a pathogen currently unknown to cause human disease'.[73] In late 2019, one such new and deadly infectious disease emerged in Wuhan, China, caused by a novel coronavirus which was given the name SARS-CoV-2.

Coronaviruses have threatened to cause pandemics before and the WHO list included severe acute respiratory syndrome (SARS), which caused an outbreak in China in 2002, and the deadlier but less infectious Middle East respiratory syndrome (MERS), which claimed several hundred lives in 2012. Both petered out and commercial efforts to find treatments fell by the wayside. After their experience with Ebola, MERS and other outbreaks, large drugmakers showed 'extreme reluctance to get involved' with the initial response to Covid-19, says Peter Hale, the founder of the Foundation for Vaccine Research, a Washington DC-based advocacy organisation. 'Some of the big players have been burned by developing vaccines for tropical diseases or neglected diseases only to have the vaccine not pan out or [to find] a very small market where the ability to make a profit is very small or negligible.'[74] As a result, 'they're not prepared to take the risks' of committing resources to emerging pathogens.

Hale is a seventy-six-year-old former advertising executive who had been an activist in Los Angeles during the AIDS epidemic in the 1980s, spurred into action after he contracted HIV himself and witnessed friends and his then-partner die of the disease. He was communications director of Search Alliance, which worked to try and develop AIDS treatments, and subsequently took jobs in the same field in Paris and Stockholm. In the early 2000s he became involved with helping to set up the Global Fund to Fight AIDS, Tuberculosis and Malaria, which uses billions raised from governments and donors to combat the spread of the three deadly infectious diseases. Hale subsequently spent years in Africa, helping countries to apply for funding from the organisation.

'After each trip I came back even more distressed that all these countries in Africa have a need for vaccines and they don't have them,' he says. These concerns led him to set up a foundation in 2011 to push for more vaccine research.

'The big picture is drug companies make their money developing drugs and treatments for chronic diseases that go on and on and on like diabetes [and] cardiovascular disease, where people have to take medicine every single day,' Hale says. 'And there are even more profits in biological [therapies] for cancer and other diseases, especially autoimmune diseases. There has not traditionally been huge profits to be made in vaccines.' The result is that research into new vaccines has largely been left to university academics, funded with whatever can be secured from grants from governments or non-profit organisations. There was even less commercial incentive to research new vaccines and vaccine technologies for tackling those diseases with potential to cause future outbreaks. When drug companies like MSD had picked up the baton and responded to previous public health crises, they had found that outbreaks had been controlled by other means before they were able to complete clinical testing on potential treatments or vaccines to market. Having committed resources and diverted scientists away from other projects, there was no revenue to show for it.

Fortunately, the public and non-profit sectors stepped in. After the delays in producing vaccines for Ebola and Zika, the Coalition for Epidemic Preparedness Innovations (CEPI) was established in early 2017 with funds from governments and private donors to try and intervene where the pharmaceutical industry was failing by funding the development of vaccines for emerging infectious diseases.

Elsewhere, scientists at several universities had heeded the WHO's warnings about 'Disease X'. Among them were two University of Oxford professors, Sarah Gilbert and Adrian Hill, who had been working on technology which could rapidly be used to make a vaccine for a previously unknown virus. When the novel Wuhan coronavirus's genetic code was first published in early January 2020, Gilbert and her team sprang into action. They inserted the genetic sequence for the distinctive spike protein of SARS-CoV-2 into a modified adenovirus which is harmless to humans. Once injected into a patient, the adenovirus infects cells and inserts DNA instructing them to produce the spike protein seen on the surface of the coronavirus. This induces an immune response, producing protective antibodies. The vaccine was ready for animal testing by the middle of February but raising funding proved difficult. 'Getting money was my main activity until April, just trying to persuade people to fund it now,' Professor Gilbert would later say.[75] The University of Oxford ended up having to underwrite the costs of producing a quantity of the potential vaccine in Italy before the British government and CEPI handed over several million pounds.[76]

Meanwhile, some large drug companies continued to prevaricate about whether to deploy their own resources. 'One of the very largest [pharmaceutical] companies kept on fighting and arguing for almost two months before they decided to get involved,' Hale says. 'It got to the point where a couple of middle-level executives . . . threatened to resign unless the company got involved.'

Ultimately, governments stepped in with huge investments and spending commitments and really got things moving. Public funding de-risked the whole process of developing a Covid vaccine, from covering research costs to buying huge numbers of doses on an at-risk basis, even before the first trial results were in. 'It wouldn't have happened without public funding,' Hale says. The US government's Operation Warp Speed handed out more than $12 billion to vaccine makers, including $1.2 billion to fund a Phase III clinical trial and accelerate the development of the Oxford team's vaccine.

The billions committed would eventually bring dramatic results, with several vaccines developed, approved and ready to be administered within a year, far quicker than the previous record of four years for a mumps vaccine in the 1960s. These included two revolutionary vaccines of a completely new type. The mRNA vaccines developed by Pfizer and BioNTech and, separately, by Moderna, introduce the genetic instructions needed to coax cells into producing the same spike protein seen in the Covid-19 virus, which in turn prompts the body to produce antibodies which protect against a future infection. The efficacy of these new vaccines – as high as 95 per cent – stunned scientists and led to renewed optimism about the potential for the technology to revolutionise the whole field.

The involvement of public funds and university researchers provided leverage over the pricing of some vaccines, as did drug-makers' fear of being seen to be exploiting a public health crisis. Early on in the pandemic, Gilead had faced these accusations over its handling of a failed Ebola drug called remdesivir, which became the first regulator-approved coronavirus treatment after securing an emergency-use authorisation in May 2020. Gilead had sought orphan status for the drug two months earlier, prompting accusations from a consumer group that this was 'an unconscionable abuse of a programme designed to incentivise research and development of treatments for rare diseases'.[77] After an outcry, the company asked the regulator to drop the designation just two days after it had been granted.[78] Gilead priced remdesivir at more than $3,000 for insured patients and $2,340 for governments for a five-day treatment course even though studies would ultimate conclude it had relatively modest benefits, with the drug shortening the recovery time for hospitalised Covid patients by five days.[79] The drug generated almost $2 billion in revenue in the fourth quarter of 2020 alone, helping to push the company's overall sales up by 26 per cent.[80]

By contrast, some vaccine makers agreed to sell their products on a non-profit basis during the pandemic. Scientists at the University of Oxford had made this a condition of any deal when seeking a manufacturing partner for its vaccine. When the pandemic hit, the team at the Jenner Institute in Oxford 'had projects on twelve different emerging infections, none of which would have made any commercial sense', says Sir John Bell, regius professor of medicine at the university and the man brought in to help broker a partnership with a large drugmaker. 'They were just chipping away at them based on philanthropic donations.'[81]

As part of a research organisation 'focused not on making money, but on achieving scientific outcomes that are good for people all over the world', the scientists working at the institute were 'committed to not exploiting the presence of a pandemic for financial gain' and were adamant that it should be sold on a not-for-profit basis.[82] They also wanted to ensure it would be available in developing countries.

Asking a large drugmaker to sell the vaccine at cost could have been hugely problematic. 'If you're a pharmaceutical company that has shareholders, it's quite a complicated conversation to have internally,' Sir John says, but AstraZeneca 'didn't shy away from that at all'.[83] Pascal Soriot, AstraZeneca's chief executive, told him: 'My kids would kill me if I didn't do this.'[84] The company agreed to make several billion doses of the vaccine available at cost and to supply lower-income companies at that price indefinitely. Johnson and Johnson's pharmaceutical division Janssen, which received $1 billion in funding for the development of its vaccine from the US government, also announced that it would make the product available on a non-profit basis while Covid infections raged.

However, the US government funding didn't come with any strings attached on pricing and not everyone was prepared to abandon sizeable profits by selling them at cost. The US biotech Moderna, which received around $1 billion in development funding and advance orders worth $3.2 billion from Operation Warp Speed, has taken a resolutely profit-driven approach. While AstraZeneca's vaccine was sold for a couple of dollars a shot, Moderna said it would charge $64 to $74 per two-shot course for smaller orders of its vaccine.[85] This made it the most expensive available, although it offered significant discounts for large orders, charging the European Union and the United States around half that amount per shot for orders running into hundreds of millions of doses.[86] Even then, the company said this was 'pandemic pricing', with prices expected to shoot up further once the company deemed the crisis to have passed.[87] Its executives had already benefited from selling stock as the company's share price soared while its vaccine was still in testing and analysts predicted the company would enjoy vaccine sales topping $13 billion in 2021 alone.[88] On top of that, the government-funded development of an mRNA vaccine helped validate technology which Moderna could now seek to apply to other diseases.

Pfizer, which set a US price tag of $39 for its own two-shot course and charged just under $30 in Europe, was predicted to enjoy even higher sales of at least $15 billion in 2021, with pre-tax profits potentially topping $4 billion.[89] The company had stood alone in not taking grant money from Operation Warp Speed but had nevertheless benefited from an early agreement for the US to pay $2 billion for 100 million doses if it secured regulatory approval, with an option for up to 500 million more. Pfizer's biotech partner, BioNTech, received up to $445 million from the German government to help fund the vaccine's development and boost manufacturing capacity there.

For all the companies involved, including those that made the vaccine available on a non-profit basis while the pandemic rages, there remains the prospect of significant financial rewards in future if, as expected, Covid-19 becomes a seasonal illness like flu requiring populations to receive regular booster shots.

The coronavirus pandemic can be seen as a victory for the pharmaceutical industry's innovative capacity, and the individual scientists involved deserved all the plaudits that came their way; but it also served as a demonstration of the shortcomings of the current business model. For drug companies, the lesson is clear: there is no need to risk funds during public health emergencies because governments have shown they will intercede and cover the costs. 'We've reached a point where industry wants government to fund their vaccine research and development,' Hale says. 'It's that simple.'[90]

The decline in commercial interest in vaccines contributed to huge manufacturing challenges in seeking to scale-up production while the success of developing several vaccines was also tempered by a failure to address the inequality of access which typifies the development of new medicines and treatments.

As the pandemic crippled economies and filled hospitals around the globe in the spring and summer of 2020, the world's richest countries moved fast to secure large quantities of the different vaccine candidates, often hedging their bets and agreeing to buy quantities amounting to several multiples of the country's entire population.

The United Kingdom began administering the first approved vaccine by December 2020, with the United States and major European nations rapidly following. Meanwhile less well-off countries faced a years-long wait before they could secure enough vaccine for their citizens. While some vaccine developers and manufacturers made laudable moves – AstraZeneca partnered with an Indian manufacturer to produce a billion low-cost shots for low- and middle-income countries and Imperial College London sought to bypass the industry altogether, setting up a social enterprise to deliver its vaccine to the developing world – wider efforts to secure a fairer distribution were hindered by an inability to obtain sufficient vaccine doses after rich countries tied up the initial manufacturing capacity. COVAX, an initiative run by CEPI, the WHO and the Gavi Vaccine Alliance, set a goal of securing two billion shots by the end of 2021 with the intention of distributing them equally to all members including dozens of low- and middle-income countries. It received significant funding but struggled to secure supplies from drugmakers who had already sold most of their capacity to richer bidders. Overall, high-income countries accounted for just over half of the vaccine purchases agreed before they received regulatory approval despite making up less than 15 per cent of the world's population.[91] By January 2021, the WHO was warning that 'the world is on the brink of a catastrophic moral failure – and the price of this failure will be paid with lives and livelihoods in the world's poorest countries'.[92]

One way of averting this crisis and relieving the pressure on vaccine supplies would have been to widen the pool of manufacturers but drug companies proved reluctant to share their expertise widely. The WHO set up a 'technology access pool' in May 2020, encouraging companies to share their intellectual property and knowledge on Covid-19 treatments and vaccines. But nearly a year later, even as several large factories around the world said they could start producing coronavirus vaccines if drugmakers shared their know-how and waived patent protection, the WHO's pool remained unused.[93] A separate proposal to suspend patents relating to Covid-19 drugs and vaccines during the pandemic was put forward at the World Trade Organization by India and South Africa in October 2020. It won support from more than 100 countries but was blocked by the US, UK and European Union, who argued that many countries lacked the capacity to produce the vaccines and that even a temporary suspension of intellectual property protection could hinder innovation, including efforts to adapt vaccines to tackle coronavirus mutations.[94] The US's opposition remained steadfast for more than six months but in May 2021, with India suffering a devastating second wave of coronavirus cases while rich Western countries were well on their way to vaccinating entire populations, President Biden made the decision to reverse this position. With India facing a humanitarian crisis and health officials warning that the uncontained outbreak could lead to the emergence of a vaccine-resistant strain of coronavirus, Biden's administration backed proposals to temporarily waive patents on Covid-19 vaccines in an effort to ramp up production and end global supply shortages. The move was strongly opposed by powerful US drugmakers but US Trade Representative Katherine Tai said that that 'extraordinary circumstances . . . call for extraordinary measures.'[95]

Jayasree Iyer, the executive director of the Access to Medicine Foundation, is critical of the number of countries who prioritised their own populations over global solidarity when striking deals to buy vaccines. She blamed 'vaccine nationalism' and companies' willingness to prioritise large early bids from wealthy countries for 'jeopardising COVAX's ability to raise enough money to purchase vaccines and to negotiate a larger production capacity from these companies'.[96]

'Like in most treatments . . . the people living in low- and middle-income countries, especially in countries that do not have a manufacturing base of their own, are the last in line.'

The coronavirus pandemic hit drug companies' bottom lines even as it challenged their moral responsibility to societies; after all, it's hard to sell as many expensive cancer drugs if far fewer patients in locked-down cities are making it to the doctor's surgery to be diagnosed. Yet, just as with the lacklustre response to rising antibiotic resistance, the threat of the next pandemic remains. While scientists rushed to find treatments and develop vaccines for Covid-19 once the consequences for the West became apparent, there remains alarmingly little work developing potential responses to other emerging infectious diseases like SARS and Zika.

A year after the first Covid-19 cases had emerged, the Access to Medicine Foundation examined research efforts into sixteen diseases identified by the WHO as posing a serious epidemic risk. It found that the largest pharmaceutical companies had no projects in the pipeline for ten of these pathogens, just as the same firms had had no coronavirus projects underway in 2018.

'These are sixteen defined pathogens that are already costing lives and economies around the world,' says Iyer. 'We have to realise that these threats are real threats.' Diseases like Rift Valley or Lassa fever are already affecting patients in specific regions but drug companies are reluctant to commit resources. 'I think the belief is, "Is this truly going to become a pandemic?",' she says. 'And even if it does become a pandemic, will this truly affect patients who will be able to afford treatment and pay for treatment.'[97]

Without sustained investment by large pharmaceutical companies with the capacity to manufacture treatments and vaccines at scale, as the report warns, global populations 'will remain worryingly vulnerable to pandemics and epidemics, particularly those that mainly affect low-income countries'.[98]

CHAPTER TEN

Hard science

At the heart of the pharmaceutical industry today is a paradox. On the one hand, companies are making more money than ever before. Many have cut down on in-house R&D and are reaping the benefits from work done by others, all the while charging higher prices and enjoying longer monopolies than previously thought conceivable. And yet, beneath the surface, all is not well.

Even with this unprecedented pricing power, there remains a longstanding problem, a nagging weakness which threatens to topple the whole enterprise. It is not just that the current business model is no longer working for patients and healthcare systems, it's also struggling to keep up with the demands of the investors and shareholders it has become in thrall to. As Jack Scannell puts it: 'The worst situation is an industry where the shareholders think they're making lousy returns and the customers think they're paying too much.'[1]

A wiry, sharp-witted man in his early fifties, Scannell has spent his career straddling the worlds of science and commerce. He started medical training and completed a PhD in neuroscience before moving to Sanford Bernstein as an equity analyst, looking deep into the drug pipelines of pharmaceutical and biotech companies as he tried to predict their future profitability.

Now living with his wife and children in Edinburgh, where he spends his spare time climbing the Cairngorms, he is perhaps an unlikely harbinger of doom. But for many years the pharmaceutical

industry, in his analysis, has borne all the hallmarks of an industry
in decline.

The price rises of the last decade or two have, he says, far exceeded
the industry's expectations. 'You start this project and fifteen years
later the drug comes to market and what you can actually get for it
is two, three or four times more than you thought you'd get,' he says.

This pricing power has allowed executives to pacify shareholders
who might otherwise have been expected to react to a problem which
strikes at the heart of the industry's purpose. Despite the colossal
leaps forward in scientific understanding over the last seventy years,
discovering new drugs has become harder and dramatically more
expensive over time.

Scannell laid out the problem in a short paper published in a
specialist journal called *Nature Reviews Drug Discovery* in March 2012.
It included a small graph under the heading 'overall trend in R&D
efficiency' which plots how many new drugs have been approved
each year for every $1 billion (adjusted for inflation) spent on research,
as declared from the financial filings of the largest companies.

The chart, which goes all the way back to 1950, is jagged and
messy, as though it has been drawn by hand in a moving vehicle.
But the trend the sharp downward slope depicts is unmistakable: a
long-term decline in research productivity indicating that, for all the
advances in technology and understanding of science, the cost of
developing new drugs has continued, seemingly irreversibly, to rise.

Specifically, Scannell and colleagues at Sanford Bernstein found
that, for the same amount of money, the number of new drugs
reaching the market was falling by half every nine years. The trend
was dubbed Eroom's Law, a reversal of Moore's Law, which came
from the observation made by Gordon Moore, the co-founder of
Intel, that computer chips were becoming twice as powerful for the
same price every two years.

The graph was a favourite of executives at Valeant, who used it
to buttress their argument that it was foolish for a pharmaceutical
company to spend money on research and development and its findings helped justify the rush of investment capital towards companies

following a similar model in the early 2010s. After all, in this context, Valeant's approach was a rational response.

The trend Scannell identified was particularly puzzling because of technological advances which had allowed the industry to industrialise its approach to drug discovery. In the early decades of the pharmaceutical industry, a limited understanding of molecular biology meant that drug discovery relied on observing the effects of potential drugs on animals and humans. Successful drugs were discovered serendipitously and launched without scientists understanding why they worked. Gradually, researchers moved towards tests on specific biological entities which had been identified as likely to be linked to the disease being targeted. Tests, known as assays, would be developed to see if drug compounds were able to bind on the target and produce the desired effect.

It was a slow and labour-intensive process, limited by how many compounds and Petri dishes a scientist could work through each day. Starting in the early 1990s, however, technological advances transformed the process of screening compounds against potential drug targets. The development of combinatorial chemistry allowed chemists, aided by computer software, to synthesise tens of thousands of new molecular compounds in the time they would previously have been able to make hundreds. A technique called high throughput screening then made it possible for these vast compound libraries to be tested on drug targets, using robotics to automate the process so that huge numbers could be tested each day.

Meanwhile, another major scientific breakthrough, the genomic revolution, promised to unlock the mystery of what causes a host of common diseases, increasing and improving the targets available. The Human Genome Project, which was largely complete by 2000, laid out the sequence of three billion or so base pairs, the building blocks of the DNA molecules that make up genes. As the doctor and medical historian James Le Fanu explained: 'Genes code for proteins, so it is then only a matter of working out how these proteins are malfunctioning in diseases like cancer or multiple sclerosis to find ways of putting them right.'[2]

Armed with the ability to test millions of compounds against millions of targets, many magnitudes more than had previously been possible, drugmakers anticipated being able to identify a vast array of new, clinically important drugs. Yet by the late 2000s it was becoming clear that the results were not living up to the promise. All of the inputs were getting massively cheaper. The cost of sequencing a human genome, crucial to identifying promising gene targets, fell from $10 million to around $1,000 in the space of a decade.[3] But the output, the cost per new drug, was getting significantly more expensive. It just didn't seem to make any sense.

As an equity analyst, Scannell would regularly speak to the people running drug companies and their R&D divisions. But when he asked what the problem was, 'the dominant answer you would get is a shrug of the shoulders and people saying we've picked the low-hanging fruit'. The individuals giving this answer were spending a few billion dollars a year on R&D. 'And if that's the true answer, well, the fruit ain't gonna get any lower,' Scannell says.

They were suggesting that the drugs already discovered had been the easy ones and the drug targets left were those higher up the tree, harder and more expensive to reach. It is the same explanation some executives continue to offer. 'Discovering new drugs is getting harder,' Jennifer Taubert of Janssen Pharmaceuticals told a congressional hearing in 2019. 'The easy diseases have largely been solved,' she said. 'It gets harder and harder as we go after new treatments and new cures for ever more challenging diseases.'[4]

Back when Scannell was working as an analyst, many in the industry appeared reluctant to vocalise the problem. 'If you're running a biomedical charity trying to get money from governments, you don't want to advertise to people that there seems to be a big slow down in the rate of innovation,' Scannell says. 'And similarly, drug companies don't want to advertise to their shareholders that actually it seems to be harder and harder to get stuff out of all this money we're spending on R&D.'

The 2012 paper was an attempt by Scannell to flush out some of the other reasons for the industry's productivity problems. There appeared to be some truth to the low-hanging fruit problem, even if earlier discoveries were not necessarily easy. The therapeutic areas with few drugs are undoubtedly those that represent a huge scientific challenge. Prominent among them are the neurodegenerative diseases like Alzheimer's and Parkinson's, which have already had vast sums thrown at them but have proved stubbornly resistant to scientific breakthroughs. The scale of the failure in these fields has led some drug companies to abandon their efforts altogether. In 2018, Pfizer announced that it was ending its attempt to find drugs to treat Alzheimer's disease and Parkinson's disease, cutting 300 jobs in the process. Funds were to be re-allocated to other more immediately profitable areas.[5] Another untapped area is the lack of any drugs to treat the so-called negative symptoms of schizophrenia – things like a chronic sense of apathy and a difficulty making social connections, which can have a hugely detrimental effect on someone's quality of life.

But there was, Scannell suggested, another problem within those therapeutic areas which already have an array of treatments. It was one created by the success of several decades of previous endeavour. When the market for generics is working as intended, cheap and effective treatments are readily available for many common diseases and doctors are happy to keep prescribing them. He called this the 'better than The Beatles' problem.

'Imagine how much new music would be published if the following factors were in play,' he says. 'One, every new record that was released had to be better than The Beatles. Two, people could download old Beatles records [at low cost]. And three, people never got bored of listening to Beatles songs.

'If you had those three factors, it would be very, very hard to commercialise new music.'[6]

For drugmakers looking to pursue genuine innovation, this is the challenge they face. Each new drug raises the bar that others in that therapeutic area will have to clear to be considered an improvement on what's already available. The 'better than The Beatles' problem helps push drug discovery activity into 'those therapy areas where, over the last fifty years, the drug industry hasn't been able to come up with much,' Scannell says. 'There's no point having yet another drug to cure stomach ulcers because we've got a whole bunch of great drugs to cure stomach ulcers and they're generic.'

As drugs get better, regulators are also likely to get more demanding, and meeting these demands through clinical tests becomes more expensive. 'As you get more and more good drugs in the therapy area, regulators get more cautious about the newer ones,' he says. The hurdles a new treatment must clear to secure regulatory approval get higher and more numerous over time, placing further obstacles and costs in the path of any successful drug launch.

The scientific challenges that have hindered R&D productivity laid out by Scannell are real. But companies have also played a significant role in their own research failings. The move to high throughput screening turned out to be based on a false premise. Industrialising the drug discovery process resulted in a numbers game. It created a mentality that 'we need to identify more targets, we need to produce more compounds, we need to screen more stuff', Scannell says.

This emphasis on quantity ignored the role of something far more important in drug development: how well success in the tests used to assess whether a compound is a promising candidate actually correlates with whether it will work against a particular disease in humans. When scientists set out to develop a new drug, there are a variety of ways to test for potential biological targets linked to the disease, and subsequently to test different compounds for their ability to interact with these putative targets. These range from cell-based tests, perhaps examining whether a compound will bind to a particular protein, to animal testing and the use of computer modelling. Whatever the test used, the extent to which it can help to identify good drug candidates is far more dependent on whether it is a good representation of how the drug will ultimately work in humans, rather than how cheaply and efficiently it can be replicated on a large set of compounds.

Scannell likens the ability of a test to predict a drug's efficacy to the role of a compass in steering a boat. Being able to travel at a faster speed won't help you get to your destination quicker if you're going in the wrong direction. And, just like a compass, small changes can have an outsized influence. Companies believed that the sheer number of compounds being tested would help create better results without realising the extent to which unreliable tests would lead them in the wrong direction. 'Changes in the validity of models that most scientists would regard as small or unknowable can have as much effect on R&D productivity as 100- or 1,000-fold changes in brute force efficiency,' he says. Good testing methods for particular diseases, such as testing potential stomach acid drugs on dogs, fall out of use once they have led to the successful development of drugs for that problem. At the same time that the best existing tests were rendering themselves redundant, the focus on brute-force efficiency meant there was an under-investment in the quality of new tests.

In 2011, the British-Swedish company AstraZeneca, aware that its own R&D productivity was below an already low industry average, launched a wholesale review of what had gone wrong. In a paper published by several AstraZeneca scientists and executives three years later, they catalogued the damage that the move to an industrialised approach had wrought. It wasn't simply that the volume-based approach hadn't brought the gains the company had hoped from speeding up the drug discovery process. They concluded it had actively damaged the research culture and the 'underlying scientific curiosity' of its staff. Instead of trying to develop a deep understanding of diseases and potential therapeutic opportunities, scientists at the company had 'instead moved towards meeting volume-based goals and identifying an unprecedented level of back-up and "me too" drug candidates'.[7] They were being rewarded for the number of new compounds brought through into clinical testing and so were churning out drug candidates which were too similar to one another. In one case, a lead candidate and seven back-up molecules all had the same toxicology problem. When one later failed in testing, the others followed suit.

The move to an industrialised, target-based approach removed the opportunity for doctors to make serendipitous discoveries as they experimented freely without specific biological targets in mind.

In the late 1990s, Bernard Munos, the long-time Eli Lilly executive, decided to study how innovation happens. 'We spend tens of billions of dollars a year trying to produce innovation and we don't even know where it comes from,' he says. 'To me, that was mismanagement on a grand scale.'[8]

His conclusion, nearly a decade later, was that innovation occurs in waves as breakthroughs in basic research around a particular disease or biological target are translated into a flood of new drugs. In the 1950s, there were revolutionary new drugs for psychiatric conditions including benzodiazepines, lithium, antidepressants and antipsychotics which 'emptied the mental asylums' and allowed the mentally unwell to return to their homes. In the late 1970s and 1980s came beta-blockers and ACE inhibitors, drugs for patients with hypertension and heart conditions. The 1990s brought SSRI antidepressants and other neuromodulators. Then, when the breakthroughs have been fully explored, the drugs in that area dry up and science moves on to something else. 'This is basically the game you have to play in drug R&D,' Munos says. 'You have to ride those waves and you have to be agile enough to jump from one to another.'

The business-minded drug executives who had sought to reduce risk and improve R&D efficiency by constraining how their scientists worked, committing them to targets and directing the precise treatment areas they should be focusing on, missed the fact that 'you cannot schedule eurekas', Munos says. 'Science proceeds at its own pace [and] takes you in a direction that is often unexpected.' Drug discovery is a creative act and so trying to apply the regimentation encouraged when running a business in another industry, as taught in business schools, was ultimately counterproductive. A failure to recognise this at Munos's own former company, Eli Lilly, brought a decade in which it brought a single drug – itself a commercial disappointment – to market.[9] Companies over-invested in areas where they were strong without realising they were 'mining ground that is exhausted'.

'We had an enormous amount of money invested pursuing innovation in areas that weren't really ready to deliver it,' Munos says. Meanwhile the firm under-invested in other fields, delaying 'exploring and taking advantage of new opportunities elsewhere that happen to be in unfamiliar territory'. It was a criticism echoed by Jürgen Drews, the former Roche research chief, who in 2003 decried that the search for blockbusters had led to the industry narrowing the scope of its research efforts, even though 'blockbuster status was in the past often obtained against the predictions of marketing departments'.[10] Trying to identify blockbusters as they were being developed was a fool's errand. They often emerged unexpectedly, from the fifth drug in a new class of cholesterol-lowering statins, or from a heart drug which became a billion-dollar erectile dysfunction treatment.

One former Big Pharma chief executive reached the same conclusion about the need for individual scientists to have the freedom to explore when confronted with the disappointing results generated by high throughput screening, where running millions of compounds against millions of targets produced drugs which ultimately failed to demonstrate basic efficacy.

'What we learned is it really takes the passion and the commitment of a lead scientist, somebody who believes in the science and, against all odds, finds a compound [that] blocks the targets that he's identified and develops a drug,' he says. 'That's more important than the scale of high throughput screening and very large-scale research.'[11]

Allowing financial rewards to dictate where R&D efforts are focused can contribute to poor productivity, with potential rewards preventing a clear-eyed assessment of the chance of success. This is particularly true when a potential drug's commercial prospects are judged in the early stages of drug discovery, years before it will hit the market and before clinical usefulness and the number of patients it might benefit are really known.

'In our experience, across a variety of companies, projects can be mistakenly driven by an overemphasis on commercial potential,' wrote researchers at AstraZeneca in a 2018 paper which looked at the lessons the company had learned from changing its R&D strategy. Projects, they said, had 'moved forward based on commercial confidence rather than scientific confidence and unsurprisingly failed in mid-stage and late-stage development'.[12]

These scientific challenges and self-inflicted errors have all helped to drive up the cost of research and development. At the same time, because all drugs get the same twenty-year patent regardless of their clinical value and new drugs enjoy a pricing floor set by previous products in the same area, companies are incentivised to pursue incremental improvements over game-changing therapies. These twin pressures have helped to make the industry as a whole more risk-averse in the kind of drugs it brings to market.

Truly breakthrough drugs have long represented a relatively small proportion of the new drugs the pharmaceutical industry develops. The US regulator has a 'breakthrough' designation which, by its determination, typically applies to only between one-fifth and one-quarter of new drugs each year. Of course it would be overstating the case to claim that this is all by design. Companies regularly pursue promising new compounds or biologics, only to find after funding clinical trials that the drug is somewhat less revolutionary than had been hoped. In fact, the true usefulness of many drugs hasn't become apparent until long after their launch, once doctors have had years to observe how patients respond. Nonetheless, there are choices to be made during the development process on how novel an approach is to be pursued and what level of risk will be tolerated in more experimental candidates.

In France, an independent scientific committee appraises every newly approved drug to assess both its clinical benefits, with five options from a rating of one for 'major' to five for 'insufficient to justify being reimbursed', and how it compares to existing treatments. These judgements are then used to set the price at which the country's universal healthcare system will reimburse the manufacturer, something which, in the eyes of the drug industry, leads to an unfairly critical approach.

Margaret Kyle, an American economics professor living in Paris, has taken these assessments and looked at the correlation between the usefulness of a drug and the price it commands. There was no meaningful link to be discerned, leading her to conclude that 'we're paying too much for those [drugs] that are not bringing a lot of added value'.[13]

That in turn encourages companies to pursue less useful drugs. 'If it's easier to do a four or five because it's a minor change to something that's already existing, then essentially we're tilting the incentives for companies to develop more me-toos rather than important breakthroughs,' she says.

The problem remained consistent across several countries Kyle looked at, including Australia, Canada and the United Kingdom. Predictably, it is particularly pronounced in the United States. Although the tiny handful of drugs deemed the most important manage to generate higher revenues over the decade after launch, there was little difference between the vast mass of medicines given scores between two and five.

Of 220 newly developed drugs launched between 2000 and 2016, ninety-two were assessed by France's National Authority for Health (an agency set up to assess the clinical value of drugs independent of their price) to offer no advantage at all over existing medications. Another fifty-four represented only a minor improvement, the fourth-lowest option on the five-point scale.[14]

'My concern is that maybe the companies aren't allocating R&D towards the areas where we would have the highest social benefits. Instead, they're allocating towards areas where they see the greatest private rate of return,' Kyle says.

Josh Krieger, the Harvard Business School assistant professor, has studied just how similar new drugs are to previously launched products and found a similar pattern. 'The percentage of drugs that are me-toos is rising over time,' he says. 'And we're measuring me-toos using molecular similarity. So we're not just saying drugs treating the same disease, or drugs that are looking at similar molecular targets. We're seeing the actual chemical composition, on average, is getting less creative over time.' Historically the most successful drugs in a new drug class are not always the first to launch, as Lipitor demonstrated in the statin market, and so Krieger says the system rewards a 'fast follower' rather than an 'explorer' developing first-in-class drugs.

This exacerbates a problem that has always existed with the way innovation is incentivised. As companies' R&D efforts cluster around certain high-value disease areas and, often, the same druggable targets, they duplicate the same research work that is being carried out elsewhere – or perhaps has already been tried and ended in failure. Some of this duplication is driven by the way in which intellectual property (IP) law works. As our levels of understanding about how to tackle complex diseases have grown, it has become increasingly clear that a single pharmaceutical intervention is unlikely to be sufficient and that the answers likely lie in combinations of drugs. This incentivises companies to pursue their own version of new classes of drug in order to avoid having to license a rival's and share the profits from any successful product.

These licensing fees have themselves played a major role in driving up the costs of R&D. Jamie Love, an economist and NGO director who has spent his career focusing on IP issues, believes that for newer treatments in particular, the cost of licensing patents from universities and other companies now makes up a majority of the funds recorded as research and development costs. The cost of buying these IP rights is directly linked to 'the price you think someone else is going to pay for the products, so IP has become very expensive', he says.[15] It is those footing the bill for treatments who ultimately pay for the tens of billions in research money wasted by inefficiencies and mistakes in how drug development is pursued.

Eroom's Law and falling R&D efficiency contributed to many of the big changes in the industry over the last twenty years. The difficulty of finding novel drugs when there is now a significant back catalogue of generic drugs available helped encouraged the push towards oncology, where even minor improvements can be commercially successful, and rare diseases, where there are usually no existing treatments that must be improved upon.

It helps explain other trends, too. Share buybacks and dividends help to keep investors happy, but they are also an economically rational response to the inefficiency of the in-house R&D efforts. As the number of new blockbuster drugs fell, price rises for existing drugs provided a way to make up for a lack of new treatments with mass-market appeal.

Above all, falling R&D productivity was wielded in support of the industry's chief rebuttal to proposals for price controls and regulation in the key American market: drugs are not just very costly to develop, they're getting more so, and so, it is argued, any attempt to squeeze profit margins will have a disastrous effect on innovation. It allowed the industry to make the case that, even as pharmaceutical spending was rising, there was little slack to accommodate lower prices.

Every decade or so, Joseph DiMasi, an economist at Tufts University, produces an estimate of the cost of bringing a new drug to market. In a paper published in 2016, this estimate stood at $2.6 billion, up from $1.2 billion in 2007 and around $800 million in 2003.[16] The numbers, like the R&D figures put out by drug companies, have been treated with scepticism. They rely on confidential data for a small proportion of drugs and include allowances for the cost of failed projects as well as the opportunity cost of locking up funds in long-term research projects at rates which some academics believe are far above average. A 2020 study using US financial filings rather than confidential data estimated an average cost of $1.3 billion after allowing for failures and using the same cost of capital rate as DiMasi.[17] It doesn't help that the industry treats the details of its R&D spending as a state secret, and that companies can take wildly different approaches to what they disclose. Most inflate their R&D costs by including Phase IV studies done after a drug is approved – which make up at least one-eighth of declared spending – and the cost of monitoring for adverse effects.[18] Some record part of the costs of acquiring a drug in their R&D spending and more than 21 per cent is now declared as 'uncategorised' by the industry's American trade body, up from 0.5 per cent a decade earlier.[19]

Nevertheless, whatever the quibbles over the specific methodology, few experts dispute that drug discovery is a very expensive process which has got even more expensive over time. These increased costs without an attendant increase in the number of new drug approvals each year created the long-term slump in R&D productivity and the return on such investment. It got so bad that some estimates even suggest that it reached the point where the return on investment was at, or even below, the cost of capital.

When weighing up potential investments, investors and companies do not simply assess the prospective returns against the prospective costs. They also take into account the cost of tying up the invested money over the duration of the project, comparing it to what could have been made had it been deployed elsewhere or earning interest as savings in a bank. If the return does not exceed the cost of capital, then an investment is not worth making.

As long ago as 2009, the consultancy firm McKinsey calculated that the return on investment from small molecule drug research had fallen to around 7.5 per cent, which it said was below the average capitalisation rate of 8.5 to 11 per cent. Deloitte's annual assessment of R&D returns at the largest drug companies placed the internal rate of return at just 1.8 per cent in 2019, down from 10.1 per cent as recently as 2010.[20] Average figures can disguise significant variation between rival companies but only one of the twelve companies the report examined had a rate of return above 5 per cent. Smaller companies are doing better, but the returns are diminishing in the same way. With these figures, as the previous year's report had concluded, the industry requires 'a transformational change in the way R&D is conducted'.

'Blockbuster costs without corresponding blockbuster sales or volume of assets is not an equation that will drive sustainable returns from the investment in innovation,' the authors wrote in 2018, warning that the industry needed to reduce the cost of developing a new drug by two-thirds to have a sustainable future even with the current high prices.[21]

'It's pretty remarkable that despite the fact that the drugs are so expensive that the health systems of developed countries are struggling to pay for them, you still can't make [enough] money doing it,' Scannell says. 'For the pension funds, hedge funds or sovereign wealth funds who own the big drug companies, high profit margins do not necessarily mean that the company is getting good financial returns on its research spending,' he explains.

'R&D money is tied up for years, decades even, and investors want returns on that money at least equivalent to the compounding "interest" it could have earned if invested in a different industry. Since drug R&D takes many years, the compounding effect is huge. Decent returns require very high profit margins.

'Today we are in an ugly situation where health systems are horrified by the price of new drugs, where industry profit margins are really high, but where R&D is so expensive that many investors think it is losing them money.'

Fortunately, in recent years, there have been the beginnings of a crucial change: Eroom's Law has been broken. In April 2020, Scannell and several colleagues published a new article in the same journal as the 2012 paper. It concluded that the high rate of failure in late-stage R&D had levelled off and then, in 2015, began to improve, 'driving the turnaround in R&D productivity'.[22] The number of new drugs approved in the United States and Europe has recovered from the nadir reached in the late 2000s. In the US, a record fifty-nine drugs were approved in 2018, compared with a low of twenty-two in 2009.

It remains to be seen if this is truly an indication that R&D productivity has improved in a sustainable way, or whether this is more of a short-term blip caused by the large number of orphan and cancer drugs which companies are currently incentivised to launch. 'Unfortunately, this is not a prediction that the underlying forces that caused the prior decline, such as the "better than The Beatles" problem, have gone away', Scannell and his fellow authors wrote. 'We believe they persist and will again take hold once the effects of the recent improvements in understanding of disease biology and decision making wane.'[23]

Even if Eroom's Law has been permanently broken, an improvement in R&D productivity does little to help patients in a system in which the whole business model for drug companies remains predicated on ever-higher prices, with no motivation for companies to pass on any efficiency savings to consumers. Escalating prices are needed in order to meet the expectations baked into a financialised model: without them, there is no way to maintain the same level of revenues from drugs with far smaller markets than the blockbusters of a previous generation.

The problem is particularly pronounced because the coming generation of targeted and personalised medicines exacerbate the pressures which have created the current predicament, with far smaller markets and far higher prices.

Advances in scientific understanding of diseases and new technologies are combining to produce a new generation of highly specialised drugs, some of which offer up the possibility of curing previously untreatable conditions. They hold huge promise for those facing devastating diseases, but these developments are of limited use if they remain out of reach for a large majority of patients. The recent focus on orphan and oncology drugs is already driving up healthcare spending and yet the six-figure prices of those treatments pale in comparison to the prices companies are demanding for the next generation of drugs. With the decline of mass-market blockbusters, drug companies are trying to squeeze an increasing proportion of their profits out of smaller and smaller groups of patients in a way that is unsustainable for both sides.

These new treatments include gene therapies, which seek to fix genetic disorders by manipulating genetic material. At the moment, this typically involves using a modified virus to deliver a normal copy of a faulty gene into cells. However, gene-editing technologies such as CRISPR-Cas9 raise the ethically fraught possibility of altering DNA in human embryos. There have only been a handful of gene therapies launched on the market so far but the collapsing cost of genome sequencing brings an era of personalised medicines ever closer.

On its own terms, each individual drug or treatment might be cost-effective over the lifetime of the patient when compared to the high prices already established for other, less effective options. But this is often simply a product of the overheated pricing environment which pharmaceutical companies have created, as well as the huge inflation in the cost of surgeries and hospital stays in the United States. Taken together, the growing number of incredibly expensive drugs threaten to bankrupt health systems, particularly when so many are biologics without the prospect of rapid genericisation to bring down the costs when their patents expire. Publicly-funded payers can't meet the huge spending the treatments require, while insurers are understandably unwilling to make such payments for patients who might move to another company with a year or two.

Even when health systems have been willing to pay for the drugs, perhaps after securing a sufficient discount on the asking price, the upfront cost has frequently led to restrictions on how many patients can be given the drug. In 2019, a revolutionary gene therapy treatment for spinal muscular atrophy called Zolgensma was launched. With a price tag of $2.1 million, the orphan drug became the world's most expensive drug, taking the title from another gene therapy, Luxturna, a treatment for patients with a rare inherited eye disorder costing $850,000. Zolgensma fell just within the upper bound of one independent US body's cost-effectiveness assessment after its manufacturer, the Novartis-owned AveXis, avoided a mooted price tag of up to $5 million.[24] The company, wary that the high cost would scare off insurers and health systems, offered to spread the cost of the treatment over five years. But even with this concession, the scale of the outlay required led to restrictions on access in several wealthy countries while the drug remains resolutely out of reach for health systems in less well-off nations.[25]

In other cases, the issue is not simply one of cashflow, but of whether the enormous prices demanded match up to the benefits the drugs provide. One of the biggest breakthroughs in cancer treatment is in immuno-oncology, where the body's own immune system defences are bolstered to help attack cancer cells. These IO-therapies, as they are known, include checkpoint inhibitors, a class of drugs which stop the body from limiting its own immune response, and CAR T-cell therapies, where a patient's immune cells are collected and genetically engineered to target and kill cancer cells before being reintroduced.

'The analyses we've done and every analysis I've seen by others suggests that the costs of the treatments almost universally are outstripping the magnitude of benefits,' says Peter Bach, who has studied the diminishing returns from cancer treatments. 'So you can be astounded by all these gains, I am personally, but if each gain costs more money than the gain before, you're on that diminishing returns curve. It matters because that's money that can't go for something else.'

One CAR T-cell therapy, Yescarta, which Gilead bought Kite Pharma to acquire, was deemed too expensive for the benefits it offered by NICE and was only made available when the manufacturer cut a secret deal with the British national health service. In the US, Medicare decided it would only partially cover the cost of the treatment.

These price tags for personalised medicines have proved problematic for the companies selling the products as well. The first gene therapy to receive approval in Europe was Glybera, a treatment for an extremely rare blood disease. Developed by an Amsterdam-based company called UniQure, the €1 million treatment launched in October 2012. It was a commercial failure and was withdrawn from the market five years later because of a lack of sales.[26] Another gene therapy, Strimvelis, was used for just four patients in the three years after its approval in Europe in 2016.[27]

The fact that many of these treatments are cures or one-time interventions poses another problem for their manufacturers under the current system. Investors prize long-term growth and the golden age was built on pills for chronic conditions which created a captive market of patients who would take the drug for life and which could be expanded by reaching more people through promotion and marketing. If a drug is a cure, the cash flow looks very different.

In April 2018, Goldman Sachs published a report with the title: 'Is curing patients a sustainable business model?' With each cure, a drug's success is reducing the pool of future patients and so 'while this proposition carries tremendous value for patients and society, it could represent a challenge for genome medicine developers looking for sustained cash flow', the investment bank warned.[28] Wall Street has shown a strong preference for less clinically useful drugs which will be taken by a large patient group for life over a breakthrough cure, even if that cure itself has a large market. Gilead discovered this to its cost when it launched its high-priced hepatitis C drugs. Sovaldi and Harvoni were enormous money-spinners, initially driving the company's stock to record highs. The revenues they brought in transformed the size of the business, bringing in sales of $58 billion over five years.[29] Yet, within a couple of years of their launch, Gilead's share price began to fall steeply because they weren't delivering the level of growth investors had expected. The high prices had prompted huge scrutiny and a rival – though less effective – treatment from AbbVie had also gone on sale earlier than anticipated, forcing Gilead to offer average discounts of 46 per cent.[30] Gilead's executives began talking up the strength of sales for their HIV drugs instead. 'Here you've got a company that's come up with this revolutionary treatment through public and private investment and yet ultimately it's their HIV treatments that they're looking to be their saviour in the medium term because it's a treatment that patients need to take for their entire life,' Victor Roy says.[31]

There is a final problem which this new era of scientific possibility brings. The wider changes in where drug research is carried out has left society more vulnerable than before to investors pulling out because of price regulation or other market shocks. Gene and immuno-therapies are being advanced in large part by biotechs, with big pharmaceutical companies cutting down on early-stage, in-house research and instead reducing the risk in R&D by acquiring biotechs with products at a later stage. These biotechs don't have the legacy infrastructure of Big Pharma. There are no large research facilities with thousands of salaried scientists or huge, expensively constructed factories to keep busy. If the expected rewards on offer fall, the venture capitalists who fund them have little incentive not to pull the plug and put their money elsewhere – into new dating apps or social media networks or whatever else is the latest flavour of the month in Silicon Valley.

It is crucial for society that we continue to push the frontiers of science and develop new and better treatments for the conditions and diseases which afflict humankind. And it is no less important that those treatments are accessible and affordable.

The forces that have rippled through the industry, from financialisation to falling R&D productivity, have placed these two things in opposition. The great fear for the pharmaceutical industry is a significant change in their ability to charge high prices, particularly in the United States. 'I think most people in the industry think that they're pushing the pricing lever as hard as they possibly can and are worried that it's not sustainable,' Scannell says. 'Venture-capital funding for small companies and shareholders' tolerance for relatively high levels of R&D spending in big companies is absolutely dependent on their view that prices are going to remain relatively high.'

Without the ability to continue raising prices, Scannell sees an industry in relative decline. Kelvin Stott, who oversees the drug development pipeline of a Swiss pharmaceutical company, believes that 'pharma literally doesn't have a choice' in following its current approach.

'It is pushing up drug prices as much as payers will bear; not only because it can, but because it can't afford not to. Otherwise the industry would enter a rapid decline due to diminishing return on investment, and investors would eventually walk away.'[32] And yet, a reckoning is surely coming.

For years, the industry enjoyed a lack of significant push back from other players in the health system. Doctors were unlikely to know the cost of a medicine, and in any event their responsiveness to peppy sales reps and the results of carefully constructed clinical trials was far more important in driving prescriptions than the price of a drug. Meanwhile, insurance companies and PBMs were happy to play the game and take their cut.

This era of mass ambivalence has come to a juddering halt. As prices rose and US insurers tried to push more of these costs on to patients in higher deductibles, co-pays and premiums, the impact on patients and the increasing burden on health budgets became impossible to ignore for everyone from doctors to politicians. And if the annual price rises and soaring launch prices of large companies were only slowly drawing attention, along came Martin Shkreli and the predatory pharmaceutical model he embodied to grab the spotlight and leave no doubt that something had gone very wrong when it came to drug pricing.

The industry's willingness to push prices higher and higher in a bid to satisfy shareholders has justifiably alienated the public. The decades-long defence that prices were a carefully calibrated means of recouping manufacturing and R&D costs has fallen apart. The 'value-based pricing' approach in which the industry justifies incredible prices by pointing to the high costs of leaving someone untreated won't work either. The professed savings are often no more than a mirage, with companies seeking to exploit excessively high costs in other parts of the health system to justify their own prices.

The prices that result are not simply excessive in the scale of the personal windfalls they can bring to biotech investors or drug industry executives. They are excessive because they are no longer affordable in even the richest countries.

Ultimately, the price and cost of drugs cannot continue to rise indefinitely. Ageing populations and growing life expectancy mean demographics are already placing a heavy burden on Western healthcare budgets and the demands on public spending will only grow in the aftermath of the coronavirus pandemic. The proportion of GDP spent on healthcare – of which pharmaceuticals represent a significant share of 10 or 20 per cent – has risen substantially and each increase comes at a cost to other services.[33]

Political pressure in Washington DC has been building for years with Republicans and Democrats in agreement that medicines have become unconscionably expensive. The pledge of several drug companies to sell a potential coronavirus vaccine at cost during the pandemic may buy some goodwill, but the structural pressures are not going anywhere. Change must come.

In the meantime, as millions who need drugs they can't afford are waiting for political and business leaders to take action, a brave few have taken matters into their own hands. Often acting at substantial personal risk, they are fighting back against the scourge of high drug prices.

CHAPTER ELEVEN

Fighting back

May 2015. As he picked his way through a curry with one eye on the door, Greg Jefferys tried to push away the trepidation rising in his stomach; the nagging doubts that his visitor wouldn't come, or that he wouldn't bring what he'd promised. The growing fear that this wasn't going to work out and that the 5,600-mile round trip was to have been in vain. He was in India to try and buy three bottles amounting to eighty-four pills. One bottle was stored safely away in his hotel room upstairs, but without the others the treatment wouldn't work and his flight home was now less than forty-eight hours away. The clock ticked loudly on the restaurant wall. Maybe the visitor wasn't coming after all.

August 2018. The two middle-aged women approached the US–Canadian border with the drugs carefully packed on ice in a cooler in the boot. Sitting in the passenger seat, Deidre Waxman was expecting trouble. The boxed vials she was bringing back were in what she thought was at best a 'grey area' legally speaking and Waxman and her friend were worried they were going to be stopped. She knew she was supposed to declare it, but when the border guards asked whether she was bringing anything back, Waxman, a social worker with jet-black hair and red lipstick, was deliberately vague. She smiled and told them that she had 'some stuff for her grandson, which I did, and nothing else'.[1] The second part was a lie, but she didn't dare risk them confiscating the insulin lying in the back.

September 2019. Ellen De Meyer had become obsessed with

checking the numbers. Each time she logged in and clicked refresh, the little counter jumped up. A few hundred this time. Now another thousand. It had seemed such a long shot, trying to persuade almost a million people to send a text message costing a couple of euros. But they were desperate. For their nine-month-old daughter Pia to be able to live a normal life, they had to raise nearly €2 million as soon as possible. And somehow, against the odds, it seemed to be working.

Three people, on three continents, waiting. Each one desperate that they should succeed in getting hold of something that could be the difference between life and death for themselves, their baby daughter, or a complete stranger.

Drug companies will go to great lengths to protect their products and defend their ability to charge high prices, even if that leaves some who need the medicine unable to get it. They wield huge power, with highly-paid lawyers, corporate lobbyists and governments willing to put their diplomatic weight behind efforts to protect their right to charge what they want for medicines, protected by legally-enforced monopolies.

But even in the face of such power, when lives are at stake there are brave and compassionate individuals prepared to do whatever it takes to get hold of the drugs they or others need. Individuals who refuse to accept a seemingly unyielding system or their own apparent powerlessness. Individuals willing to fight back.

Greg Jefferys had expected to spend his sixties living a quiet life at home in the south Australian island of Tasmania, spending his time researching colonial history, playing with his dog and fishing for trout in the Huon River. Now he found himself thousands of miles away in a bustling metropolis, sweating in the forty-degree heat. A tall, lean man with a mid-length white beard and the weather-beaten skin of a former farmer, Jefferys' trip to Chennai had been set in motion by a diagnosis he'd received nine months earlier. Shortly after a bout of flu while on holiday on the mainland in Queensland, he returned home and found himself so fatigued that one morning he was unable to get out of bed. He'd noticed an alarming change to his urine, too: it was darker than usual and had an unpleasant smell which reminded him of rotting meat.[2]

A trip to the doctor followed and tests revealed the culprit: he was infected with hepatitis C. Left untreated, hepatitis C, which many sufferers unknowingly carry for years without any symptoms, can lead to liver failure or cancer. In his late teens, while living in north Sydney, he'd been one of thousands addicted to heroin. A near-fatal overdose in 1975 had allowed him to kick the habit, but shared needles are the most common way in which hepatitis C is spread and the virus can lie dormant in the bloodstream for decades.

Jefferys was told that the only treatment offered in Australia relied on interferon, a harsh regimen with a success rate no better than 50 per cent. As he researched the disease, he discovered a new drug, Sovaldi. The first of Gilead Science's breakthrough hepatitis C treatments, it was being launched in the United States with a cost which was the equivalent of $100,000 Australian dollars. It was clear it wasn't going to be affordable. 'I had no savings or anything like that and I thought I'm not going to sell my house to cure this disease,' Jefferys says.[3]

His enzyme levels were elevated and although an ultrasound had shown no signs of tumours on his liver his doctor pushed him to start the interferon treatment. But, aware of how punishing that could be, Jefferys instead decided to try to manage the virus with lifestyle changes, giving up drinking and sharply reducing his consumption of coffee and red meat. At the same time, he sought other ways to get hold of Sovaldi. A clinical trial due to start on the mainland in Sydney offered hope, but, after flying there to meet the doctor running it, he was turned down. Places were in high demand and he wasn't sick enough yet. Adding to his disappointment, the trial doctor said he expected the Australian government would limit access to Sovaldi once approved in Australia because of the cost.

After first receiving US regulatory approval in December 2013, Sovaldi, also known as sofosbuvir, was gradually being launched around the world. The company ran into problems in India, a country with a history of not complying with Western drug patents. Until 2005, it had not permitted patents on medicines and, although that had now changed, a US-based non-profit was challenging Gilead's attempt to patent Sovaldi. In September 2014, Gilead elected to head off that problem by signing agreements with several Indian generics manufacturers. They would be allowed to make cheap versions of the drug, on which they'd pay Gilead a royalty, but could only distribute them to a designated list of mostly low-income countries. However, there was nothing to stop them from selling these generic versions to anyone willing to travel to India to pick them up.

A few months later, a friend of Jefferys called with news. He'd found out that Indian generics manufacturers had already started selling the drug. With a price tag of around $1,000 for a twelve-week course, these generic versions were a fraction of what Sovaldi cost in the West. Jefferys bought a plane ticket to Chennai immediately, afraid that Gilead would be moving to close this loophole. In January 2015, the Indian patent authority had rejected Gilead's application, claiming that the drug wasn't sufficiently innovative to patent, but the company was appealing the decision and the Australian wasn't sure what would happen if they won.

When he landed that May, he didn't have much of a plan. On the first morning, waking early, he took a stroll around the streets near his hotel and noticed some chemists and doctors' offices nearby. None of them were open yet but, returning a little later, he began knocking on doors and asking if they knew where he could buy the generic hepatitis C medicine. No one could help. Somewhat dispirited, he returned to his hotel room to try an alternative approach. During the flight over, he'd been sent a message from someone who had been reading the blog Jefferys was keeping to chronicle his experience since being diagnosed with hepatitis C. The correspondent had offered to put him in touch with a friend who lived in Chennai and was currently taking a generic version of Sovaldi. Jefferys met them the next day and was pointed towards a local gastroenterologist.

So it was that on the third day of his trip Jefferys found himself at the Apollo Hospital, a modern facility in what appeared to be an affluent suburb. After navigating a system which required him to register at several different desks, each one requiring a small fee and yet more paperwork, he was eventually able to get an appointment with the doctor. The gastroenterologist who saw him was about to go on holiday to Greece and wouldn't be back before the Australian flew home. Once Jefferys had explained his situation, however, he agreed to write a prescription in exchange for a promise to get a particular test done the next day.

He had the crucial bit of paper, but Jefferys would quickly discover that exchanging it for the pills he needed was not going to be straightforward. Over the next few days, he tried to call distributors working for several generic drug companies but found communications difficult. Eventually he arranged to buy the drug from a salesman working for Mylan, a large multinational generic drugs manufacturer. The drugs were due to arrive at 11 a.m. in the morning on the penultimate day of Jefferys' trip but when the salesman showed up – a couple of hours late – he only brought one of the three bottles of pills needed for the treatment to be effective. After several calls and arguments, the remaining pills were promised for delivery that evening.

He was still waiting as he ate a curry and watched the clock tick past six. Finally, a delivery man arrived. Alerted to his visitor, Jefferys ran upstairs from the hotel's restaurant and gathered bundles of rupees from his room. After the deal was done, he returned to look at his purchase.

'It seemed totally absurd,' he wrote in a travel diary. 'Three little plastic jars, each with 28 little tablets in them. I had travelled halfway around the world, spent nearly a week jumping through seemingly endless burning hoops, all for these three little jars. Ninety thousand dollars worth in Oz. It just seemed too absurd. These little jars held the difference between health and sickness, life and death, years of good life or years of suffering.'[4]

He returned home and started taking the pills. Soon, liver function and viral load tests administered by his doctor showed the treatment was working and by mid-August, three months after he started taking the drugs, tests showed he had been cured.

Since starting a blog, Jefferys had been inundated with emails from people from around the world wanting advice on how to buy the drugs in India and he decided he wanted to help them. The Australian government would eventually strike a novel agreement with Gilead which allowed widespread access for all adults with hepatitis C. But other countries' citizens were less fortunate, with extensive rationing by health services who were paying for the drug on a per-patient basis. Jefferys set up a website offering advice to others on how to buy generic versions. Over time, he built up connections with Indian manufacturers which allowed him to take advantage of personal importation rules to arrange delivery of the treatments to anyone in the world on a non-profit basis. Jefferys initially worked with an Australian doctor, James Freeman, who set up his own buyers' club, FixHepC, to offer the same service. Together, the two men have helped thousands of people from around the world.

Among them are 'Demir', who lives in a small town in Bosnia. He prefers not to use his real name because there is 'total stigma' around hepatitis C. 'People just don't know about it,' he says. 'They think it's the plague and they think if they breathe the same air in the same room they can get it.'[5] Born in 1973, he contracted the virus during the vicious civil war which fractured the country along ethnic lines in the early 1990s. 'It was wartime, doing drugs, having no future,' he says. 'I was addicted to heroin.' After the war, 'when life started again', he went to a drug rehab clinic in Medjugorje, a small town near the Croatian border which had become a popular pilgrimage site for Catholics. It was here that blood tests revealed the diagnosis. 'At that time I wasn't thinking about it too much,' he says. 'They said you can live with it, there is no real cure, so it's not like I paid too much attention about it.'

Demir moved on with his life. He had a series of jobs, got married and divorced, found a new partner and had a daughter. It was nearly two decades after his diagnosis when he visited a doctor to discuss treatment for hepatitis C. When Demir asked about the new Gilead treatments he was told there was no prospect of being able to access them. 'He told me we live in Bosnia so it's going to take many years until something like that comes to us.' Interferon was available, but Demir had seen the harsh side effects on others who'd taken the treatment at the rehab clinic in Medjugorje. He forgot about getting treatment again until, two years later, he experienced liver pain and took it as a signal that he had to do something.

Demir had been active in a Facebook group for hepatitis C patients and he'd noticed that the same name had come up again and again as they responded to people's questions – Greg Jefferys. He went online, found his way to Jefferys' website and sent him an email. Jefferys talked him through how he could acquire the drug. First, he needed to undergo testing to establish which genotype he was carrying and how long he would need to take the drugs for.

There was a laboratory nearby but it was expensive. 'I don't have much money,' Demir says. 'I earn 350 euros a month and the test is 200 euros so it's more than half of my monthly income so it was a lousy month.' He couldn't afford the pills themselves but Jefferys said he would pay and arranged for the medication to be sent to a friend of Demir's in Croatia to avoid any problems with the Bosnian authorities. Twelve weeks after taking them, a test confirmed that there was no longer any trace of the hepatitis C virus in Demir's blood.

'It was deeply emotional,' he says. 'It's so much burden off your back. With that kind of disease it's like you are always expecting something. There could be something in front of you. Whatever plans you make you have "What if?", "What if liver cancer appears?".

'I thought hepatitis C was something that was going to stay with me for all my life.'

Deidre Waxman, a Massachusetts mother of two, has been battling the rising price of insulin since being diagnosed with type 1 diabetes at the age of sixty in 2011.

The cost of the injections which keep her alive weren't very noticeable at first; she was covered by health insurance and the portion of each prescription she was required to pay remained modest. Unbeknown to her, however, the price of insulin in the United States was rising sharply. In 2016, she hit her sixty-fifth birthday and moved to Medicare, the American health insurance programme for the elderly, and suddenly found herself much more directly exposed to the price of the medications. Waxman's co-payments for the two types of insulin she needed went up to nearly $200 a month and, having spent time helping her elderly social work clients get on Medicare, she was acutely aware of a danger that lay in store. For years, Medicare set a threshold over which patients were required to cover the full cost of medicines until they reached a second, higher threshold known as the 'catastrophe limit', after which they were fully covered again. The gap between the two thresholds became known as the doughnut hole and by 2019, when the system was changed, this difference amounted to nearly $1,300.[6]

Waxman, who only works part-time, didn't have the money she would have to pay if she hit this limit, so she came up with an alternative plan. She had friends in Canada who were also diabetic. 'I checked with them about the prices and they were radically different,' she says. The drugs were widely available to American citizens in Canada at up to one-tenth of their price back home.

On that first trip, after making the six-hour drive from her home in Newton to Montreal and nervously navigating the border checks, breathing a sigh of relief when they didn't look inside her car, she had only brought back enough for a few months. On later trips the haul expanded as she brought back insulin for friends. A box of five vials which might cost the best part of $1,000 in the US cost just $67 at Canadian pharmacies. Later, Waxman's husband's job took him to Canada for six months and he would return home with more vials packed into his suitcase, hoping the medication, which usually requires refrigeration, had remained sufficiently cool.

Every year, tens of thousands of Americans drive across the northern border to access the life-saving vials of insulin they need at an affordable price. Although it is technically illegal to import most prescription medicines, customs officials tend to look the other way for those bringing back up to three months of supplies for personal use. Canada doesn't require prescriptions for insulin.

For Americans living within close range, a twenty- or thirty-minute drive into Canada has long been an easy way to save hundreds of dollars on drugs for arthritis, high cholesterol or other common ailments. In the early 2000s, three towns in Michigan even organised free trips for their citizens to pick up cheaper Canadian medications.[7] More recently, politicians and activists have organised several insulin 'caravans', driving buses across the border to highlight the high cost of insulin in the United States. Bernie Sanders, the veteran left-wing politician, led one such trip in 2019 during his campaign to be the Democratic party's presidential candidate, using it to call the disparity in prices a 'national embarrassment'.[8]

Waxman believes the pricing is 'unadulterated greed', with a vial costing $6 to $8 to make being sold for twenty or thirty times that. She also questions why the only three manufacturers of insulin in the US 'raised their prices in lockstep' with one another. In recent years, she has become involved in activism through the non-profit Right Care Alliance, moved to action by her own situation and the plight of friends. 'There's been a lot of people that I know personally that have lost their adult children to insulin rationing,' she says.

On a frigid day in mid-November 2018, Waxman and dozens of others took part in a 'die-in' outside Sanofi's offices in Cambridge, Massachusetts, echoing the actions of activists who challenged the price of the AIDS drug AZT. The cremated ashes of two diabetics who died while rationing insulin were brought to the protest by their parents. One of the mothers, Antoinette Worsham, told a Boston radio station that her daughter, Antavia, just twenty-two, hadn't been able to afford the $1,000 monthly cost of the insulin she needed. 'It's either pay your rent, pay your car payment or get your medication,' she said.[9] A year later, during a protest which saw blood poured on the pavement outside an Eli Lilly research building, Waxman took the microphone:

'We call on Eli Lilly and the three-legged monopoly to cease and desist killing our fellow diabetics with their appalling greed,' she said.

'We call on them to put patients over profits and we call on them to do it now.'[10]

As well as joining protests, Waxman has also been involved in helping other diabetics access the medication they need to keep them alive. Through a series of Facebook groups and Internet forums, Waxman and as many as sixty other civic-minded volunteers co-ordinate what amounts to an underground insulin network, linking up those with vials to spare with those desperately in need. 'We put the word out to each other in the diabetes online community,' she says. It is a network built entirely on good deeds, with no money changing hands.

Until she turned sixty-five, Waxman's private health insurance and low co-pay allowed her to build up a stash of insulin which she would mail out to needy diabetics in places like South Carolina and California. 'Before I was on Medicare I gave away thousands of dollars of insulin to people who were going to die without it,' she says.

Now she acts as a conduit for diabetics desperate for help, sometimes breaking the law to do it. Each morning and throughout the day she regularly logs onto her laptop or checks her phone for new messages. 'Unless I'm asleep, I'm on it,' she says.

'I had one person caught up in a very messy divorce and on social security disability and she couldn't get on government assistance for two years. It's hard to get on government assistance here, even if you deserve it. So she couldn't afford insulin and she was absolutely willing to take anything from anybody. I'm talking expired drugs, or [types of] insulin that she'd never used before, or pens, vials, just anything. Really it breaks your heart,' Waxman says. The woman was sent $2,000 worth of insulin in the mail.

On another occasion, a friend of Waxman had unused insulin to give away after his daughter died unexpectedly. 'I got information about somebody in Colorado who was really on edge about not having enough insulin and I went to the post office and sent her $6,000 worth of insulin . . . Now that is really scary,' she says. 'Going to the US post office and sending insulin, which is illegal unless you have a DEA licence, with your name as the return addressee. Every time I do it, I go and bite my nails and think, "Oh my God, I hope that this person gets it and that [postal workers] don't look in it," you know? But I've done it many times . . . because you can't just sit there and watch people die,' she says.

For a while, much of the coordinating was done through Facebook groups, but it became more difficult in 2019 after the social media giant decided this breached their terms and conditions. 'At this time Facebook has shut them down so it becomes harder to help people online lately. Sometimes, when we put down what we have or what we need, we'll scramble the letters so Facebook won't pick up the key words but we all know what we're talking about,' Waxman says. Volunteers have also turned to other, more secure messaging services.

Pia was only a few months old when her mother noticed something was wrong.

'At first everything was just great, a normal baby,' Ellen De Meyer says. 'And then when she was about three and a half months old, I started to notice that she wasn't holding her head up. And when I laid her down on her belly she wasn't moving.'[11]

Pia was quieter than usual too, able to make only a faint sound even when she was crying, so De Meyer, thirty-three, took her to see a local doctor close to where she and her husband, Tim Boehnke, thirty-seven, live in Antwerp, Belgium.

De Meyer, who also has a young son, Briek, who is three, was told not to worry, that some babies were just a bit slower to develop than others. But she was sure it was more serious than that and persisted. A second doctor diagnosed floppy baby syndrome and referred her on to a specialist to find the cause. After several tests, the neurologist had the answer. 'OK, she probably has SMA,' she told Pia's parents. 'It will be the end.'

SMA stood for spinal muscular atrophy, an inherited muscle-wasting condition caused by a faulty gene. Until very recently, a diagnosis of type 1 SMA was effectively a death sentence, with most infants unable to ever speak or walk and rarely making it beyond their second birthday.

As they returned home and despairingly searched the internet for information on the disease, they read about a recently launched drug which appeared to offer some hope: Spinraza. Approved by the European medicine regulator in May 2017, Spinraza was the first treatment to target the underlying cause of SMA and trials suggested it could slow, or even stop, the condition's progression. At €88,000 a dose – with four needed initially, and then three more every year for life – it was extremely expensive but it offered hope, even if the regular administering of an injection into her spinal cord would be far from comfortable for Pia.

When Spinraza was launched, several European countries had deemed it unreasonably expensive and refused to offer it to patients. Fortunately, as Pia's parents discovered when they went back to hospital a week later to receive the results of a DNA test which confirmed their daughter's diagnosis, Belgium's national health system had reached an agreement with the manufacturer in 2018 and would cover the cost of the drug, at least until Pia turned two. They could start the treatment the following day.

The new neurologist also mentioned another breakthrough treatment: a gene therapy called Zolgensma. 'I haven't seen much before that renowned scientists would call a miracle,' the neurologist said, 'except for this drug.' Zolgensma wasn't quite a cure – it's still too new for any detailed evidence of its long-term effects – but it had proved highly effective in clinical trials. A one-time dose uses a virus to add a working copy of the SMN1 gene which is defective in babies born with SMA and promises to stop the disease in its tracks. The treatment seemed likely to be more effective than Spinraza, potentially allowing Pia to walk one day, and, as a single shot, there would be no need to worry about whether it would continue to be covered by Belgium's health system throughout her life.

Like many novel drugs, the gene therapy has its origins in publicly funded work, in this case by US academics and a French charity. During its development, several American charities raised millions to allow the research to continue.[12] It was licensed to AveXis, a Chicago-based firm co-founded by a medical researcher, Brian Kaspar, which was bought by the Swiss drugmaker Novartis for $9 billion in 2018, shortly before the drug was ready for launch. The breakthrough drug came with a breakthrough price tag: more than $2.1 million, making it the world's most expensive drug.[13]

It hadn't yet been approved in Europe, and so the Belgian government wouldn't cover the cost. But, in a stroke of apparent good fortune, a clinical trial for the drug was due to begin in Belgium a few weeks later. Pia's neurologist promised to do everything she could to get her enrolled but she was too late; the trial was full. De Meyer and her husband turned to the manufacturer, Novartis, instead, firing off emails to executives to see if there might be another way to get the drug. They were told they'd have to pay the full market price.

'I think the first thing we said was, "OK, it ends there",' De Meyer says. 'But then you don't give up. I literally went to bed every night thinking we need to do whatever it takes. To know the drug is out there and it's just a matter of money to get it, it was really difficult for us.' They decided to get into 'battle mode'. If the health service and the manufacturer wouldn't help, they would have to get the money together themselves.

De Meyer is a law clerk and her husband works in sales. Neither had any experience in raising funds on this scale but with help from relatives they set up social media pages and a website for 'Team Pia'. Friends held wine sales and cheese-tasting events and they solicited donations through the crowdfunding website GoFundMe. All told, in the space of two months they had raised nearly €100,000, a sizeable haul but nowhere near enough to pay for the drug. It was now July and they knew that, because Zolgensma is more effective the earlier it is given, every day that passed came with the permanent loss of motor neuron cells.

Then a friend came up with a new idea. Why didn't they set up a campaign where people could send a text and automatically donate? It need only be a small sum — two euros, say — but with enough people they could raise the money they needed.

The campaign launched on a Wednesday evening in September 2019. 'At first it was just our friends who shared it and their friends and family. And then we noticed that here in Antwerp it started to live a little bit.' De Meyer was regularly checking in on the numbers. By Sunday evening they had received 20,000 text messages. The next day, a friend who worked for a big electronic music festival asked two well-known musicians, DJs Dimitri Vegas and Like Mike, to share it on Facebook. Things quickly snowballed. De Meyer spent her lunch break doing interviews with radio stations and fielding questions from print reporters. She gave her login details to a reporter at the country's biggest-selling newspaper, *HLN*, so they could check the latest text message count and soon a banner was emblazoned across the paper's website homepage giving the latest updates.

The whole country was gripped. 'I could refresh every few seconds and another 500 or 1,000 have come in. It was crazy,' De Meyer says. That evening they reached 300,000 and the number had doubled again by Tuesday afternoon. The publicity had also drawn attention to the charges being levelled by telecoms companies on each dona-tion but a torrent of angry social media users quickly resulted in these being dropped, ensuring that Pia's fund would receive the full two euros from every text.

Two news crews joined the family that evening as the counter ticked past 850,000, eager to capture the moment they reached their goal. De Meyer had spent the past two days worried that they might raise a huge sum – €1m or €1.5m perhaps – but still fall hundreds of thousands of euros short of what they needed to actually buy the medicine. It was only then she realised it was going to succeed.

The TV crews wanted to stay all night but by 11 p.m. De Meyer had had enough. She announced that she was going to bed and kicked them out, promising they could come back first thing. So it was on her own, at 3 a.m. in the morning when she got up to make a bottle for Pia, that she checked and saw they'd done it. More than 950,000 texts – the equivalent of almost one in ten Belgians – had been received.

Three weeks later, on a grey autumn day, De Meyer and Boehnke accompanied Pia as she was transferred from the paediatric wing to the intensive care unit at Antwerp University Hospital.

There they entered one of the hospital's 'clean rooms' and watched nervously as, over the course of an hour, doctors dressed in scrubs and masks injected the contents of six small bottles into a tube inserted into one of Pia's veins. Just over 50ml of a clear liquid, purchased at a cost of €1,945,000 by wiring a bank transfer to Novartis.[14]

In early November, a few weeks after the gene therapy had been injected, they began to notice improvements. Pia could pick things up with her hands and her ability to control her head improved. 'When she cried, she cried like a real baby,' De Meyer says, and a week or two later she started to roll over by herself. 'That was a milestone because that was something that she would never have been able to do without the drug.'

Pia lies behind De Meyer, babbling in her cot as her mother speaks. The physical therapist reports that she is starting to use her muscles more and her parents are hopeful that, thanks to Zolgensma, she'll be able to live an independent life, even if she has to use a wheelchair.

De Meyer is grateful for the opportunities Zolgensma has created for Pia but she is sharply critical of the price. Biogen's Spinraza had been the first treatment for an otherwise fatal rare disease and had exploited that pricing power. Novartis in turn used that benchmark to justify its own price. It represented good value, Novartis argued, because it was just half the cost of ten years of Spinraza. 'I don't think the price is fair in any way,' De Meyer says. 'I understand they need to make a profit but making a therapy that can help children who are suffering from a terrible disease and asking $2.125 million for it is in my opinion in no way justified.'

If Pia's case shows both the promise and the failure of the drug industry – an incredible scientific advance, but one out of reach for so many who would benefit – then Greg Jefferys and Deidre Waxman show that drug companies, however powerful, cannot prevent individuals from fighting back. Even while governments' responses are inadequate, a few brave and resourceful individuals can make real headway in resisting the pursuit of maximum profits at the expense of access for patients.

Buyers' clubs, like the one set up by Jefferys, have sprung up for a number of high-priced breakthrough drugs as patients help one another to obtain the medications they need. The benefits these efforts can offer go beyond the patients directly helped, adding to pressure on a drugmaker to strike a deal to sell the drug on a more affordable basis in order to avoid losing future sales in that country from patients going online and obtaining it themselves. When the British health service failed to reach an agreement with Vertex over the price of a new cystic fibrosis treatment, patients gathered together to share information and travelled to Argentina to buy the medication. After a long stand-off, Vertex eventually agreed to a price cut which allowed the NHS to cover the drug.

Patients can have a real impact on the pricing of specific medicines, as Peter Staley and his fellow activists had shown in the late 1980s, and, increasingly, doctors have also taken a prominent role in challenging the state of affairs. Much of the pricing behaviour of the last twenty years has relied on the silent complicity of participants in the healthcare system, but some companies remain responsive to the spectre of bad publicity.

In 2012, Dr Leonard Saltz, the gastroenterology specialist at Memorial Sloan Kettering Cancer Center in New York, was getting ready to approve the use of a new cancer drug, Zaltrap, at the hospital. 'I was writing up the paperwork to put it on the formulary because it's a new FDA-approved drug and one of the pharmacists I worked with emailed me and said, "Are you aware of the cost?"'[15] Despite initial hopes it could represent a major therapeutic advance, clinical studies had shown Zaltrap to be no more effective than a drug that was already on the market, Avastin.[16] When Saltz opened the email from the pharmacist, however, he was in for a shock. 'The cost of Zaltrap was more than double the cost of Avastin,' he says. 'We're talking many thousands of dollars per month difference.'

He wrote to seventeen other doctors at the hospital. 'You all know the efficacy level of this drug,' he wrote. 'What I just learned is this price issue. Given this, I don't have any plans to use the drug. Do any of you?' When his colleagues all replied to say they didn't, Saltz took the then unprecedented decision not to put it on the formulary because of its cost. After discussions with Peter Bach, who worked upstairs, they decided to take another novel step, penning an op-ed for the *New York Times* denouncing the price of the drug. 'Soaring spending has presented the medical community with a new obligation,' they wrote. 'When choosing treatments for patients, we have to consider the financial strains they may cause alongside the benefits they may deliver.'[17]

Bach believed that the only restraint on pricing was shaming companies when their prices were too high. Sure enough, three weeks later, stung by the outcry, Sanofi cut the price in half.[18] 'It showed just what a fiction these prices are; that the company could come out with one price and within a few weeks just decide to sell the drug for half,' Saltz says.

By helping people navigate personal importation laws, buyers' clubs serve to undermine or manoeuvre around the monopoly power granted by patents. Activists have also advocated a more direct challenge to the way in which drug companies divide up global markets and concentrate on the wealthiest countries. When a situation demands it, some even go as far as calling for the protections granted by intellectual property rights to be tackled head-on.

In the late 1990s, as Americans enjoyed the benefits of combination antiretroviral drugs which had turned a previously fatal disease into a manageable chronic condition, sub-Saharan Africa was in the grip of an AIDS epidemic. In South Africa alone, half a million people were becoming infected with HIV each year while across the continent the total number of HIV-positive patients had reached 20 million. Western drugmakers sold the pills for the same price in South Africa as they charged in the United States, amounting to $1,000 a month.[19] It was just about affordable for white middle-class professionals, but was unthinkable for the vast majority of the population in a country with an average income of $2,600 a year. Meanwhile, the government-funded public health system couldn't afford to pay even the reduced rates drug companies were demanding.

In December 1997, the South African government passed legislation which would allow them to buy cheaper versions of antiretrovirals from abroad. The South African government insisted that this wasn't a challenge to international agreements on patent law as these didn't prevent imports of cheaper medicines, but the pharmaceutical industry construed it as a direct threat to their patent rights and responded by filing a legal challenge in February 1998. The case would become an international sensation.

The drugmakers' challenge was backed up by the US government which, at the urging of the industry's powerful trade association, tried to force the South African government to reverse course. The US ambassador wrote a strongly worded letter to officials and South Africa was put on a watch list and threatened with trade sanctions. As the legal action dragged on, activists fought for access to the drugs that would save their lives. One group, calling themselves the Christopher Moraka Defiance Campaign after a colleague who had died of AIDS, arranged to buy 3,000 capsules of a generic version of a Pfizer drug.[20] They brought the pills back from Thailand, where they had cost 7 per cent of what the drug company was charging the South African government, but the shipment was confiscated by police as contraband.

By this point in 2000, US policy had changed and President Clinton promised not to challenge efforts by developing countries to access AIDS medicines. The manufacturers' legal case was paused and would eventually be dropped a year later, with the thirty-nine companies involved agreeing to pay the South African government's costs.[21] In the meantime, however, little was changing for South African AIDS patients. The government still viewed the combination drugs known as the 'AIDS cocktail' as too expensive, even at the lower price available abroad, and it didn't help that Thabo Mbeki, who had been elected as the country's president in 1999, was an AIDS denier.[22] In July 2000, an annual international AIDS conference was held in South

Africa for the first time. The opening speech was given by Nkosi Johnson, an eleven-year-old boy who had been born HIV-positive. He recounted attending his mother's funeral and called on the government to start providing AZT to pregnant mothers 'to stop the virus being passed on to their babies'. 'I think the government must start doing it because I don't want babies to die,' he added.[23] Mbeki walked out of the conference hall during Johnson's speech.[24]

Into this stalemate came Yusuf Hamied, an Indian chemist who ran Cipla, a generic drug manufacturer founded by his father. Since the early 1970s, in response to what it deemed excessively high prices, the Indian government had refused to recognise patents on drugs, leaving Hamied and others free to make low-priced copies of blockbuster medicines.[25] India had finally been reined in when it signed up to a 1995 international trade agreement on patent rights, but the terms of the deal included a lengthy ten-year transition period during which manufacturing of generic versions of drugs which were patent-protected elsewhere could continue.

One night in August 2000, several men gathered at Hamied's London flat for a clandestine meeting. Among them were two Americans: Bill Haddad, a former investigative journalist turned campaigner for generic drugs, and Jamie Love, the intellectual property activist. Love and a colleague were the first to arrive, and he hit it off with Hamied almost immediately. 'What I liked about Dr Hamied was he was sort of a cowboy,' Love says. 'I was used to dealing with corporations where they would retreat and discuss things. With Dr Hamied you could just sit down and get something done with him.'[26]

Love had a question. 'I said, "Let's be quite open", you know, we're really trying to figure out what it would actually cost if he didn't have to worry about patents or anything like that. What would it cost to actually make the drugs?' Hamied had already given it some thought and decided that Triomune, a combination of Nevirapine, 3TC and D4T, was the AIDS cocktail with the cheapest active ingredients. He told Love that, taking into account distribution and other costs, he could sell it to the government for $800 a year per patient.

'So I said, "Suppose I just drive a truck up to your factory and

load it up and pay you with cash, then what would the price be?"'
Love recalls. Hamied said in that case he could do Nevirapine for
65 cents a day, 3TC for 35 cents and D4T was so cheap he would
throw it in for free – a price of $1 a day.

A month later, Hamied was invited to speak at a conference
organised by the European Commission. There, before health minis-
ters and pharmaceutical bosses, he announced plans to offer one of
the triple-drug cocktails for $800, well below 10 per cent of the price
multinational drug companies were charging. He invited other drug
companies to follow his lead and drop their prices. 'It is up to you,
the international community, to grasp this opportunity . . . to alleviate
the suffering of millions of our fellow men who are afflicted with
HIV and AIDS,' he proclaimed.[27]

Several months later, in February 2001, Love wrote to Hamied to
push him on the price; could he do it for the $1 a day he'd mentioned,
he asked. This was the price of the active ingredients alone, meaning
Cipla wouldn't recover its own costs, and Hamied was initially reluctant. 'He said no because then everyone will want it and that's a price
based on the idea that you take care of the distribution and you pay
cash and that's not what's going to happen elsewhere,' Love says. He
suggested Hamied could describe it as a charitable gesture purely for
the non-profit Médecins Sans Frontières. What was important at this
point was not that drugs would immediately be available at this price
on a mass scale, but to show that a dramatic reduction in price was
possible; that treating patients in Africa needn't cost a couple of
thousand dollars a day, it could be just a few hundred. 'I said, "I
need something that isn't incremental. I need to capture people's
attention." So he trusted me on that,' Love says. Hamied agreed to
do it. 'We said we are making so many drugs, if we lose on one or
two drugs, what difference does it make?' he later told an interviewer.
'It's a cause. It was a humanitarian approach.'[28]

His offer to supply Médecins Sans Frontières at $350 a year, slightly
below $1 a day, made the front page of the following day's *New York
Times*. 'It was dramatic, it was shocking, it completely changed everything,' Love says. 'It had a bigger effect than I expected.' Drugmakers

had claimed that these AIDS drugs could never be sold so cheaply but Hamied's offer would demolish that argument.

As well as driving down costs, the landmark price tag helped to fundamentally shift the scope of policy debates. If 30 million people could be kept alive for $1 a day, it created a moral imperative for international organisations and Western governments to act. Until that point, some efforts to tackle the AIDS epidemic in Africa had been focused on persuading large drug companies to cut the price of their brand-name drugs. It was now clear that generic drugs would provide the answer. Love says it was a 'game changer', transforming the Bush Administration's approach and prompting UN Secretary General Kofi Annan's call for a global fund to battle AIDS. The Clinton Foundation was also instrumental in taking advantage of generic versions of antiretroviral cocktails to help developing countries secure the drugs for a price which eventually fell below $100 a year. These programmes saved millions of lives.

The legal dispute over South Africa's attempt to explicitly allow so-called 'parallel imports' of cheap AIDS drugs centred around a 1995 agreement which saw the adoption of minimum standards of patent protection around the world. It was this deal, the TRIPS agreement, which meant patents for medicines became obtainable in India a decade later in a major victory for drug companies. But lingering concerns from developing countries over the ability to afford new medicines meant that the agreement also included a facility for countries to allow the manufacture of a patented medicine without the consent of the owner in certain circumstances. Intended as a push-in-case-of-emergency option, compulsory licensing allows a generic version of a drug to be produced for the domestic market, with a fee paid to the patent-holder.

Although South Africa's government had always insisted it had no plans to use compulsory licensing to access AIDS drugs, this tool has been used by other countries to make cheap antiretrovirals. Compulsory licensing originally required countries to manufacture the relevant drug domestically, rendering the provision useless for poor countries without the factories or expertise. But the 2001 Doha declaration recognised and removed this obstacle. It came into effect in 2006, allowing developing countries to issue a licence and for another country to manufacture a drug on its behalf. The provisions have been successfully used since then, although only on a handful of occasions. In 2007, Brazil used compulsory licensing to obtain cheap versions of a number of AIDS drugs while the following year the government of Rwanda granted a compulsory licence to a Canadian generics manufacturer to make three batches of an anti-retroviral.[29] More recently, Russia granted its first compulsory licence, for the cancer drug lenalidomide, in 2018, while two years later, the Israeli government granted a licence allowing a drug undergoing testing as a potential coronavirus treatment to be cheaply imported as a generic from India despite its patent-protected status.[30]

Drug companies are quick to seek the support of Western governments in trying to dissuade other countries from using compulsory licences. Nevertheless, the mere threat of issuing a compulsory licence can be an important tool in negotiations for fairer pricing for drugs. This has been demonstrated by the United States, which threatened to use the rights to obtain a treatment for anthrax in October 2001. The American government wanted to stockpile the antibiotic ciprofloxacin, which was covered by a patent owned by a German drugmaker, and warned it might issue a compulsory licence to make its own version if the price didn't come down. The manufacturer, Bayer, swiftly lowered the price.[31]

Compulsory licences give countries an opportunity to take matters into their own hands and several non-governmental organisations are strong advocates of issuing them, believing them to be vital to challenging drug companies' monopolies. However, for anything more than the occasional use, they are no substitute for much needed global reforms since the routine granting of compulsory licences would severely hamper the incentives for companies to fund innovative research. It is this conundrum, and the reforms required, to which we now turn.

CHAPTER TWELVE

A reckoning

'I think there's pretty universal agreement that the rising cost of healthcare in general and the rising cost of drugs in particular is unsustainable,' says Dr Leonard Saltz, the oncologist who sounded the alarm over the price of cancer drugs from a Chicago conference stage in 2015.

'It's a bubble, okay. All bubbles eventually burst. Whether it's, you know, tulip bulbs in Holland or ostrich feathers in South Africa or the internet around the turn of the millennium, bubbles burst if no one finds a way to rationally let the air out.'[1]

The transformations in the pharmaceutical industry over the past four decades have left a business model built on the premise of ever-higher revenues and, invariably, ever-higher prices. Global spending on prescription drugs after discounts and rebates is predicted to increase by up to 5 per cent a year, closing in on $1.2 trillion by 2024.[2]

But health budgets and insurance premiums are already higher than they've ever been and above-inflation increases in pharmaceutical spending must come at the expense of other priorities. Eventually, a tipping point at which society is no longer prepared to pay the sums demanded for drugs will surely be reached, and with the growing public outcry over drug prices and the enormous economic upheaval wrought by the coronavirus pandemic, there is good reason to believe that time is fast approaching.

The truth is the structure that has prevailed for decades is no longer working. Drug companies have exploited the loopholes and misaligned incentives that market failures, legislation and government regulations have created to hike the prices of old drugs and bring out hugely expensive new drugs in areas which are the most lucrative but not necessarily the most clinically useful. We need reforms to free up the funds to pay fair prices for genuinely innovative new drugs and prevent the price-hiking abuses which have plagued wealthy countries in recent years. Spending on drugs must be better aligned to clinical value – not on the industry's terms, as a means to justify ever-higher prices, but on terms which benefit the wider public. In the process, these changes must start to address the flaws in how research is currently incentivised and the inefficiencies created by a system predicated on patent rights and trade secrets. The goal is clear: we need to ensure that the drugs we get are the drugs we need at prices we can afford.

The founding social contract – a set period of monopoly power followed by the rapid entry of cheap generics – has been distorted almost beyond recognition by decades of bad behaviour and must be restored to its original terms. There is a legitimate debate to be had on the delicate balance between the rewards required to incentivise innovation and the need for drugs to be reasonably and affordably priced, but that needs to start with restoring control over the size of the rewards available. Central to this, and to solving access to medicine issues globally, is the importance of proper competition when a drug goes off patent; whether that be from traditional generics or biosimilars for biological medicines.

If companies can enjoy far longer exclusivity periods than the twenty-year patent term originally envisaged by deploying a toolkit of trickery and litigation, the additional revenue extracted serves no productive purpose beyond plumping up profits. There was already sufficient incentive for companies to undertake the risky research needed to bring them to market. Governments must use existing competition law or new legislation to crack down on evergreening and other attempts artificially to extend a drug's period of monopoly pricing such as by limiting access to samples needed to demonstrate the generic drug's equivalence or locking up the only source of the active ingredient of a drug. These practices harm consumers and patients by allowing R&D-led companies to continue selling their products at artificially high prices for far longer than would otherwise be possible.

Alongside this should come changes to how orphan drug status is awarded so that these benefits – including substantial R&D tax credits and an additional exclusivity period – are not simply boosting the profitability of blockbusters. There are now far too many orphan drugs, many of which stray far from the legislation's original intention to incentivise the development of products which would otherwise be abandoned on a laboratory shelf because there was no prospect of recouping the costs of bringing them to market. At minimum, orphan status should be limited to genuinely new drugs, excluding those already on the market for other indications, and, as others have suggested, the exclusivity period they provide should be curtailed once a drug reaches a certain revenue threshold – perhaps annual sales of $1 billion.[3]

These changes would help to enforce limits on how long a drug enjoys exclusivity, and with it monopoly pricing power. This power ends when a new drug which is at least clinically equivalent (if not better) is launched by a rival who elects to compete on price, or when copies of the original drug are launched by generic manufactures. Older medicines which have lost patent protection and gone generic are crucial to reducing pharmaceutical spending and improving access to medicines. When the generics market functions properly they are the industry's greatest gift to humankind, making the innovative drugs of a previous generation widely available as cheap commodities. But, as we have seen, a cadre of business executives have proven adept at taking advantage of market failures to increase the cost of drugs long after their patents and any other legal protections have ended.

Fines and other regulatory action can help to punish those who break competition laws but the basic practice amounts to exploiting

a market failure rather than anything unlawful. Abuses in pricing old
medicines are often reliant on a manufacturer having something close
to a monopoly. What is required, therefore, is to improve competition and, where the market is ailing, offer a credible threat of an
alternative source for generic drugs if prices get out of hand. To
achieve this, there is a strong case to be made for non-profit generic
drugs manufacturers, most likely funded by national governments.

Encouraging a national health system to produce some of its own
drugs harks back to an earlier era when hospital pharmacists would
regularly compound drugs for patients. In fact, in the Netherlands
the government has recently endorsed a return to this approach as
part of efforts to reduce the cost of expensive new drugs. A law
change in 2019 allows pharmacists to prepare patent-protected medicines as long as this is only for small numbers of people.

The British health service already has a small generics manufacturing facility of sorts. On the outskirts of a seaside town, workers
at Torbay Pharmaceuticals make several dozen injectable solutions
at a £26 million facility which opened in 2017. In the United States,
several large hospital owners, fed up with drug shortages and price
spikes, joined together in 2018 to create a new non-profit generic
manufacturer called Civica RX.

These possible solutions are never going to produce drugs as
cheaply as large multinational generics manufacturers, even if they
are operating on a non-profit model. But they are there as a backstop
rather than as a replacement; for emergency use when normal market
forces are not working.

They can also help another, antithetical problem. When generic
markets do function and there is adequate competition, there have
been cases where the buying power of large purchasers, particularly
national health systems, has driven down prices so far that manufacturers have struggled to turn a profit. The result in some cases is
companies pulling out of the market, causing supply problems and
creating the conditions ripe for the predatory price-hiking model.
State-owned pharmaceutical manufacturing facilities could step in in
such situations, even if only on a temporary basis, while modest

prices rises are allowed to restore incentives for private generics manufacturers. As the coronavirus pandemic has shown, the ability to make medicines within a country's borders can also serve as an important national strategic asset.

The use of generics still varies wildly between different countries, with the United States, where generics account for around nine in ten prescriptions, among the best, while Switzerland, with 17 per cent, is among the worst.[4] The picture is reversed on biosimilars – competing versions of biological drugs – where, as we have seen, the US has been very slow to encourage their introduction. Removing these barriers is vital, particularly as the industry focuses its resources on developing more and more biologics. Not only are biologics among the most expensive medicines, this lack of competition means healthcare systems have to bear these heightened costs for far longer than the typical period of patent protection. If efforts to encourage biosimilars to launch in sufficient numbers to compete on price don't work, an idea proposed by Peter Bach has merit. He suggests mandating price cuts once the original twelve-year US market exclusivity period for biologics ends. At this point, the price of the biologic would be required to be reduced to a level guaranteeing 10 per cent profit above the cost of producing and distributing the product, thereby ensuring significant savings for consumers without being reliant on the entry of biosimilars.[5]

Reasserting limits on a drug's period of exclusivity and encouraging the use of cheap generics and biosimilars are important steps in reforming society's bargain with the pharmaceutical industry. Without competition, and the ensuing significant fall in prices usually seen with generics, funds are not freed up for healthcare systems to use to pay for new medicines and the social contract simply doesn't work.

Tackling the high cost of new drugs, and balancing this with the desire to continue to incentivise privately-owned companies to pour billions into drug research, is a more complicated problem. The key question – the trillion-dollar conundrum – is how much slack is there in the current system? How quickly would drug companies need or want to cut their investment in drug development if sales revenues were squeezed; and if they did so, just how many potential new drugs would be lost?

That question goes to the heart of a long-running dispute between industry executives, academics and activists. On one hand, there are pharmaceutical bosses and lobbyists who argue that even the slightest hint of US price controls or other means of exerting significant downward pressure on drug sales will have a devastating effect on innovation. They would have you believe that there is no slack at all in the current system. The arguments used to buttress this – that R&D costs are enormous and rising and drug discovery very difficult – are genuine issues even if it doesn't follow that cuts to current profit levels would necessitate immediate and drastic swingeing cuts to R&D.

On the other hand, there are many critics who believe that R&D figures produced by the industry are not merely exaggerated, but are overstated by several orders of magnitude. The truth lies somewhere between these two extremes. It is undoubtedly the case that drug discovery is very expensive and, at least until very recently, had been getting dramatically more so. But it is also true that the expectations of biotech investors and large drug companies have reached perilous heights and there is scope for reducing rewards and readjusting expectations.

In any event, rising drug discovery costs are not reason alone for health systems to pay significantly more for each new drug. No other industry demands consumers pay for something simply because it has been expensive to produce, effectively asking the public to write a blank cheque for any failures, miscalculations and wasted money in its research efforts. It is up to drug companies to produce products with significant clinical value – and, crucially, to share that economic value with the purchaser – so that they can earn back enough money to cover the cost of failed projects and make a profit.

Even if the industry's pleadings were true, we are reaching the point where there is little choice; high drug prices are already causing grave consequences in access and inequality around the world.

'This comes across the wrong way from a Republican and someone who supports the drug industry. But I really believe we have to get to a point where we say, we give these patents as a society; they're not inalienable rights, we are granting that. In return, we expect responsible behaviour,' the former analyst David Maris says.[6]

'When you think of it from a broad economic standpoint, taxing the sick to pay for buybacks and dividends is really sickening. I think at some point you have to realise there are people that are showing up at the pharmacy who get told their bill and they walk away from the counter, from the medicine they need. They just walk away because they can't afford it.

'I'm not a bleeding heart liberal, I'm not, but I think of it as we give you patent protection, you have to act responsibly. If you're not going to act responsibly, then we have to do something more.'

As has become abundantly clear, prices are not as high as they are out of necessity but because companies believe they can get away with those levels. The deliberations of executives at Gilead as they debated where to set the launch price of their hepatitis C medicines are a clear example of this. Nor is there much to suggest pharmaceutical companies have slashed unnecessary costs to the bone. Drug industry executives remain lavishly rewarded for their efforts. Big Pharma's headquarters are invariably sprawling and spectacularly well-appointed campuses. And drug companies have been handing back vast sums for years in the form of legal settlements and fines. The opioid epidemic is just the latest example of this, with Purdue Pharma alone agreeing to hand over more than $8 billion in late 2020.[7]

Even Alex Azar, the former executive at Eli Lilly who was named secretary of health and human services in Trump's White House, has taken a sceptical view of the suggestion that there is no room at all for drug companies to accept lower profits without having to implement major cuts.

'Drug companies have insisted we can have new cures or affordable prices, but not both,' he said in 2018. 'I've been a drug company executive – I know the tired talking points: the idea that if one penny disappears from pharma profit margins, American innovation will grind to a halt. I'm not interested in hearing those talking points any more."[8]

If we accept that there is at least some slack before R&D has to be cut in a damaging way, it then becomes a question of behavioural change – weaning drug companies off the idea that every new drug must be substantially more expensive than those it seeks to replace, that share buybacks and other cash disbursements are the best way of growing a company for the long-term – and of practical ways of exerting downward pressure on drug prices and profits.

The biggest impact on growing drug prices comes from the US market, where the government won't negotiate prices and insurers can't drive the kind of hard bargains for cancer drugs and other pricey treatments that would be possible if they were able to walk away from the table and decline to provide drugs deemed too expensive. Recalibrating drug prices around the globe must therefore centre around changes to the US system. Prices for new drugs in the US cannot continue to race upwards, regardless of the relative clinical value of these products. The lack of push back during years of relatively minor advances in some areas has created a situation where genuinely breakthrough drugs can command six- or seven-figure sums. There are no hard and fast rules on the maximum percentage of GDP modern economies should commit to healthcare spending, but given the access problems that already exist it is a trajectory that is clearly unsustainable.

An easy first step is to end the habit of drugmakers imposing regular price rises for branded, patent-protected drugs which are already on the US market. These costs are almost never justified by new R&D costs or a sudden increase in manufacturing expenses; drugmakers are simply taking advantage of their market power. They've become addicted to these increases. A recent study of price rises associated with nine commonly prescribed drugs in America could find no evidence to justify the price increases of seven of the drugs which had together added $4.8 billion to spending over two years.[9]

Another relatively straightforward reform is to empower Medicare to directly negotiate the price of drugs covered under the Part D benefit for non-hospital drugs. An indication of the savings possible comes from the Department of Veterans Affairs, which routinely achieves savings of up to 50 per cent on those prices paid under Medicare Part D.[10]

Parts of the American healthcare system are already very effective at driving down prices. The eventual emergence of competition for Gilead's hepatitis C drugs showed how insurers can demand significant savings when they have a strong hand to play. But in other disease areas, particularly for the cancer drugs and treatments for rare diseases which, as we have seen, make up so much of the pipeline of new drugs, the push back has been almost non-existent. Instead, an increasing proportion of costs are transferred on to patients in the form of co-payments calculated as a percentage of a drug's list price, high deductibles which must be met before insurance kicks in and restrictive formularies (lists of drugs an insurer will cover) which limit access. It is this transfer of costs back to patients – a reversal of the growth in insurance which helped fuel drug spending growth in the 1990s – which has prompted the public outcry in the US as high drug prices leave more and people unable to afford their prescriptions.

The growing gap between list prices and net prices after discounts and rebates shows the scale of savings being achieved in some areas, but the opaque web of wholesalers, insurers and pharmacy benefit managers means that these savings are not consistently passed on to consumers. Insulin is a classic example of this problem. After years of bloviating, insulin manufacturers finally slashed prices but much of the savings have been absorbed by the middlemen. Fixing this will require transparency – so those in the system can see how money is flowing – and new rules to require savings to be passed on to patients.

Applying downward pressure to US drug prices is necessary given how pumped-up the market has become and the devastating consequences for many sick Americans, but it is also fraught with danger for other wealthy nations. From the industry's perspective, European countries benefit from a situation where America pays higher drug prices and subsidises R&D for everyone else. In reality, the overheated pricing environment has pulled up prices for everyone so far that European systems are struggling to control costs even as they pay less than their American counterparts. The air needs to come out of the bubble everywhere.

Some of the proposals which have found favour in American politics over the past decade or so are likely to prompt drugmakers to try and recoup reduced American prices by seeking higher prices elsewhere. Simply pegging US prices to the rest of the world, as has been supported on both sides of the political aisle, is likely to drive up prices internationally, outweighing, on a global scale, the benefits of reduced American drug costs. Similarly, allowing imports from Canada can help if limited to a small number of exceptional cases, but on a mass scale would lead to a crisis there as drug companies demand higher American prices.

In the short term, US pricing reforms would force other countries to use all the tools at their disposal to resist pressure from an industry looking to recoup the scale of profits it has become accustomed to in America. But meaningful push back on the most expensive medicines in the US healthcare system will ultimately benefit everyone. It can help to reset expectations around the pricing of new medicines, ending the conveyor belt effect which sees drugs priced at or above those charged for treatments in the same therapy area, regardless of how much more or less effective they are. With the US leading the way, other countries would be even better placed to use their own negotiations to drive down prices.

A truly global effort would remove the current danger of drug companies cherry-picking the most favourable markets and walking away from those seeking a much lower price. This is one of the biggest issues facing the otherwise relatively successful British approach to paying for new medicines. As well as requiring new drugs to pass a cost-effectiveness test, the British healthcare system currently has an agreement with drugmakers which sets a limit on

the growth of spending on branded medicines. For the duration of
the current scheme, which runs until 2024, that spending bill will
not increase by more than 2 per cent. If it grows by more, companies have to pay a proportion of their sales back to the British
government.[11] The scheme is effective at limiting the increase in
medicine spending – although the country's healthcare system, which
is under immense financial strain, would undoubtedly benefit from
a more ambitious goal – but is powerless to prevent companies from
withholding their drugs if they aren't happy with the price the UK
is willing to pay.

There are also questions over the long-term sustainability of this
approach, which is echoed in France and other countries, unless
changes in the United States help to bring down drug prices across
the board. More and more drugs require significant confidential
discounts from their announced prices in order to pass the UK's
cost-effectiveness test while spending pressures meant the country
had to bring in a budget impact test which can delay coverage of
some drugs even though they have been deemed cost-effective.
Beyond that, negotiating new five-year agreements with drugmakers
is likely to become harder as new drugs skew ever more towards
high-priced cancer and rare disease treatments where officials have
been persuaded to use a much higher QALY threshold for judging
whether a price is acceptable. Each of these high-cost medicines
accepted by the system equates to a financial hit for rival companies
and as the size of these payments increase so too will the pressure
for a higher spending cap.

In the last few years, there have been the first indications that drugmakers are starting to listen to public outrage at the levels drug prices
have reached in the US. The growth in list prices for branded drugs
has slowed significantly from above 13 per cent to around 4 per cent
a year in the space of five years up to 2020. Below that, net prices
– the amounts charged by manufacturers – actually fell by between
2.2 and 2.6 per cent for three straight years from 2018 to 2020,
according to data covering more than 90 per cent of US branded

drug sales.[12] This is a welcome and encouraging sign. But undoing years of escalating prices is going to take something more dramatic.

Some industry observers hope that change can come from within: with investors pushing companies to move beyond the mantra of 'maximising shareholder 'value' and the pursuit of the largest possible profits, encouraging them to instead take a broader long-term view of the need to do good by their customers and wider society. Perhaps the coronavirus pandemic can serve as a wake-up call reminding executives of the industry's true purpose.

Jayasree Iyer, who runs the Access to Medicine Foundation in the Netherlands, believes the pandemic has encouraged investors to hold companies accountable for their societal responsibilities. She argues that persuading companies to invest in developing drugs for important but not necessarily lucrative diseases requires these investors to 'start saying we're only going to invest in companies that are ready . . . to deal with the worst problems in the world. That is a shift that a company will have to look at and they may have to compromise their profit margins in order to make that space for the greater good.'[13] There is a role here for pharmaceutical industry employees too, she argues, as staff increasingly place importance on working 'for a company that actually has a strong social impact'.

In the meantime, there is another tool which policymakers can use to help drive down prices and also shape the kind of drugs we get: a lever which governments are, inexplicably, failing to use. Governments are struggling to afford pharmaceuticals despite the huge role public financing plays in drug development. The United States pours nearly $40 billion a year in taxpayer funds into medical research while the UK spends more than £3 billion. That money pays for scientists to push back the frontiers of science, exploring the underlying mechanisms behind diseases and identifying promising targets for therapeutic intervention. It pays for researchers who create new technologies which drug companies then use to develop new types of drugs. Recombinant DNA, the ability to alter genetic material to manufacture proteins which launched the biotechnology revolution, was invented by two academics, Stanley

Cohen and Herbert Boyer, working at Stanford University and the University of California, San Francisco. And public funds pay for the discovery of new small molecule compounds and biologics which can eventually make the leap from the lab to the market. As many as one in four new drugs were discovered at least in part in public sector research institutions, including a disproportionate number of the most novel drugs.[14] Nine in ten have benefited from the public funding of basic research which laid the platform for their development.[15]

But despite this impact, public funds largely serve to bolster the coffers of drugmakers. The insights which spur new approaches to drug discovery are not patentable and governments have failed to use the leverage of more immediately practical discoveries, such as new small molecule compounds, to demand both a fair share of the rewards and affordable pricing for patients.

In the aftermath of the AZT pricing scandal, the US National Institutes of Health (NIH) introduced a 'reasonable pricing' clause allowing it to revoke licences for compounds it had developed if the prices set by manufacturers for the eventual market-ready drugs were deemed excessive. However, the clause was abandoned a few years later under pressure from industry lobbying which claimed it was making companies unwilling to work with government scientists in developing drugs. Harold Varmus, the NIH's director at the time, took the view that pricing and access to medicines should simply not be a concern of scientists, even if they had contributed to a drug's development.[16]

That argument has carried the day ever since, removing a signifi-cant potential weapon from the arsenal of those charged with negotiating the price of new medicines. It doesn't prevent the NIH from seeking royalties from drug sales, but these amount to no more than $140 million a year, representing a tiny fraction of its annual budget.[17] When it has struck deals, they've rarely been viewed as securing favourable terms for taxpayers. In 2003, the NIH was censured for a deal involving the cancer drug Taxol, such was the paucity of returns the organisation had agreed to. The drug was developed with almost $500 million in public funding and licensed to Bristol-Myers Squibb, who launched it on the market in 1993. Over the following decade, the manufacturer paid $35 million in royalties while racking up sales of more than $9 billion.[18]

Universities have also been able to secure a cut of the profits when they've played a major role in developing the drugs but only a proportion of these windfalls go back into scientific research. Unlike the NIH, which sets a $150,000 per year cap, universities have not restricted the amount the individual researchers involved can receive and so their rewards can be vast – as when $210 million was split by three scientists after Emory University sold royalties for the HIV drug FTC for $525 million in 2005. In another large deal, UCLA sold its future royalties from Xtandi, a prostate cancer drug, for $520 million in 2016.[19] While the university's chemistry department and a medical institute were among the beneficiaries, UCLA said half the money would be put into an investment portfolio to fund future scholarships – an admirable scheme, but not one which contributes directly to future drug development or lower prices.

Meanwhile, countries have struggled to afford drugs they helped fund. The US drugmaker Janssen, the pharmaceutical arm of Johnson & Johnson (J&J), launched Zytiga, a new prostate cancer drug, in 2011 and it rapidly became a blockbuster. The drug works by interfering with testosterone production to slow the growth of cancer and a clinical trial found it extended the lives of patients with advanced prostate cancer by an average of four months. It originated from work done by scientists at the publicly-funded Institute of Cancer Research (ICR) in Sutton, south London, in the 1990s. A team led by Professor Mike Jarman wanted to find a way to suppress a testosterone-producing enzyme called cytochrome P17 which existing treatments couldn't reach. They had noticed that a substance called ketoconazole helped to inhibit this enzyme and sought to find a similar but more effective drug.[20] The compound they eventually alighted on was called abiraterone acetate. A team from ICR compiled a dossier for the first patent but, as a condition of the institute's government funding, had to assign the intellectual property to the

British Technology Group, a successor of two national bodies set up to help commercialise publicly-funded innovations. In 2004 the drug abiraterone acetate was licensed by BTG to Cougar Biotechnology, an American start-up. The clinical trials which followed were funded with significant contributions from cancer charities, the British Medical Research Council and direct funds from the government.[21] In 2009, with Phase III trials underway and showing significant promise, J&J bought Cougar Biotechnology for $1 billion.

Although public money had paved the way for the development of abiraterone at every step, when it came to setting a price it was entirely at the discretion of its new owner, J&J. The pharmaceutical giant opted for a price so high it initially failed the cost-effectiveness test carried out by NICE, meaning it wasn't recommended for use by the British health service.[22] It was only with a return to the negotiation table and another, larger, confidential discount on the list price that it was approved in 2012. Even then, there were restrictions, with patients required to be treated with chemotherapy first. It would be another four years, with further pricing discussions and demands for more clinical trial evidence, before this would change.

To the frustration of the ICR, the drug is still not available for newly diagnosed patients with advanced prostate cancer in England and Wales because it hasn't been deemed cost-effective for this group at the price the manufacturer is offering. The institute has criticised both sides for the stand-off and said it believed 'the price of new cancer drugs generally is too high and we want to see [them] come down' but the cost of clinical trials meant it had no choice but to partner with commercial organisations.

Abiraterone is not the only drug developed with public funds which that same country has then had difficulties accessing for financial reasons. Keytruda, a cancer drug which was developed with extensive funding from the Dutch government, was initially withheld from Dutch patients by the Ministry of Health because of its high cost. It was only after three months of negotiations secured a sizeable discount on the €100,000-a-year asking price that it was made available.[23] These examples highlight concerns that taxpayers are paying even more for drugs than the amount negotiated by a health-care system since they are effectively paying twice: first through funding its development, and then again when paying for the pills or injectable solutions.

The same dynamic has played out in the race to produce a Covid-19 vaccine. Governments poured huge funds into a range of attempts to develop a treatment to end the global pandemic. As we have seen, Moderna, one of the many biotech companies clustered around Harvard University and the Massachusetts Institute of Technology in the affluent city of Cambridge, was the biggest winner, receiving $1 billion in funding and a further $3.2 billion in advance orders. Scientists at the NIH's Vaccine Research Center played key roles in the development of the drug and Moderna agreed to pay undisclosed royalties, but there were no restrictions on pricing and the company's chief executive made it clear to investors he intended to maximise revenues.

The failure to attach pricing stipulations to publicly-funded drug development grants ultimately falls on politicians. The US govern-ment has long had the power to intervene. Legislation passed in 1980 includes a provision which allows the government to grant a licence to another manufacturer if a product which has emerged from federally-funded research is not made available to the public on 'reasonable terms'. Campaigners have suggested this phrase incor-porates the pricing of a drug and could therefore be invoked in a situation where a licence has been used to produce a drug which is not available at a reasonable price. The US government, however, has never tested it and other countries funding scientific research have similarly failed to attach conditions to their own contributions. Whatever the exact wording or form these take, it represents a powerful opportunity to require drug companies to open their books, to set reasonable limits on prices or profits, and even to use it as leverage for more radical reforms.

Some activists and academics propose a new model in which public funding replaces private capital and takes over all the costs of drug development. They cite the high levels of public spending on basic research and argue that, without a profit motive, government-run pharmaceutical R&D would be able to develop new drugs at a lower cost than the private sector. Handing over the role of taking discoveries through from ideas to products is, for the time being at least, unrealistic and undesirable. As long as the costs and risk of failure of clinical trials remain as high as they currently do, no government could be expected to gamble tens of billions of public money when they may ultimately have nothing to show taxpayers for it and there is little to suggest there would be major efficiency gains from a system which would have far fewer participants. Whilst there is more scope for public funding to step in to cover particular market failures – such as with antibiotics, or when there is a global emergency on the scale of Covid-19 – overall it is in society's interest that private companies remain incentivised to invest heavily in pharmaceutical R&D.

There is, however, much to be said for a big increase in public funding for bodies like the US National Institutes of Health, which carry out the basic science that eventually leads to clinical breakthroughs. This research doesn't have to be fixated on direct clinical use in the way industry-funded efforts are and, as history shows, novel drugs and other therapeutic interventions don't happen until scientific advances help create the understanding of a disease and viable drug targets. Public funding allows governments to shape research priorities and, in turn, help ensure we get the kind of drugs we need.

Better negotiation of drug prices in the United States and attaching conditions to public funding can help to drive down drug costs, while clamping down on the exploitation of patent laws and old generics will also help save money. But we shouldn't just be looking to bluntly cut costs; healthcare systems can also be smarter about how they allocate the funds they do spend.

At a global level, the present system has become skewed by the way in which high prices and sales can be disconnected from the clinical value of a drug. The solution is to create a clear and rational framework to show drugmakers what society deems useful and will pay for, and what it won't. If healthcare systems are smarter about how they use their limited resources, choosing which drugs are funded and in what circumstances, there should be more than enough money to reward companies who bring through the drugs we truly need even if we might end up with fewer new drugs each year.

'There's this concept [that] every drug is so useful that we cannot bear to live without it,' says Dr Leonard Saltz.[24] It is a myth that needs exploding. The current system, with indiscriminate high pricing, encourages drug companies to develop a steady stream of new drugs based on their perceived commercial rather than clinical value. The same twenty-year patent term applies to a 'new' drug which is little more than a minor change to the chemical structure of an older product just as it does to a truly revolutionary innovation. It is fuelling, particularly in the United States, huge amounts of unnecessary spending on drugs. 'We've created this artificial situation that allows for drugs with the most mediocre sleight-of-hand advancement to get on the market and then be priced at an absurd level,' Saltz says. 'If you only had the budget to develop the drugs that were looking the most [clinically] promising, you'd kill an awful lot of drugs earlier in development and save your development costs for those drugs that are making more substantial advantages.' Saltz argues that drugs which represent only minor improvements cost more to develop, requiring huge trials to show an effect of statistical significance. 'When you have a really good drug, you can get a definitive trial with under 100 patients,' he says. By adopting a European approach which seeks to assign a clinical value to drugs and to use that to determine a reasonable price, the American healthcare system can become more selective about the drugs it chooses to pay for. The tools for such a change are already in place.

When Steve Pearson founded the grandiose-sounding Institute for Clinical and Economic Review (ICER) it was little more than a name on a letterhead. 'It was kind of a joke,' he says. '"Institute" was just me.'[25]

After training as a doctor, Pearson had won a fellowship which allowed him to spend a year at Britain's cost-effectiveness body, NICE. He returned to the United States determined to set up an independent body which would take a similar approach – seeking to establish a fair price for medical treatments. In Europe, it is perfectly normal for debates about healthcare to discuss how best to deploy limited resources but he knew that in the United States attitudes were very different. 'We didn't yet have that kind of system in which that kind of . . . honesty would be able to be politically viable,' Pearson says. Nor are there public budgets for healthcare in the same way, 'but the same kind of tensions around evidence and around how to allocate resources certainly existed'.

ICER was set up as a grant-funded research project at Harvard Medical School, where Pearson works. 'I wanted to . . . experiment with ways to do evidence reviews, weaving in all the broader contextual and ethical issues, talk about costs and cost-effectiveness, but figure out how to do it in a way that could advance the public dialogue on these issues in the United States,' he says. Fifteen years later, ICER has offices in the heart of Boston's financial district, employs thirty staff and already plays an important role in national conversations about drug pricing.

ICER started by examining healthcare costs in general and its first reports looked at radiation therapy and surgical robots. It turned its focus firmly onto drug pricing in the wake of the public debate around Gilead's hepatitis C drugs in 2014, when its report on Harvoni drew significant attention as individual US states grappled with the enormous costs of this new cure. Gilead's drugs brought the kind of conversations ICER had been seeking to provoke out into the open.

'It created tremendous tension in the US healthcare system that was completely ill-equipped to deal with the idea of [rationing],' Pearson says. 'Should we try to pick just the sickest patients and treat them first in order to smooth out the budget impact so that we don't do damage to other parts of the health system? . . . Legally [and] culturally, it's very hard for us to talk that way.'

The body works by reviewing the evidence around a drug's

effectiveness and canvassing for views on additional benefits or disad-
vantages which are not captured by clinical trial data – issues around
the severity of the illness, for example, or whether the drug is the
first ever available for a particular condition or patient group.

ICER requires a drug's benefit over existing treatment options to
fall into the range of $50,000 to $150,000 per year of good health
to be deemed cost-effective. This threshold is significantly higher
than Britain's NICE, which typically requires drugs to fall within
£20,000 to £30,000 per QALY. Even with the higher threshold, only
around a quarter of the US drugs ICER has examined have been
deemed reasonably priced. In Harvoni's case, ICER determined that
the price was cost-effective for the benefit it provided over the existing
interferon-based treatments but nevertheless represented 'low value'
to health systems because of the budgetary impact. It suggested the
price should be cut by more than 50 per cent, to between $34,000
and $42,000 per course of treatment, in order to allow insurers to
provide the drug to all those who needed it.[26]

ICER now includes a recommended price in all its reports and
Pearson says these figures are already being used by insurers and
other payers, including the US Department of Veterans Affairs, in
negotiations with drug companies. 'I think one of my favourite terms
was "it stiffened my spine when I went into the room to negotiate
a price",' he says.

When he set up ICER, Pearson was under no illusions about the
difficulties he would face. The body was challenging powerful corporate interests. 'Would any industry welcome an outside entity saying
here's what a fair price would be when you have a monopoly? There's
no reason that they would welcome this,' he says. 'We instantaneously
became kind of public enemy number one.' Patient groups were
sceptical too. After all, high prices for drugs treating one particular
condition can help to attract more investment. Some of the skirmishes
have been ugly. 'When we get attacked it can get very personal,'
Pearson says. He's been called a eugenicist and accused of wanting
old and disabled people to die. One of his colleagues was involved
in a heated public meeting to discuss the value of a cancer drug and

was then the subject of social media attacks telling them 'I hope your kid gets this condition'. Like the New York cancer doctor Peter Bach, Pearson has been a regular target for an industry-funded organisation called Patients Rising which claims to offer a voice to 'people living with chronic and life-threatening illnesses' and presents the pair as a threat to innovation and access to drugs. The non-profit's argument that 'every patient deserves access to the best healthcare' comes with the unwritten conclusion that this should be regardless of the cost and it is little surprise it is bankrolled by large drug companies.[27]

Still, Pearson understands some of the concerns. 'Cost-effectiveness can be used in an inappropriate way to say that if we have a limited resource, we should give it to people who are running around, as opposed to people who are in a wheelchair.' Pearson argues that society has to make a judgement on what it values, allowing, as with Britain's NICE, for different cost-effectiveness thresholds for rare diseases and end-of-life care.

ICER's approach helps to restore rationality to spending decisions and could lead to some immediate savings. If the most commonly used drugs in America were re-priced according to ICER's definition of a fair price this alone would save billions, Pearson says. Encouraging insurers and other payers to say no to over-priced or ineffective drugs would also free up funds, while creating a clear framework for what is deemed valuable innovation can guide drug companies towards focusing R&D on the most beneficial areas.

Health technology assessments (HTAs) help to decide if a drug is worth using. By experimenting with different QALY thresholds they can also help to control spending, ensuring it is aligned with budgetary pressures. Some argue that the threshold should be no higher than the figure that has effectively been attached to expenditure in other parts of a healthcare system. Researchers at the University of York led by the health economist Karl Claxton have shown that approving new drugs which cost more than around £15,000 per QALY does more harm than good by reallocating funds away from other healthcare spending. The true threshold should therefore be half of the figure typically used to assess new medicines.

'When NICE approves a new drug at £30,000 per QALY, then the health benefits we get from that drug are more than offset to a factor of two by the harms in terms of QALYs lost elsewhere in the healthcare system,' he says.[28]

Professor Claxton, who is in his early fifties with close-cropped hair and a punkish hooped earring in his left ear, argues that NICE has become too close to the pharmaceutical industry and too susceptible to political pressure when making decisions as to whether to approve a drug as cost-effective. 'Instead of fulfilling its primary mission, which was to look after all NHS patients, it sees its primary job as making sure we get some kind of approval for the next oncology drug,' he says. Research has shown that NICE has approved a number of drugs even though their cost-effectiveness was deemed to be above the thresholds the watchdog has set.[29]

The professor, who was involved in NICE's establishment in 1999 and spent more than a decade on the cost-effectiveness body's appraisal committees, also questions why society has deemed it fair to set much higher QALY thresholds for end-of-life treatments and drugs treating rare diseases.

'There's very little out there that empirically justifies placing a greater weight on the health gains in a rare disease . . . than the same health gains in a disease that just happens to be more common,' he says.

Doing so has incentivised the investment in rare-disease treatments, and in slicing up common diseases so they can be deemed rare, producing the flurry of high-priced drugs which have emerged. A partial reduction in the higher QALY thresholds granted to certain types of drugs could help rebalance the whole system. As Claxton argues, health systems need to 'stop paying more than we can afford for new oncology drugs because if we did that, all of a sudden, other areas of research would look a lot less risky and a lot more lucrative . . . At the moment [if] you can get a return [on investment] by successfully getting the next oncology drug – with no evidence of overall survival benefit – through the FDA then why wouldn't you do it?'[30]

Health systems using cost-effectiveness tests must include all alternative treatments for a disease, including any cheap generics available, when making determinations. If drugs are only compared to high-priced patent-protected medicines, drugs can be made to look cost-effective for a health service even when they're not. It is important too that payers are not afraid to walk away if a drug is deemed too expensive; and to hold that line notwithstanding the lobbying and patient group pressure which may be leveraged in an attempt to change the decision.

We should give healthcare systems the resources to be as proactive and aggressive as possible in pushing back against manufacturers in drug negotiations. Doing this effectively means using new tools like adding stipulations to publicly-funded work but it also means knowing as much as possible about how different drugs compare. As Jack Scannell and others have argued, payers can benefit hugely from running head-to-head trials between rival products of the sort that drugmakers go out of their way to avoid.[31] If rival drugs are deemed sufficiently similar, a tendering process can be used to award the contract to the lowest bidder, in much the way many vaccine prices have been driven down. Further reforms can also help to strip out the noise generated by drug company efforts to influence doctors and, in the US, by pharmaceutical advertising. There is a genuine need for educating busy medical professionals on the relative merits and uses of new drugs but this should be taken out of manufacturers' hands, perhaps through the establishment of new, independent organisations funded by a levy on drugmakers as a condition of having their drugs reimbursed.

Alongside this, there are arguments to be made for introducing far more transparency to the pharmaceutical market in order to help those negotiating prices. In the current system, countries can end up paying wildly different prices for the same drug on the basis of their relative negotiating success. This pricing secrecy is of as much benefit to those individual countries who secure the biggest discounts as it is to drugmakers who don't have to offer the same price cuts else-where. It allows drug companies to declare a list price for use as a reference price whilst secretly agreeing to significant discounts. More transparency around pricing, as is being advocated by the World Health Organization, could lead to a more equitable solution for all. However, there is also a risk that it instead leads to higher prices, particularly if the political response in the US is that it is unwilling to continue paying higher prices than other Western nations. More research on the potential impact is needed and any change would have to acknowledge the need for a tiered system globally, with middle- and low-income countries necessarily paying less than their richer counterparts.

A more unambiguously useful change is in exploring new ways of structuring payments so those paying the bills are equipped with more information about the clinical value of what they're buying – something which also benefits those companies who produce genuinely useful and innovative products. Medicines have generally been sold to large patient groups with limited data on their therapeutic value. It is only after a few years of regular use that doctors begin to learn more about a new drug and which patients are best placed to benefit. 'The problem with the current system is that we pay up front for a drug that has a 30 per cent probability of working in any specific patient, and so we waste a lot of money by setting a high price for all patients,' says Margaret Kyle, the professor of economics in Paris who has studied pharmaceutical pricing.[32]

If drug price negotiations are a one-off before launch, healthcare systems and cost-effectiveness bodies like ICER are hampered by the limited information available. It is therefore sensible for drugs to be regularly reappraised – ICER revisit drugs after a year on the market and seek to revisit the most important after two years – but there's also scope for health systems to strike more innovative payment deals with drugmakers, ones which share the risk and rewards a little more evenly. 'If you change the system so that the company gets paid if its drug turns out to work in a patient, then they have incentives to develop drugs that work for a larger number of patients and they have incentives to develop tests to screen which patients it's most likely to work for,' Kyle says. 'That's a way I think to realign incentives in a way which is good for innovation and good for society.'

Novel payment terms can also help to reduce drug costs. Australia was among many countries which had to impose strict rationing on Gilead's hepatitis C drugs when they were first launched. But it then reached a deal which saw it pay a lump sum of several hundred million dollars for unlimited access to Gilead's drugs for all Australian patients who needed the treatment. This so-called 'Netflix model' allowed Australia to pay an estimated one-seventh of what would have been expected under normal purchase arrangements.[33] The benefit for Gilead was a guaranteed upfront sum, removing any commercial risk or the prospect of a rival product gaining ground and negating the need for marketing costs in that territory. With low manufacturing costs, many drugs lend themselves to a subscription-style model which can allow healthcare systems to fully leverage their bulk-buying power and give both sides confidence in what the costs or revenues will be. For patients, such deals remove restrictions on access and ensure use can be determined by clinical need instead of budgetary requirements.

For personalised medicines with their huge upfront costs, striking agreements for outcome-based payment terms spread over many years may be the only way of persuading health systems to use the products. This approach avoids the cashflow issue multi-million-pound drugs can cause by spreading out their cost and also ensures payments are linked to how effective the drug proves to be. Of course, as with all pharmaceuticals, this must all be on health services' terms, with the usual cost-effectiveness assessments and need for hard negotiations required lest it become a means for drug companies to try and extract excessively high sums simply by allowing them to be paid over a number of years.

More radically, changes could be made to set a ceiling on revenues from an individual drug – even after it has passed a cost-effectiveness test – in order to prevent excessively large rewards. Jamie Love, the intellectual property activist, is an advocate of reducing patent lengths once drugs have generated significant sales. For drugs which have received public funding, he suggested that 'after the first billion dollars in global revenue we'd like you to reduce the exclusivity by one year for every additional $500m which is generated'.[34]

'We're saying charge whatever you want for the first billion, you've got a monopoly. And if you never reach a billion we're not going to mess with you. But once you hit a billion dollars we're going to start looking your way.' Creating what is in effect a kind of revenue cap encourages companies to improve their profit margin through internal efficiencies and reduced marketing spend, although it requires close scrutiny to avoid incentivising companies to push up the declared cost of R&D. This approach could also be used to set different revenue caps for different therapeutic areas, if desired, in order to increase research investment in underdeveloped areas. Doing so would require companies to be compelled to open their books to governments and to agree on how broad spending on R&D is allocated or divided up among projects but it is far from unworkable.

Love's idea is one of several which seek to de-link the incentive for investors to put up funds for drug research from the prices of drugs and the monopoly grants which patents represent. In another version of this approach, prize funds have been proposed as a way of incentivising the discovery of antibiotics. The idea is that, instead of rewarding companies with a monopoly period, a fund raised from governments and philanthropic donors would be awarded and patent rights would then be handed over for public use. The 'Netflix' model can help here too. The United Kingdom has proposed paying for new antibiotics on a subscription basis – paying for access rather than by volume used – in order to incentivise companies to bring their products to market without affecting the need to reduce antibiotic use in an effort to combat growing resistance. As with so much in the pharmaceutical sector, however, one country cannot go it alone. For this approach to work and provide sufficient financial incentives it must be adopted globally.

The changes outlined so far would create a more rational market for drugs: allowing limited resources to be deployed where they are most effective, encouraging companies to develop the most useful products and punishing medicines with minor advantages and high price tags. They represent a re-balancing of the existing model. Companies might have to weather lower profit margins than they enjoy today, but rewards would still come in the form of a patent-protected monopoly period during which prices would need to be high enough to incentivise continued investment in other drug discovery projects. What these changes would not achieve is solving the challenges brought by spiralling drug discovery costs even if they buy more time for solutions to arrive.

'A central tenet of economics is the law of diminishing returns. In this case, additional resources going into innovation inevitably yield fewer important breakthroughs,' two prominent American health economists wrote in 2017. 'At some point, perhaps already reached, the yield from additional resources going into [pharmaceutical] R&D no longer justifies what society is paying in the form of higher prices to support this.'[35] To put it another way, 'if we can't afford to develop new treatments in a cost-effective way, there are going to be better uses of our money, like paying for the treatments we already have', Bach, the New York epidemiologist, says. For him, the key question for policymakers is where public money is best spent in terms of shared social goals. If healthcare spending can only grow at the expense of education, defence or social security, is that a price worth paying? These judgements are not easy, but Bach is all too familiar with the reality of what these choices mean for dying patients or those diagnosed with currently untreatable ailments; he lost his wife to metastatic breast cancer in 2012.

'We have a lot of really effective drugs already that people don't have access to and we're spending half a trillion dollars on drugs [at invoice prices in the US] today,' Bach says. 'And I would wager that if we had to trade a five-year pause in new drug development for universal access to what we currently have, our health gains would be larger and we could put the money we would save to other things that would also improve health.'[36]

The industry is structured around finding new chemical molecules or biological medicines because of the commercial incentives to develop things which are patentable and can be sold at a high price. But, as Jack Scannell, the former equity analyst, and others argue, this comes at the expense of other potentially useful innovations. 'People want improvements in technology that make them healthier and live longer and feel better,' he says. 'But I think to a certain extent, the investment has been skewed towards novel chemical matter, because that is the easiest kind of innovation to monetise.'[37]

Professor Claxton, the British health economist who worked closely with NICE for many years, agrees: 'There is a tendency to fetishise technologies which claim disease modification over other things that we can do to improve people's wellbeing, quality of life, dignity [and] to make them feel like there's care and compassion in society,' he says. 'Branded pharmaceuticals that claim a biological effect on disease action are not the only way for society to care for people. In my opinion, there are probably better ways to ensure people are cared for and looked after and feel care and compassion . . . without spending money on a drug.'[38]

Other, medically useful developments are more difficult to generate rewards from under the current model. 'It's very hard to make as much money out of cognitive behavioural therapy as it is out of a new pill,' Scannell says. The same issue applies to finding new uses for generic medicines which are likely to be long out of patent. Demonstrating an old drug's effectiveness against a new disease still requires an expensive clinical trial but with scant reward for any company willing to fund it because of the lack of patent protection.

If the future is ultimately one in which we must accept fewer new drugs because of limits on what society can afford, it paves the way for a large role for alternative sources of finance, including philanthropic funding or charitable fundraising on a not-for-profit model, and for alternative approaches to finding new drugs.

It is not realistic to argue that public financing can take on the huge risk private industry bears under the current model, but nor does drug development need to remain the exclusive purview of large pharmaceutical companies. In 1999, the Nobel Peace Prize was awarded to Médecins Sans Frontières (MSF), an aid organisation which employs doctors and nurses sent to war zones and humanitarian crises. MSF decided to use the prize money to address diseases neglected because of a lack of commercial potential. A few years later, this funding led to the creation of the Drugs for Neglected Diseases initiative (DNDi).

The organisation doesn't seek to discover completely new drugs but instead looks to take advantage of discontinued research, improving existing out-of-patent compounds. It strikes deals with drug companies who agree to manufacture the resulting products and sell them at cost. As a result, it has been able to develop six drugs, each one costing a fraction of the drug discovery costs reported by large drug companies for new compounds.

Perhaps its biggest success has been fexinidazole, a drug which had been languishing in the library of the German company Hoechst when it was dusted off by DNDi. Fexinidazole is a treatment for sleeping sickness, a potentially fatal disease endemic in sub-Saharan Africa. Bernard Pécoul, who set up DNDi in 2003, spent the preceding twenty years with MSF and he recalls having no choice but to treat patients with a derivative of arsenic, 'knowing that in using this we were killing one out of twenty of the patients due to the toxicity of the product'.[39] Recent advances had improved treatment but required patients to be hospitalised. Fexinidazole replaces that with a simple ten-day course of pills and has been approved by the European medicines regulator and for use in the Democratic Republic of Congo. Among other projects, DNDi is currently working on an affordable hepatitis C drug, challenging the market dominated by Gilead and AbbVie.

If health systems decide they cannot afford to continue to give treatments for rare diseases the special status – and ability to demand higher prices – they currently hold, that will inevitably lead to less industry investment in this area but there are other sources of funding. Two decades ago, dismayed by the lack of interest in funding research into drugs that could target the underlying cause of the disease, the Cystic Fibrosis Foundation went looking for a drug company to partner with. It eventually gave Vertex more than $75 million towards research and development costs, and helped promote patient awareness after the first treatment launched in 2012.[40] The charity received royalty payments but made a mistake in not ensuring it had a say over the price set for the treatment by the for-profit drug company Vertex. This led two dozen researchers involved with the development of the drugs to write to Vertex's chief executive to express their 'dismay and disappointment' at the 'unconscionable price' of the first treatment.

Commercial drug discovery relies on intellectual property and trade secrets but the solution to the hardest scientific problems may lie in an open, collaborative approach. 'Right now you have legal barriers from developing products because of the way that patent protection plays out,' Love says. 'That drives up the cost of doing research and also it legally eliminates a lot of people that could be working on it.' Dementia, and its most common form, Alzheimer's disease, has been a graveyard for experimental treatments, with a failure rate of 99.6 per cent for drugs which entered clinical trials.[41] Only a tiny number of drugs have been approved and none have yet been found which can halt or even have a meaningful effect on the disease. This failure rate, matched with the high cost of clinical trials – which must last years to capture the slow deterioration caused by the disease – has made drugmakers very cautious about committing funds to research in this area. The financial rewards for even a moderately effective treatment could be enormous, but even then only a small number of major drug companies continue to invest significant sums in neuroscience.[42] In these circumstances, a collaborative approach between scientists in different institutions and from different disciplines may be the only path to success.

These proposed changes are not the only options for altering the system by which drug discovery is incentivised and paid for but whatever precise course is chosen, we should accept trade-offs in access and innovation and allow health systems, and ultimately patients and the public, to dictate the terms of engagement – shaping which drugs are developed and how much we are willing to pay for them. A future in which power is more evenly distributed and profits more fairly won.

Inaction is not an option unless we are willing to accept a dystopian society in which inequalities of access become even more pronounced. In December 2019, perhaps mindful of the disquiet the price of Zolgensma had caused, Novartis announced a solution: a new initiative to give the gene therapy away to 100 children for free, randomly selecting the lucky recipients in a lottery.[43]

'My first reaction was, wow, that's great, because other children this year will receive it without having to pay for it,' Ellen De Meyer, the mother of baby Pia, says. 'Then of course you start thinking about it more and you realise it's just a drop on a hot plate, as we say.

'There are tens of thousands of children all over the world who will actually need it so 100 is just very, very small.'[44]

De Meyer says she would find the lottery draws unbearable. 'The idea you'd get your hopes up every two weeks and then have to realise that, again, your child has not been drawn and another month passes, or another two; I think it's even more heartbreaking than knowing you can't have access to it.'

EPILOGUE

Concordia's fall

Concordia's descent was even swifter and more spectacular than its rise.

When the company bought AMCo in September 2015, time was already running out for the get-rich-quick approach of debranding old drugs and hiking the prices.

Three years earlier, government officials at the UK Department of Health had lodged a complaint with the competition watchdog over the pricing of phenytoin capsules, the epilepsy drug which leapt in price after Pfizer struck a deal with Flynn Pharma.[1] The price increase had caught the attention of doctors who feared that patients who had been stabilised on the drug would lose control of their seizures if they were forced to move to a different treatment. By the time the AMCo deal was announced, there was reason to believe that the British government was becoming aware that debranding was a wider problem. Buried in the text of a consultation document quietly released by the health ministry earlier that month was a reference to cases where drugs previously sold under a brand name had been re-launched as a generic 'and a large increase in price has been applied due to lack of regulatory control and lack of a competitive market for the product'.[2] It sought views on whether the government should intervene. This development was not flagged to investors when the AMCo deal was announced.

The private equity buyout which had held so much promise for Concordia in late April 2016 never materialised. Instead, press scrutiny over its pricing practices grew on both sides of the Atlantic culminating, six weeks later, in a series of investigative reports in *The Times* which laid out how AMCo and several other companies had adopted the debranding trick as a business model, allowing them to push through large price increases for dozens of drugs. The scale of the problem became undeniable and a series of front-page stories, which also showed how health service officials had waved through the price rises unchallenged, forced the government to act.

At the same time, several of Concordia's North American acquisitions were unravelling. When the company acquired Donnatal, it had believed that 'no new products could enter the market and exclusivity for Donnatal could be maintained indefinitely'.³ Instead, it was subject to unexpected generic competition in 2016, which an appeal to the regulator failed to block. Meanwhile, insurers were waking up to the price rises for other drugs and beginning to refuse to cover them. Slumping prescriptions in the United States left the company increasingly dependent on AMCo's portfolio but the scrutiny those drugs were now under made further price rises impossible. In August 2016, Concordia issued a press release acknowledging the problems facing several of its drugs in the American market as well as currency exchange losses caused by a fall in the value of sterling in the wake of Britain's vote to leave the European Union. It warned investors that revenues for the year would be lower than previously anticipated.

In mid-September 2016, the British government announced that it was tabling new legislation to crack down on pricing abuses which had driven up the cost of old medicines. Concordia was one of the companies singled out for criticism by members of Parliament. Speaking from the green benches of the House of Commons, politicians lambasted the company's 'unusually high increases in prices' for depriving the country's NHS of much-needed revenue. Jeremy Hunt, the then-health secretary, decried 'companies that appear to have made it their business model to purchase off-patent medicines for which there are no competitive products. They then exploit a monopoly position to raise prices,' he said. 'We cannot allow this practice to continue unchallenged.' His opposite number in the Labour party added to the criticism of those who 'make themselves extremely wealthy by using loopholes in the law to prey on the sick and the vulnerable and extract obscene profits from our health service'.[4]

At the start of June 2016, Concordia's share price stood at around $26, well down on the heady days before investors turned on the AMCo deal and Hillary Clinton's social media post prompted a sell-off across specialty pharma stocks, but still in reasonable shape. By October that year, it had plummeted below $5, and would fall further still. That month, the company announced that its founder and chief executive Mark Thompson had resigned. A year later, Concordia filed for debt restructuring. The move would allow it to reduce its debts by more than $2 billion but meant investors who had bought shares were all but wiped out. For the short-seller Marc Cohodes, who had ridden the company's share price all the way down, it represented vindication – and time for some new trophies. He named a horse after Concordia and a rooster after the former CEO, Mark Thompson, although neither remained at the farm for long. 'I sold the horse and made some money . . . and that rooster was killed and eaten,' he says.[5]

On both sides of the Atlantic, the party was ending and when the music stopped some were better off than others. Pharmacy benefit managers were now scrutinising older medicines, identifying the worst offenders among price-hiked medicines and taking them off their formularies, which meant insurers no longer covered them. Some companies had showed up too late. During 2015, Novum Pharma, a new company set up by several former Horizon Pharma employees, bought the rights to several skin medications which had no generic alternatives and increased prices ten-fold. Over the following months, there were two more rounds of price rises. Although it was a simple combination of two cheap ingredients, the list price of one of the drugs reportedly rose from $226 to around $9,500 a tube.[6] For patients with insurance, Novum offered co-pay coupons so they faced no out-of-pocket charge but the business quickly ran into the headwinds hitting the predatory pricing model. The health insurer CVS kicked the drugs off its formulary in 2016, and a few years later Novum called it a day and filed for bankruptcy. In the filings, a Novum executive said the prices had 'led to public scrutiny regarding [Novum's] business model and further increased prescription rejection rates'.[7] Among the creditors left behind was a pharma executive who claimed he was owed $5 million for introducing Novum to the drug company it had bought the skin medicines from and an outstanding bill of more than €50,000 owed to the five-star Four Seasons Hotel George V in Paris.[8]

Regulators and other government agencies in the US and the UK began to open inquiries into a wide range of alleged abuses, from drug-pricing to marketing practices. Margrethe Vestager, a former Danish politician who had been appointed as the European Union's antitrust commissioner, fixed pharmaceutical companies firmly in her sights. Her targets included Aspen Pharmacare, which was subject to an investigation into its apparent attempt to hold a series of European countries hostage over the price of cancer therapies. In response, Aspen agreed to cut the price of six cancer drugs by an average of nearly 75 per cent as part of a settlement deal.[9]

After he left Concordia, Mark Thompson set up a new drug company. Seeking a rebirth, he called it Lazarus Pharmaceuticals. The company manufactured a treatment for irritable bowel syndrome similar to Concordia's Donnatal. It was so similar to Donnatal, in fact, that Thompson and other Lazarus executives were sued by his old company, which alleged they had stolen trade secrets in order to create a 'knock-off' version of the bowel drug.[10]

The hedge fund savant Bill Ackman walked away from his investment in Valeant in March 2017. Over a two-year period, his company, Pershing Square, had lost nearly $4 billion. The chief executive who had pushed through Valeant's price-hiking strategy, Mike Pearson, resigned in March 2016 and was last seen squabbling over how much he was owed by his former employer.[11]

Four companies including Valeant and two run by Martin Shkreli were eviscerated in a 2016 US Senate report into the 'hedge-fund model of drug pricing'.[12] Shkreli was jailed on unrelated charges of securities fraud in 2017 and the overnight increase in the price of Daraprim from $17.50 to $750 finally caught up with him and his former company, Turing, in early 2020. The Federal Trade Commission filed legal papers accusing Turing, now renamed Vyera Pharmaceuticals, of orchestrating 'an elaborate anticompetitive scheme to preserve a monopoly for the life-saving drug'.[13] The case alleged that the company had broken the law in its efforts to stop would-be generics manufacturers from getting hold of samples of Daraprim which they needed to secure regulatory approval for competing versions of the drug. Turing had also banned data companies from selling information on the sales of the drug in an apparent effort to dissuade generics from deciding to enter the market. Shkreli has personally been named as a defendant in the case, with several US states joining as complainants.

The names of many of the companies that became most synonymous with price-gouging old medicines have disappeared. Some have rebranded in a bid to shake the damaging headlines and Google search results. Others have been absorbed into larger companies or closed down altogether. The industry has tried to show that it has cleaned up its act. In 2017, the main US trade body for the industry, the Pharmaceutical Research and Manufacturers of America, updated its membership rules to require all members to spend at least 10 per cent of revenue on R&D. Two price-hiking companies, Mallinckrodt and Marathon Pharmaceuticals, were thrown out.

After the restructuring, Concordia adopted a new name – Advanz Pharma – and a new business model. Sanjeeth Pai, who became chief executive of Concordia's North American business in August 2017, said he found a debt-laden business whose 'operating model was previously to just raise prices, which is not sustainable', he says. 'I was trying to change that so it became more of a pharmaceutical company rather than a company that just raises prices.'[14]

Valeant has also rebranded, becoming Bausch Health in 2018 and beginning to invest in research and development. The aftermath was nevertheless a messy one, with a flurry of lawsuits from aggrieved investors and insurance companies to add to the regulatory investigations. In 2019, Bausch Health handed over $1.2 billion to settle a class action lawsuit over the previous collapse in the company's share price.[15]

Advanz Pharma settled a number of class action claims of its own after the restructuring but paid far less, at around $23 million.[16] Mallinckrodt was sued by the city of Rockford near Chicago, Illinois, over price rises for Acthar. The city paid the health costs of its own employees and their families directly and in 2015 had to stump up nearly half a million to pay for nine vials of Acthar after two babies were diagnosed with the rare condition for which the drug is the best treatment. The lawsuit, filed in 2017, also accused a middleman, the PBM Express Scripts, of failing to drive down the cost and helping Acthar to protect its monopoly by signing an exclusive deal to supply the drug.[17]

In the UK, the British competition watchdog, at the urging of government officials, opened a succession of investigations into the pharmaceutical market. Concordia alone would find itself embroiled in nine separate probes.[18] By this point, some owners had already sold their businesses and walked away before things went awry, leaving others to carry the can. Cinven had overseen AMCo's price increases but sold up to Concordia before the backlash began in a deal worth more than $3 billion, several times what it had paid to put the company together.[19] Questcor, the California company responsible for increasing the price of Acthar Gel, had been acquired by Dublin-based Mallinckrodt in 2014 for $5.6 billion. The founders of Auden Mckenzie, Amit Patel and his sister Meeta, sold their business in early 2015 for more than £300 million.

The deal allowed Patel to fulfil his desire to sell up before turning forty and he and his wife set out to enjoy their wealth, buying an eighteenth-century English castle, a mansion on a golf course in south-east England and a five-bedroom villa on an artificial island on the coast of Dubai.[20] Some of the properties featured in the pages of glossy interior design magazines, while Patel was the cover star of an issue of *Asian Wealth Magazine*, posing for photographs in the grounds of the castle and lauded in the accompanying article for his 'phenomenal success'.[21]

The sale meant that it was Actavis and Teva, who had acquired the company, who were largely left to deal with the consequences when Auden Mckenzie was caught up in several regulatory investigations – under the codename Project Silver – over the following years. However, Patel would nevertheless find himself drawn back into the fallout after being named as a party in one of those cases while Cinven, which had so lucratively flipped AMCo to Concordia, would feature among the parties in at least two Competition and Markets Authority (CMA) investigations.

Despite his wealth, Patel did not retire from the industry altogether. After selling his shares in Auden Mckenzie, he set up a consultancy firm, Amilco. It had no website or public presence but details of its activities emerged when the CMA revealed that it had earned several million pounds by helping to broker a deal between the South African drug company Aspen Pharmacare and a Dutch manufacturer, Tiofarma, in 2016. Under the agreement, Tiofarma and Patel's company stayed out of the UK market for a treatment for Addison's disease called fludrocortisone acetate. In exchange, Amilco was granted a 30 per cent cut of the increased prices that Aspen could charge in the absence of competition. Those price increases reached 1,800 per cent.[22] In June 2020, he accepted a five-year ban from serving as a director for his involvement in the fludrocortisone case, and in a separate market-sharing case involving an antidepressant.[23] It also emerged that while running Auden Mckenzie he had padded his earnings by arranging for the company to spend millions on fake 'research and development' expenses. UK tax inspectors got wind of the fraudulent scheme and Patel handed over nearly £15 million after striking a confidential settlement agreement with HM Revenue & Customs.[24]

As regulators picked over how the price-hiking business model had worked, raiding pharmaceutical company offices and interviewing former employees and whistleblowers, they realised that some companies appeared to have worked together in an effort to rig the market and keep competition at bay. Before Concordia bought AMCo, the British company had struck a deal with another drug company, Morningside, to carve up the market for an antibiotic called nitrofurantoin, the CMA alleged.[25] The companies agreed not to compete in price when selling to a major wholesaler over a period during which the cost of a packet of 50mg capsules rose five-fold. In another case, the CMA provisionally ruled that four drug companies had colluded to force up the price of a drug used by cancer patients, which rose from around £6.50 to £51 a packet.[26] Auden Mckenzie was also accused by the regulator of breaking competition law to protect the profits from the inflated price for hydrocortisone. The drug had already risen from £1 to £45 when, in 2011, Auden Mckenzie agreed to pay a competitor owned by the brothers who sold Amdipharm to Cinven to stay out of the market.[27] One of those brothers was later awarded an OBE for services to business and philanthropy.

It wasn't just on the pricing front that things were pushed further and further in the pursuit of profits. In the US, some companies have been accused of bribing doctors in order to persuade them to prescribe their expensive drug over a cheaper alternative. Two lawsuits brought by whistleblowers alleged that Questcor and Mallinckrodt rewarded a small group of physicians responsible for the majority of prescriptions of Acthar Gel with spa treatments and trips to Las Vegas.[28] Mallinckrodt paid $15.4 million to the US Department of Justice to settle the claims without admitting liability but is still fighting legal action filed by a US health insurer.[29] Other companies were accused of breaking US law by using what were purportedly independent charities to pay patients' co-pays for drugs covered by government health programmes, and handed over more than $120 million to resolve the claims.[30]

The UK legislation designed to tackle pricing abuses was passed in April 2017.[31] Yet, four years later, politicians still haven't used the powers to reduce prices.[32] If they thought it would be sufficiently effective as a deterrent alone, drugmakers have called their bluff. Only just under one-third of the seventy or so generic drugs affected by huge price hikes have seen their prices come significantly down.[33] In many cases, the market is still not working because even when generic manufacturers have launched rival versions they elected not to launch at a much cheaper price. Liothyronine tablets, which some thyroid patients consider life-changing, still cost the NHS around £5 a pill in early 2021 – having cost 16 pence a few years earlier – even though two other companies have obtained UK licences and launched competing versions since AMCO's actions saw prices peak at more than £9 a pill.[34]

The CMA has secured around £10 million in payments to the NHS and several cases are still open but it remains to be seen whether the British government will use the eventual conclusion of these and other investigations to take legal action to recoup the extra funds spent on price-gouged drugs.[35] In the meantime, drug companies haven't stopped their efforts to profit from price increases for older medicines. In mid-2020, during the height of the coronavirus pandemic, a firm called Essential Pharma announced it would no longer be selling Priadel, the bestselling brand of the bipolar drug lithium. The decision, taken a few months after the company had been bought by a Swiss private equity firm, would push patients towards a much pricier alternative version also sold by Essential Pharma. This alternative was more expensive because, a few years earlier, it had had its price increased from £3.22 – close to the price of Priadel – to £87 a packet. In this case, an outcry from mental health professionals and a swift referral to the competition watchdog, which opened an investigation, prompted the company to announce it was rethinking the plan.

Though politicians rushed to condemn pricing practices in the United States as well, price-hiked drugs have also remained costly there. During a congressional hearing in early 2016, Valeant's then-chief executive apologised for being too aggressive in taking price hikes and the company promised to drop the price of two heart drugs. They eventually came down – though it took months – but other Valeant drugs remain far more expensive than they were before the price hiking began. In 2018, Teva launched a competing version of Syprine, which had risen from around $650 to more than $21,000, according to list prices. The Israeli generics company adopted a list price of more than $18,300 for a bottle of 100 pills, still far above what the drug had cost a few years earlier.[36] Other drugs, like Horizon Pharma's Vimovo, continued to have their prices hiked for years.[37]

Among the previously price-hiked drugs which have become much cheaper after more manufacturers entered the market is dexamethasone, a common steroid sold in 2mg and 500mcg doses. It was fortunate that it had because in the summer of 2020 the drug was the first to show a significant benefit as a treatment for Covid-19 patients. For some of the sickest patients, those on ventilators in intensive care units, administering 6mg a day of dexamethasone reduced deaths by one-third.[38]

For all the efforts to clean house, price hikes for old drugs haven't disappeared for good, even if companies have been scared off implementing increases of 1,000 per cent or more. The former analyst David Maris thinks there is a 'one hundred per cent' chance of a price-hiking model returning. 'There are charlatans in every market and it doesn't appear that there's any enforcement action increase that's ferreting these out in any better way, shape or form than they did before. So, of course it will happen again,' he says. 'There are people whose whole retirements were in those stocks. In Valeant, in Concordia. And very few people [involved] have seen their own fortunes go away. It's really sad that people's lives have been ruined and the executives get away scot-free.'[39]

Even if some of the worst price-hiking companies have been halted, the deep-seated problems with the pharmaceutical industry's business model remain – for old and new drugs alike.

In many ways, Valeant, Concordia and other companies pursuing a similar strategy were the antithesis of everything the pharmaceutical industry purports to be. So why were they able to gain such traction, to grow so fast and send their share prices soaring so high? The answer lies in the cultural changes and underlying forces which have transformed the industry. These companies, so at odds with the vision espoused by George W. Merck and others, were possible because they were extreme versions of the philosophy many drug companies and investors were articulating: they had an aversion to R&D, a rational response to the slumping rate of return from R&D investment across the industry, and a willingness to push prices that was different only in scale to the approach being gratefully adopted by executives at some of the largest companies in the world as they looked to make up for a lack of new drugs or ability to sell more pills.

The wider view of drugs as financial assets disconnected from their societal importance is the result of the financialisation of the industry as it, like many others, adopted the maxim of maximising shareholder value: as much money as possible as quickly as possible, so that the company is seen to be growing and the all-important number – earnings per share – continues to rise.

The same forces helped create the opioid epidemic. A cadre of profit-hungry drug companies, management consultants and unethical doctors conspired to push a flood of highly addictive pills on millions of people, unleashing a torrent of addiction, overdoses and misery which has ravaged the United States and other countries. The epidemic amounts to a catalogue of the industry's worst instincts and the effects will linger far beyond the billions in settlement payments drugmakers have made as they account for their role in the health crisis.

Of course, not every company is alike. Some, among them the Swiss firm Roche and US company Merck & Co. (MSD), have remained resolutely committed to a research-focused approach and enjoyed the rewards of a string of innovative products, even as these cutting-edge treatments raise their own affordability issues because of the prices applied. Each time the record for the most expensive drug in the world is broken it sets a precedent for others and after the Novartis drug Zolgensma was priced at $2.1 million, BioMarin said in January 2020 that it was exploring a price of between \$2 million and \$3 million for a gene therapy it hoped to offer as haemophilia treatment.[40]

Valeant and Concordia have new names now, and have renounced their price-hiking ways, but whatever reckoning has come for a handful of individual companies, the fissures in the pharmaceutical industry's wider business model that they exposed remain. Prices remain artificially and unsustainably high. Drugs are still viewed as financial assets to be exploited, regardless of the impact on patients. Health services and insurers continue to be forced to make life-or-death decisions about how to use limited budgets. And at the same time, drug executives grappling with the expectations of shareholders and the rising cost of development face challenges of their own.

It is only by facing up to all this, and tackling the hard public policy debates and decisions which must follow, that we can avoid a future in which the medicines we need are not available; either because they are unaffordable or because commercial drug discovery has been abandoned. To navigate a path through the middle, those discussions must start now.

Acknowledgements

Writing this book, as with any such endeavour, couldn't have happened without the assistance and support of a great number of people and it would be impossible to single them all out but there are some I wish to highlight. My thanks go in particular to those who shared the stories of loved ones who died because of a lack of access to medicines: Mark Lindsay and Mindi Patterson. Others, including Greg Jefferys, Ellen De Meyer, Deidre Waxman, Lori Kessell, Melanie Woodcock and 'Demir' shared details of their medical histories – or in Ellen's case, her daughter Pia's – in the hope that it might help others.

I conducted well over 100 interviews for the book and so I must apologise to those whose words didn't make it into the pages of the final manuscript but whose insights nevertheless helped inform and guide the book. My particular thanks go to Jack Scannell, who, in addition to the interview quoted in the book, tolerated long conversations about issues facing the pharmaceutical industry over many months as I thrashed out some of the arguments expressed in the book and helped fill the many gaps in my knowledge. To single out a few others, Peter Staley, Bernard Munos, Leonard Saltz, Steve Pearson, Abbey Meyers, Victor Roy, Mick Kolassa, Shahram Ahari, Jamie Love, Dimitry Kmelnitsky, Marc Cohodes, David Maris, William Lazonick, Karl Claxton, Margaret Kyle, Jim O'Neill, Jayasree Iyer and Peter Hale were all generous with their time. Fran Quigley helped to facilitate an interview with Fran Leath, for which I'm grateful, Aaron Toleos put me in touch with Deidre Waxman, and Mark Harrington kindly shared documents relating to ACT UP and a chapter on the group's actions from an unpublished memoir.

Some of those I interviewed agreed to speak only if they could remain anonymous, often because they worked at companies involved in dubious pricing behaviour; I thank them too, though for obvious reasons they won't be named. As noted in the book, Mark Thompson did not agree to an interview and so I'm particularly grateful for those who worked with him for their contributions. The staff at the British Library and Wellcome Library were helpful as I conducted research and I was aided too by the reporters who penned the many newspaper reports and magazine articles from which I've drawn.

Several people looked over a draft of the book and offered helpful feedback. My brother Charlie Kenber was a very charitable early reader and I'm grateful too to Mike Sweeney for his feedback on a later draft. Jack Scannell, Andrew Hill and Jim Furniss looked over sections of the book and I am grateful to them, too. The mistakes that remain are, of course, my own. Others who've helped in various ways and whom I'd like to thank include Peter Chappell, Alice Hall, Elettra Scrivo, Georgina Turner, Harriet Whitehead, Oli Wright, Francis Elliott, Simon Harker, Harry Bradwell, who coined the title of the book, Andrew Norfolk, Ben Merriman, Naina McCann, Shoaib Rokadiya and Tom Whipple. Several people helped with sourcing some of the figures used in the book, among them Öner Tulum, Jim Yocum at Connecture, Andrew Davis at Elsevier, and Elaine Towell and her colleagues at the ABPI.

The genesis of this book can be traced back to a series of investigative reports I wrote in 2016 for the *Times* newspaper (where I still work). It was a suggestion from Alexi Mostrous that I might look into 'pay for delay' deals that ultimately put me on the path to writing about pharmaceuticals. Those stories wouldn't have been as impactful as they proved to be – leading to a change in the law and close to a dozen regulatory investigations – without the support of several colleagues at the newspaper. In particular, Jeremy Griffin and Fay Schlesinger, who edited and fought for the stories, and Brid Jordan, Pia Sharma, Pat Burge and David Hirst, who helped shepherd them into the paper in the face of legal threats from some of the subjects of the articles. I'd also like to thank the paper's editor, John

Witherow, for giving me the time necessary to pursue investigative articles and later this project.

In the wake of those stories, which were narrowly focused on price hikes for debranded generics in the UK, I realised there was an important – and much wider – story to be told about the changes that have swept through the pharmaceutical industry and their relationship to the outcries over drug prices which have become a regular fixture of the news agenda around the world. The journey to finding a publisher willing to take on this project was not always straightforward and my thanks go to my indefatigable agent Heather Holden-Brown for her help and guidance as we navigated the process.

I am very grateful for the happy home the book has found at Canongate, a free-thinking, independent publisher with a brilliant and energetic team. The book's editor, Simon Thorogood, was a patient and calm presence even as the coronavirus pandemic forced a lot of reshuffling of plans and Leila Cruickshank was a very diligent copy editor who helped tighten the prose.

The relationship between a journalist and a lawyer is not always a smooth one so particular thanks must go to Alex Wade, who, as both an author and a lawyer, was perfectly placed to assist with this book. I'm grateful for the care and time he spent on the task.

Finally, on a personal level, I'd like to thank my friends and family for their encouragement during such a lengthy project. Above all, this book, much of which was written in evenings and weekends, would simply not have been possible without the efforts of my fiancée, Sam. Without her love, support and sacrifice I would have given up long before delivering this manuscript. The book is for her.

As a journalist, I'm always keen to hear from readers. If you'd like to get in touch, I can be reached on Twitter @billykenber or by email at billy@billykenber.com.

Notes and references

Introduction

1. Pollack, A., 'Drug Goes From $13.50 a Tablet to $750, Overnight', *New York Times* (September 20, 2015). Although the price increase was reported as having taken Daraprim from $13.50 to $750, later legal filings by the Federal Trade Commission show that the price had already reached $17.50 before Shkreli increased it.
2. Interview by the author with Jack Scannell.

Prologue: A house near Lake Ontario

1. Mark Thompson appearance on Business News Network (March 10, 2015).
2. Ibid.
3. Concordia Healthcare 2013 annual information form.
4. Ibid.
5. Transcript of Concordia Healthcare Corp. at CIBC Whistler Institutional Investor Conference (January 20, 2016). Mark Thompson did not respond to multiple requests for an interview and this and later chapters draw on interviews with more than two dozen people including former Concordia employees, investors, analysts and other parties close to the company as well as company filings, transcripts of earnings calls and investor conferences, legal testimony and other documents.
6. 'M & A Machine; Mark Thompson has Concordia Healthcare on the verge of something big', *Financial Post Business* (October 1, 2015).
7. Cross-examination of Mark Thompson in *Mark Thompson* v. *Marc Cohodes*, Ontario Superior Court of Justice (January 10, 2017).
8. 'Amended and Restated Preliminary Prospectus – Initial Public Offering', Legacy Pharma Income Fund (August 15, 2005).
9. Willis, A., Reguly, E., Stewart, S., Robertson, G., 'Ottawa's move on income trusts throws sector into disarray', *Globe and Mail* (September 28, 2005).
10. 'PLIVA Terminates Agreements with Legacy Pharma', press release on pliva.com (October 3, 2005).
11. Cross-examination of Mark Thompson in *Mark Thompson* v. *Marc Cohodes*, Ontario Superior Court of Justice (January 10, 2017).
12. Ibid.
13. Filing statement for Mercari Acquisition Corp. (December 13, 2013).
14. Concordia Healthcare 2013 annual information form.
15. Concordia Healthcare presentation at RBC Capital Markets Healthcare Conference (February 24, 2015).

16. Federal Trade Commission press release and associated documents, 'Pharmaceutical Companies Settle FTC Charges of an Illegal Agreement not to Compete, which Resulted in Higher Prices for Generic Version of ADHD Drug', ftc.gov (August 18, 2015).

17. Pfannenstiel, B., 'Lenexa health company owners ordered to pay $12M settlement', *Kansas City Business Journal* (October 23, 2013).

18. Concordia Healthcare 2013 annual information form.

19. Ibid.

20. Interview by the author with Kevin Combs.

21. Interview by the author with Lori Kessell.

22. Ibid.

23. Wholesale Acquisition Cost (WAC) figures from Elsevier's Gold Standard Drug Database. WAC prices are the manufacturer's list price when selling to wholesalers but do not include any rebates or other off-invoice discounts. Smaller pharmaceutical companies like Concordia have complained that middlemen called pharmacy benefit managers squeezed profits by demanding an increasing cut from drug sales during this period as well as a minimum proportion of any price rises.

24. 'Business acquisition report – Donnatal', Concordia Healthcare (June 9, 2014).

25. Interview by the author with Kevin Combs.

26. The drug's WAC rose by 10 per cent to $865 for a bottle of 100 pills in February 2015, according to Elsevier's Gold Standard Drug Database.

27. Ibid.

28. Concordia Healthcare Corporation FY 2013 Earnings Call (March 31, 2014).

29. Moylan, T., '2 Drug Makers To Pay $214.5 Million For Off-Label Marketing Of Zonegran', Lexis Nexis Legal News Room (December 16, 2010).

30. List price figures from Elsevier's Gold Standard Drug Database recording WAC. According to figures from SSR, the net price of the drug – the cost after rebates and discounts – was around 70 to 80 per cent of the list price while under Eisai's ownership. Net price figures for Concordia were not disclosed but Mark Thompson told analysts the price increase had been 25 per cent – lower than the nearly 50 per cent list price increase recorded.

31. Shufelt, T., 'Little-known drug company offers powerful antidote to Big Pharma's patent headache', *Globe and Mail* (September 12, 2014).

32. The $160 billion Pfizer–Allergan deal was abandoned in April 2016 after the Obama administration passed new rules which made it harder for companies to benefit from tax inversions.

33. Mark Thompson appearance on Business News Network (March 10, 2015).

34. Interview by the author with Niall McGee, September 2019.

35. Batcho-Lino, S. and Lam, E., 'Valeant Clone Concordia Top Canada Stock as CEO Eyes Deal', Bloomberg News (April 7, 2015).

36. Mark Thompson appearance on Business News Network (March 10, 2015).

37. McGee, N., 'Concordia Healthcare "not done yet" with deals', *Globe and Mail* (March 9, 2015).

38. Langreth, R., 'Dealmakers Behind Soaring Drug Prices Hit the Jackpot', Bloomberg News (November 2, 2016) and 'Moody's Reviews Covis Pharma's ratings, direction uncertain', Moody's Investors Services (March 10, 2015).

39. 'Business acquisition report – Covis', Concordia Healthcare (July 3, 2015).

40. Plieth, J., 'After Turing, the industry's biggest price gougers', evaluate.com (September 23, 2015). The list was based on the national average drug acquisition cost (NADAC) of drugs, which is compiled weekly from the price paid by US pharmacies to acquire drugs but does not include likely rebates.

41. List price of Dibenzyline 10mg tablets according to Elsevier's Gold Standard Drug Database.

42. Analyst's research note on Concordia Healthcare by David Martin at Bloom Burton & Co. (May 19, 2015).

43. 'Report: Heightened Risk at Concordia', Pacific Square Research (March 11, 2016). Lanoxin was a brand name for digoxin. The unbranded generic version sold by two other companies also underwent significant price rises during this period. See 'Why are some generic drugs skyrocketing in price', hearing before the subcommittee of Primary Health and Aging of the Committee on Health, Education, Labor and Pensions, United States Senate (November 20, 2014).

44. Taibbi, M., 'The Great American Bubble Machine', *Rolling Stone* (April 5, 2010).

45. In the Matter of Concordia Pharmaceuticals Inc.; Concordia Healthcare Corp.; Par Pharmaceutical, Inc.; Par Pharmaceutical Holdings, Inc.; and TPG Partners VI, L.P., 'Analysis to Aid Public Comment', US Federal Trade Commission (August 18, 2015).

46. Management information circular filed by Concordia Healthcare (March 24, 2016).

47. Interview by the author with David Maris.

48. 'Acquisition of Amdipharm Mercury Limited – Creating A Global, Diversified Platform For Growth', corporate presentation by Concordia Healthcare (September 8, 2015).

49. Cotterill, J., 'Cinven to sell AMCo to Concordia in £2.3bn deal,' *Financial Times* (September 8, 2015).

50. In September 2015, Thompson held just over 2.1 million shares in Concordia and the stock hit a peak of $89.10 that month. He also held 125,000 share options and restricted share units, according to SEDI disclosures.

51. McGee, N., 'How Concordia Healthcare got caught in a stock market storm', *Globe and Mail* (October 2, 2015).

52. Pollack, A., 'Drug Goes From $13.50 a Tablet to $750, Overnight', *New York Times* (September 20, 2015). The drug had previously had its price increased from $13.50 to $17.50 per tablet by Impax Laboratories in June 2015, two months before it was acquired by Vyera and the price was further raised to $750 per tablet.

53. Tweet sent by Hillary Clinton @HillaryClinton (September 21, 2015).

Chapter One: Apothecaries, pills and guns

1. Le Fanu, J., *The Rise and Fall of Modern Medicine* (Little, Brown, 1999; Abacus, 2011) p.17.

2. Gaynes, R., 'The Discovery of Penicillin – New Insights After More Than 75 Years of Clinical Use', *Emerging Infectious Diseases* (May 2017).

3. Chain, E., Florey, H.W. et al., 'Penicillin as a chemotherapeutic agent', *The Lancet* (August 24, 1940).

4. Heatley, N.G., 'In Memoriam, H.W. Florey: an Episode', *Journal of General Microbiology* (July 22, 1970).

5. The scientists had previously experimented with different methods of administering penicillin on several patients. The first volunteer was a terminally ill fifty-year-old woman with breast cancer who received an injection around one month before the Oxford policeman. See Fletcher, C., 'First clinical use of penicillin', *British Medical Journal* (December 22, 1984).

6. Abraham, E.P., Chain, E. et al., 'Further Observations on Penicillin', *The Lancet* (August 16, 1941).

7. Wells, P.A., 'Some Aspects of the Early History of Penicillin in the United States', *Journal of the Washington Academy of Sciences* (September 1975).

8. Ibid.

9. Neushul, P., 'Science, Government, and the Mass Production of Penicillin', *Journal of the History of Medicine and Allied Sciences* (October 1, 1993).

10. Ibid.

11. Aldridge, S., Parascandola, J., Sturchio, J.L, 'International Historical Chemical Landmark: The discovery and development of penicillin', *American Chemical Society* (November 19, 1999).

12. Neushul, P., 'Science, Government, and the Mass Production of Penicillin', *Journal of the History of Medicine and Allied Sciences* (October 1, 1993).

13. Federal Trade Commission, 'Economic Report on Antibiotics Manufacture', US Government Printing Office (June 1958).

14. Ginsberg, J., 'Development of Deep-tank Fermentation: Pfizer Inc.', *American Chemical Society* (June 12, 2008).

15. Quinn, R., 'Rethinking Antibiotic Research and Development: World War II and the Penicillin Collaborative', *American Journal of Public Health* (March 2013).

16. Ibid.

17. Corley, T.A.B., 'The British pharmaceutical industry since 1851' in Richmond, L., Stevenson, J. and Turton, A. (eds), *The Pharmaceutical Industry* (Routledge, 2003).

18. Wertheimer, A., Santella, T., 'The history and economics of pharmaceutical patents' in Farquhar, I., Summers, K.H. and Sorkin, A. (eds), *The Value of Innovation: Impact on Health, Life Quality, Safety and Regulatory Research* (Emerald Group Publishing, 2007).

19. There is controversy over the credit for the discovery of aspirin. Hoffmann was working for, and likely under the instruction of, Arthur Eichengrün. See Desborough, M.J., Keeling, D.M., 'The aspirin story – from willow to wonder drug', *British Journal of Haemotology* (January 20, 2017).

20. Gaudillière, J-P., 'How pharmaceuticals became patentable: the production and appropriation of drugs in the twentieth century', *History and Technology* (March 7, 2008).

21. Brown, H.T., 'Chairman's Address: Patents in Pharmacy and Medicine', British Pharmaceutical Conference Bournemouth (December 1, 1959).

22. Product patents were not allowed in Germany until 1968 – nearly twenty years later than in Britain – but from the early twentieth century German manufacturers made 'massive use of process patents' to protect chemical

processes. See Gaudillière, J-P., 'How pharmaceuticals became patentable: the production and appropriation of drugs in the twentieth century', *History and Technology* (March 7, 2008).

23. Corley, T.A.B., 'The British pharmaceutical industry since 1851' in Richmond, L, Stevenson, J. and Turton, A. (eds), *The Pharmaceutical Industry* (Routledge, 2003).

24. Ibid.

25. Brown, H.T., 'Chairman's Address: Patents in Pharmacy and Medicine', British Pharmaceutical Conference Bournemouth (December 1, 1959).

26. Ballentine, C., 'Sulfanilamide Disaster', *FDA Consumer Magazine* (June 1981).

27. Lee, J., 'Innovation and strategic divergence', *Management Science* (February 2003).

28. Corley, T.A.B., 'The British pharmaceutical industry since 1851' in Richmond, L, Stevenson, J. and Turton, A. (eds), *The Pharmaceutical Industry* (Routledge, 2003).

29. Engs, R.C. (ed.), *Health and Medicine Through History: From Ancient Practices to 21st-Century Innovations* (Greenwood Publishing, 2019) p.332.

30. Clark, R.W., *The Life of Ernst Chain* (St Martin's Press, 1985) pp. 55–9.

31. Ibid.

32. The NRDC would allow the mistake to be repeated when the slow response of officials working there resulted in the failure to patent the technique for producing monoclonal antibodies in the 1970s. This technology would prove instrumental in the birth of the biotech industry and several of the world's bestselling drugs are monoclonal antibodies.

33. Merck, G.W., 'Medicine Is For The Patient, Not For The Profits', Speech at Medical College of Virginia at Richmond (December 1, 1950).

34. The American company Merck & Co. is known as Merck Sharp & Dohme (MSD) outside the US because of the continued existence of its former German parent company, Merck KGaA. The two companies have been separate entities since the US subsidiary was confiscated by the American government during the First World War.

35. Johnson & Johnson, 'Our Credo', jnj.com/credo

36. 'Administered Prices: Drugs', Report of the Subcommittee on Antitrust and Monopoly, the Committee on the Judiciary, United States Senate, US Government Printing Office (1961).

37. Waksman's own motives were not entirely pure. He has been accused of bullying postgraduate student Albert Schatz, who was involved in discovering streptomycin, into assigning his royalty rights to the trust. In doing so, Waksman failed to disclose that he had cut a deal with Rutgers to receive 20 per cent of the royalties paid by Merck. Schatz later discovered this and sued. See Rawlins, M., 'The disputed discovery of streptomycin', *The Lancet* (July 21, 2012).

38. Temin, P., 'The evolution of the modern pharmaceutical industry', Working Paper, Department of Economics, Massachusetts Institute of Technology (September 1978).

39. It would later emerge that lawyers for the National Foundation for Infantile Paralysis, which had funded the vaccine's development, had explored the

possibility of patenting it and concluded it would not be granted under the novelty requirements of the time although 'there is no indication that the foundation intended to profit from a patent on the polio vaccine'. See Palmer, B., 'Jonas Salk: Good at Virology, Bad at Economics', slate.com (April 13, 2014) and Smith, J., *Patenting the Sun: Polio and the Salk Vaccine* (William Morrow & Co., 1990).

40. Temin, P., 'Technology, Regulation, and Market Structure in the Modern Pharmaceutical Industry', *The Bell Journal of Economics* (1979).

41. Federal Trade Commission, 'Economic Report on Antibiotics Manufacture', US Government Printing Office (June 1958).

42. Temin, P., 'Technology, Regulation, and Market Structure in the Modern Pharmaceutical Industry', *The Bell Journal of Economics* (1979).

43. Federal Trade Commission, 'Economic Report on Antibiotics Manufacture', US Government Printing Office (June 1958).

44. In 1948 four of eleven antibiotics were one-company products. By 1958 seventeen of twenty-nine were. Ibid, p.90.

45. Temin, P., 'Technology, Regulation, and Market Structure in the Modern Pharmaceutical Industry', *The Bell Journal of Economics* (1979).

46. Ibid. The figures are sourced from surveys done by the Pharmaceutical Manufacturers Association.

47. Slinn, J., 'Patents and the UK pharmaceutical industry between 1945 and the 1970s', *History and Technology* (March 7, 2008).

48. Bud, R., 'Antibiotics, Big Business, and Consumers: The Context of Government Investigations into the Postwar American Drug Industry', *Technology and Culture* (April 2005).

49. The charges were ultimately dropped after a decade-long legal battle, with Pfizer required to license tetracycline more widely.

50. Greene, J.A., Podolsky, S.H., 'Reform, Regulation, and Pharmaceuticals – The Kefauver–Harris Amendments at 50', *New England Journal of Medicine* (October 18, 2012).

51. Slinn, J., 'Patents and the UK pharmaceutical industry between 1945 and the 1970s', *History and Technology* (March 7, 2008).

52. The 'freedom period' was initially set at three years and in 1964 was extended to four years. See Ibid.

53. The scheme was also designed to incentivise investment in the United Kingdom and was later altered because it fell foul of European Union rules on state aid.

54. The Crown use provision still exists in the UK but has not been invoked since Powell's actions.

55. Greene, J.A., Podolsky, S.H., 'Reform, Regulation, and Pharmaceuticals – The Kefauver–Harris Amendments at 50', *New England Journal of Medicine* (October 18, 2012).

56. Teff, H., 'Regulation under the Medicines Act 1968: A continuing prescription for Health', *The Modern Law Review* (May 1984).

57. Goozner, M., *The $800 Million Pill* (University of California Press, 2005) p.170.

58. Ibid, p.100.

59. Lee, J., 'Innovation and Strategic Divergence: An Empirical Study of the US Pharmaceutical Industry from 1920 to 1960', *Management Science* (February 2003).

60. Morgan, D.C., Allison, S.E., 'The Kefauver Drug Hearings in Perspective', *The Southwestern Social Science Quarterly* (June 1964).

61. Green, J.A., *Generic: The Unbranding of Modern Medicine* (Johns Hopkins University Press, 2014) p.85.

62. Wertheimer, A., Santella, T., 'The history and economics of pharmaceutical patents' in Farquhar, I., Summers, K.H. and Sorkin, A., (eds), *The Value of Innovation: Impact on Health, Life Quality, Safety and Regulatory Research* (Emerald Group Publishing, 2007).

63. Taylor, D., 'The Pharmaceutical Industry and the Future of Drug Development' in Hester, R.E. and Harrison, R.M. (eds), *Pharmaceuticals in the Environment* (Royal Society of Chemistry, 2016) and Le Fanu, J., *The Rise and Fall of Modern Medicine* (Little, Brown, 1999; Abacus, 2011).

64. Vagelos, P.R., *The Moral Corporation: Merck Experiences* (Cambridge University Press, 2006) p.128.

65. Hawthorne, F., *The Merck Druggernaut: The Inside Story of a Pharmaceutical Giant* (John Wiley & Sons, 2003) pp.16–7.

66. 'Over 30 Years: The Mectizan Donation Program', Merck.com (January 6, 2021).

67. McCarthy, J., 'Big Pharma Sinks to the Bottom of US Industry Rankings', Gallup.com (September 3, 2019).

Chapter Two: AZT – the first AIDS drug

1. Interview by the author with Peter Staley.

2. Blumenstyk, G., 'Missed Chances', *Chronicle of Higher Education* (August 12, 2005).

3. Ibid.

4. Naussbaum, B., *Good Intentions* (The Atlantic Monthly Press, 1990; Penguin Books, 1991) p.177.

5. Holt, N., 'Remembering Dr. Jerome Horwitz and AZT', blogs.scientificam erican.com/guest-blog/remembering-dr-jerome-horwitz-and-azt/ (September 2012).

6. Horwitz, J.P. et al., 'Nucleosides. V. The Monomesylates of 1-(2'-Deoxy-β-D-lyxofuranosyl)thymine1,2', *Journal of Organic Chemistry* (July 1964).

7. Naussbaum, B., *Good Intentions* (The Atlantic Monthly Press, 1990; Penguin Books, 1991) p.178.

8. 'HIV/AIDS: Snapshots of an Epidemic', amfAR, The Foundation for AIDS Research, amfar.org/thirty-years-of-hiv/aids-snapshots-of-an-epidemic/

9. Harden, V., Hannaway, C., 'In Their Own Words: NIH Researchers Recall the Early Years of AIDS', oral history interview with Dr Sam Broder, history.nih.gov/display/history/Samuel+Broder+Interview (February 2, 1997).

10. Harden, V., Hannaway, C., 'In Their Own Words: NIH Researchers Recall the Early Years of AIDS', oral history interview with Dr Robert Yarchoan history. nih.gov/display/history/Dr+Robert+Yarchoan+Interview (April 30, 1998).

11. Interview with Dr David Barry, ex-director of global research, Burroughs Wellcome Oral History project, Wellcome Library (April 30, 2001).

12. Interview with Dr David Barry, ex-director of global research, Burroughs Wellcome Oral History project, Wellcome Library (January 24, 2002).

13. Ibid.

14. Interview with Dr David Barry, ex-director of global research, Burroughs Wellcome Oral History project, Wellcome Library (April 30, 2001).

15. Leary, W.E., 'Outspoken and Impatient Scientist Takes Charge of War on Cancer', *New York Times* (February 7, 1989).

16. Harden, V., Hannaway, C., 'In Their Own Words: NIH Researchers Recall the Early Years of AIDS', oral history interview with Dr Sam Broder, history. nih.gov/display/history/Samuel+Broder+Interview (February 2, 1997).

17. Interview with Dr David Barry, ex-director of global research, Burroughs Wellcome Oral History project, Wellcome Library (January 24, 2002).

18. Crawford, A., 'I thought I had made a mistake', BBC News (December 1, 2007).

19. Interview with Dr David Barry, ex-director of global research, Burroughs Wellcome Oral History project, Wellcome Library (January 24, 2002).

20. Ibid.

21. Interview with Pedro Cuatrecasas, ex-head of research and development, Burroughs Wellcome Oral History Project, Wellcome Library (March 21, 2002).

22. Testimony of David Barry before the Human Resources and Intergovernmental Relations Subcommittee of the Committee on Government Operations, US House of Representatives (July 1, 1986).

23. Naussbaum, B., *Good Intentions* (The Atlantic Monthly Press, 1990; Penguin Books, 1991) p.41.

24. Ruling in *Burroughs Wellcome Co.* v. *Barr Laboratories, Inc. and Novopharm, Inc*, United States Court of Appeals, Federal Circuit (November 22, 1994; rehearing denied December 15, 1994).

25. Naussbaum, B., *Good Intentions* (The Atlantic Monthly Press, 1990; Penguin Books, 1991) p.46.

26. Arno, P. and Feiden, K., *Against the Odds: The Story of AIDS, Drug Development, Politics & Profits* (HarperCollins, 1992) p.40.

27. Ibid, p.42.

28. Harden, V., Hannaway, C., 'In Their Own Words: NIH Researchers Recall the Early Years of AIDS', oral history interview with Dr Robert Yarchoan, history. nih.gov/display/history/Dr+Robert+Yarchoan+Interview (April 30, 1998).

29. Ibid.

30. Ibid.

31. Ibid.

32. A. Kaletsky, 'Treatment for AIDS Victims To Be Distributed Free', *Financial Times* (September 23, 1986).

33. Interview with Tom Kennedy, VP Production Engineering, Burroughs Wellcome Oral History project, Wellcome Library (April 19, 2001).

34. Harden, V., Hannaway, C., 'In Their Own Words: NIH Researchers Recall the Early Years of AIDS', oral history interview with Dr Robert Yarchoan, history. nih.gov/display/history/Dr+Robert+Yarchoan+Interview (April 30, 1998).

35. Interview by the author with Jean McGuire.

36. Interview with Bill Sullivan, ex-president of Burroughs Wellcome USA, Burroughs Wellcome Oral History project, Wellcome Library (April 23, 2001).

37. Ibid.
38. Lohr, S., 'Market Place: Wellcome's Bet On AIDS drug', *New York Times* (January 12, 1987).
39. Testimony of Ted Haigler before the Subcommittee of Health and the Environment of the Committee on Energy and Commerce, US House of Representatives (March 10, 1987).
40. Naussbaum, B., *Good Intentions* (The Atlantic Monthly Press, 1990; Penguin Books, 1991) p.176.
41. AZT was often described as the world's most expensive drug, but biotech company Genentech had received approval for Protropin, a synthetic growth hormone used to treat children with a hormone deficiency, in October 1985. Dosing depended on a patient's weight, with the cost typically ranging from $8,000 to $16,000 a year. Factor VIII, a blood-clotting agent drawn from donated blood plasma and injected into haemophiliacs, was also more expensive on an annual per patient basis.
42. Interview with Tom Kennedy, VP Production Engineering, Burroughs Wellcome Oral History project, Wellcome Library (April 19, 2001).
43. 'Cost and Availability of AZT', Hearing of the House of Representatives, Committee on Energy and Commerce, Subcommittee on Health and the Environment, Washington, DC (March 10, 1987).
44. Interview by the author with Jean McGuire.
45. Penslar, R. and Lamm, R., 'Case Studies: Who Pays for AZT?', *The Hastings Center Report* (1989).
46. Interview by the author with Mark Harrington.
47. France, D., *How to Survive a Plague* (Picador, 2016) p.253. The book, an account of AIDS activism, follows a number of prominent activists including Peter Staley.
48. Interview by the author with Peter Staley.
49. Ibid.
50. Kramer, L., 'The F.D.A.'s Callous Response to AIDS', *New York Times* (March 23, 1987).
51. Interview by the author with Peter Staley.
52. Harden, V., Hannaway, C., 'In Their Own Words: NIH Researchers Recall the Early Years of AIDS', oral history interview with Dr Robert Yarchoan, history. nih.gov/display/history/Dr+Robert+Yarchoan+Interview (April 30, 1998).
53. Testimony of Ted Haigler before the Subcommittee of Health and the Environment of the Committee on Energy and Commerce, US House of Representatives (March 10, 1987).
54. Chase, M., 'Pricing Battle: Burroughs Wellcome Reaps Profits, Outrage From Its AIDS Drug', *Wall Street Journal* (September 15, 1989).
55. O'Reilly, B., 'The Inside Story of the AIDS Drug', *Fortune* (November 5, 1990).
56. Chase, M., 'Wellcome PLC Sets Price of AIDS Drug at $8,000 a Year, Higher Than Expected', *Wall Street Journal* (February 17, 1987).
57. 'Study Assesses AZT Profits', Antiviral Agents Bulletin, Biotechnology Information Institute (August 1, 1993).
58. Chase, M., 'Pricing Battle: Burroughs Wellcome Reaps Profits, Outrage From Its AIDS Drug', *Wall Street Journal* (September 15, 1989).

59. Interview with Bill Sullivan, ex-president of Burroughs Wellcome USA, Burroughs Wellcome Oral History project, Wellcome Library (April 23, 2001).
60. Interview with Fred Coe, ex-president of Burroughs Wellcome USA, Burroughs Wellcome Oral History project, Wellcome Library (undated).
61. O'Reilly, B., 'The Inside Story of the AIDS Drug', *Fortune* (November 5, 1990).
62. Interview with Sir Alfred Shepperd, ex-chairman of Burroughs Wellcome USA, Burroughs Wellcome Oral History project, Wellcome Library (November 24, 2001).
63. Testimony of Ted Haigler before the Subcommittee of Health and the Environment of the Committee on Energy and Commerce, US House of Representatives (March 10, 1987).
64. Ibid.
65. Interview by the author with Peter Staley.
66. Ibid.
67. Ibid.
68. Taken from Mark Harrington's unpublished memoir.
69. Transcript of meeting between ACT UP and Burroughs Wellcome (January 23, 1989). Courtesy of Mark Harrington and Peter Staley.
70. Ibid.
71. Interview with Dr David Barry, ex-director of global research, Burroughs Wellcome Oral History project, Wellcome Library (January 24, 2002).
72. Transcript of meeting between ACT UP and Burroughs Wellcome (January 23, 1989). Courtesy of Mark Harrington and Peter Staley.
73. Taken from Mark Harrington's unpublished memoir.
74. Zonana, V., 'AIDS Groups Urge Firm to Lower AZT Price', *Los Angeles Times* (August 31, 1989).
75. 'Editorial: AZT's Inhuman Cost', *New York Times* (August 28, 1989).
76. 'Pressure grows for Wellcome to cut price for AIDS drug AZT', *The Guardian* (September 1, 1989).
77. Hilts, Philip J., 'Wave of Protests Developing On Profits From AIDS Drug', *New York Times* (September 18, 1989).
78. Cimons, M., Zonana, V., 'Manufacturer Reduces Price of AZT by 20%', *Los Angeles Times* (September 19, 1989).
79. Interview by the author with Peter Staley.
80. Ibid.
81. Naussbaum, B., *Good Intentions* (The Atlantic Monthly Press, 1990; Penguin Books, 1991) p.320.
82. 'Decision in *People* v. *James McGrath*', published in the *New York Law Journal* (May 25, 1990).
83. Interview with Dr David Barry, ex-director of global research, Burroughs Wellcome Oral History project, Wellcome Library (April 30, 2001).
84. Kolata, G., 'US Halves Dosage for AIDS Drug', *New York Times* (January 17, 1990).
85. Haigler, T., 'Opinion: Reduced Dosage Cuts Cost of AIDS Drug', *New York Times* (September 16, 1989).
86. Mitsuya, H. et al., 'Opinion: Credit Government Scientists With Developing Anti-AIDS Drug', *New York Times* (September 28, 1989).

87. Zonana, V., 'White House Urges Pricing Restraint', *Los Angeles Times* (October 14, 1989).
88. Fabbri A., Parker L., Colombo, C., et al., 'Industry funding of patient and health consumer organisations: systematic review with meta-analysis', *BMJ* (January 22, 2020).
89. Mesce, D., 'FDA Approves Second AIDS Drug', Associated Press (October 9, 1991).
90. Recer, P., 'FDA Approves Third AIDS Anti-Viral Drug', Associated Press (June 22, 1992).
91. Naussbaum, B., *Good Intentions* (The Atlantic Monthly Press, 1990; Penguin Books, 1991) p.321.
92. 'AZT Patent Expires', *Raleigh News & Observer* (September 18, 2005).

Chapter Three: The hunt for blockbusters

1. 'Blockbuster Drugs 2006', R&D Pipeline News special report (July 6, 2007).
2. In the late 1970s, at a sample of large drug companies, 5 per cent of their products, an average of twenty-eight different drugs, made up a little over half of all sales. See Reekie, W.D., *The Economics of the Pharmaceutical Industry* (Macmillan, 1975) p.127. During the 1990s and 2000s, a single blockbuster, like Pfizer's Lipitor, could account for up to 25 per cent of much higher revenues.
3. Angell, M., *The Truth About Drug Companies* (Random House, 2004) p.11.
4. Morgan, S.G., Basset, K. et al., '"Breakthrough" drugs and growth in expenditure on prescription drugs in Canada', *BMJ* (September 2, 2005).
5. According to the European Federation of Pharmaceutical Industries and Associations.
6. O'Reilly, B., 'Drugmakers under attack', *Fortune* (July 29, 1991).
7. Interview by the author with Shahram Ahari. Ahari has written about his experiences in 'Following the Script: How Drug Reps Make Friends and Influence Doctors' published by *PLoS Medicine* in April 2007.
8. Ahari, S., Testimony to Special Committee on Aging, United States Senate (March 12 2008).
9. Saul, S., 'Gimme an Rx! Cheerleaders Pep Up Drug Sales', *New York Times* (November 28, 2005).
10. Turner, W., '"Detail men" Push Companies' Drugs in Doctors' Prescriptions', *New York Times* (June 13, 1966).
11. Elliott, C., 'The Drug Pushers', *The Atlantic* (April 2006).
12. Neurons are the cells used by the brain to communicate.
13. Singer, N., 'No Mug? Drug Makers Cut Out Goodies for Doctors', *New York Times* (December 30, 2008).
14. The billions a year drug companies spend on their relationship with doctors continues to work. A 2016 study found that doctors who had eaten a single industry-sponsored meal promoting an antidepressant were more than twice as likely as other physicians to prescribe it. See DeJong, C., Aguilar, T., Tseng, C-W., 'Pharmaceutical Industry Sponsored Meals and Physician Prescribing Patterns for Medicare Beneficiaries', *JAMA Internal Medicine* (June 20, 2016).
15. Interview by the author with Shahram Ahari.

16. Swiatek, J., 'Indianapolis-Based Eli Lilly Adds On to $1 Billion Expansion Plan', *Indianapolis Star* (July 16, 2000).

17. Goldberg, M., Davenport, B., Mortellito, T., 'P.E.'s annual sales and marketing employment survey: The big squeeze', *Pharmaceutical Executive*, cited in Fugh-Berman, A., Ahari, S., 'Following the Script: How Drug Reps Make Friends and Influence Doctors', *PLoS Medicine* (April 2007).

18. Munos, B., 'Lessons from 60 years of pharmaceutical innovation', *Nature Reviews Drug Discovery* (December 2009).

19. Gagnon, M-A., Lexchin, J., 'The Cost of Pushing Pills: A New Estimate of Pharmaceutical Promotion Expenditures in the United States', *PLoS Medicine* (January 2008).

20. Lewis, A., 'Should drug firms make payments to doctors?', BBC News (April 17, 2014).

21. Smith, C., 'Retail Prescription Drug Spending in The National Health Account', *Health Affairs* (January 1, 2004).

22. Ventola, C.L., 'Direct-to-Consumer Pharmaceutical Advertising: Therapeutic or Toxic?', *Pharmacy & Therapeutics* (October 2011).

23. This figure is for 2016. Kaufman, J., 'Think You're Seeing More Drug Ads on TV? You Are, and Here's Why', *New York Times* (December 24, 2017).

24. Lanthier, M., Miller, K.L., Nardinelli, C., Woodcock, J., 'An Improved Approach To Measuring Drug Innovation Finds Steady Rates Of First-In-Class Pharmaceuticals, 1987–2011', *Health Affairs* (August 1, 2013). The study divided new drugs into first-in-class drugs, advance-in-class drugs and addition-to-class drugs which offer 'no substantial new medical benefit'. The last category made up 46 per cent of drug approvals between 1987 and 2011.

25. Proportion of new drugs given FDA's priority review designation between 1992 and 2002. Priority review is applied to drugs offering 'Significant improvement compared to marketed products in the treatment, diagnosis, or prevention of a disease'. Standard review drugs are deemed to have 'therapeutic qualities similar to those of one or more already marketed drugs'. Figures archived from fda.gov

26. Interview by the author with Shahram Ahari.

27. DiMasi, J.A., Faden, L.B., 'Competitiveness in follow-on drug R&D: a race or imitation?', *Nature Reviews Drug Discovery* (December 10, 2010).

28. Hollis, A., 'Me-too drugs: is there a problem?', WHO.int (December 13, 2004).

29. Ibid.

30. Prokesch, S., 'Glaxo's Search: Son of Zantac', *New York Times* (October 11, 1989).

31. Lipitor was believed to be a superior statin for years but in 2005 Germany's Institute for Quality and Efficiency in Healthcare rejected Pfizer's 'claims that its drug atorvastatin was superior to other statins'.

32. Johnson, L.A., 'Pfizer's Lipitor: The Blockbuster Drug That Almost Wasn't', Associated Press (December 30, 2011).

33. Jack, A., 'The fall of the world's best-selling drug', *Financial Times* (November 28, 2009).

34. Simons, J., 'The $10 Billion Pill', *Fortune* (January 20, 2003).

35. Schmit, J., 'A winded FDA races to keep up with drug ads that go too far', *USA Today* (May 31, 2005).

36. Moynihan, R.N., Cooke, G.P.E., Doust, J.A. et al., 'Expanding Disease Definitions in Guidelines and Expert Panel Ties to Industry: A Cross-sectional Study of Common Conditions in the United States', *PLOS Medicine* (August 13, 2013).

37. Abramson, J., Starfield, B., 'The effect of conflict of interest on biomedical research and clinical practice guidelines: can we trust the evidence in evidence-based medicine?', *Journal of the American Board of Family Practice* (September 1, 2005).

38. This topic has been explored in several books including Moynihan R., Cassels, A., *Selling Sickness* (Allen & Unwin, 2005).

39. Deer, B., 'Sex drugs & rock 'n' roll', *Sunday Times Magazine* (September 6, 1998).

40. Lexchin, J., 'Bigger and Better: How Pfizer Redefined Erectile Dysfunction', *PLoS Medicine* (April 11, 2006).

41. Ibid.

42. Atkinson, T., 'Lifestyle drug market booming', *Nature Medicine* (September 2002).

43. Hawthorne, F., 'Merck's Fall from Grace', *The Scientist* (May 1, 2006).

44. Drews, J., 'Strategic trends in the drug industry', *Drug Discovery Today* (May 2003).

45. Interview by the author with Bernard Munos.

46. Psaty, B.M., Kronmal, R.A., 'Reporting Mortality Findings in Trials of Rofecoxib for Alzheimer Disease or Cognitive Impairment', *Journal of the American Medical Association* (July 17, 2008).

47. Testimony of David J. Graham to the US Senate Committee on Finance (November 18, 2004).

Chapter Four: How to price a drug

1. Meyers, A.S., *Orphan Drugs: A Global Crusade* (self-published, 2016).

2. Interview by the author with Abbey Meyers.

3. Ibid.

4. Mikami, K., 'Orphans in the Market: The History of Orphan Drug Policy', *Social History of Medicine* (August 2019).

5. Ibid.

6. Seligman, A.W, Hilkevich, J.S. (eds), *Don't Think About Monkeys: Extraordinary Stories by People with Tourette Syndrome* (Hope Press, 1992) p.45.

7. Waxman, H., Green, J., *The Waxman Report: How Congress Really Works* (Twelve, 2009) p.53.

8. Ibid, p.56.

9. Testimony of Melvin H. Van Woert, M.D., 'Drug Regulation Reform – Oversight: Orphan Drugs', House of Representatives, Subcommittee on Health and the Environment (June 26, 1980).

10. Testimony of Sharon Roubeck Dobkin and Melvin H. Van Woert, M.D., 'Drug Regulation Reform – Oversight: Orphan Drugs', House of Representatives, Subcommittee on Health and the Environment (June 26, 1980).

11. Series 6, Episode 14: 'Seldom Seen, Never Heard', *Quincy, M.E* (1981).

12. Interview by the author with Abbey Meyers.

13. This was reduced to 25 per cent in 2017.

14. It was only after an amendment in 1985 that the seven-year exclusivity period

for an orphan designation was extended to include drugs which were still under patent.

15. Sarpatwari, A., Kesselheim, A.S., 'Reforming the Orphan Drug Act for the 21st Century', *New England Journal of Medicine* (July 2019).

16. Waxman, H., Green, J., *The Waxman Report: How Congress Really Works* (Twelve, 2009) p.67.

17. Rosin, J., *Quincy M.E., The Television Series* (BearManor Media, 2014) and Waxman, H., Green, J., *The Waxman Report: How Congress Really Works* (Twelve, 2009) p.67.

18. Russell, C., 'Victims of Rare Disorder Get New Relief – "Orphan Drug" wins US Approval', *Washington Post* (August 8, 1984).

19. Letter from Thomas G. Wiggans, president, Serono, Hearing before the Subcommittee on Health and the Environment of the Committee on Energy and Commerce, US House of Representatives (February 7, 1990).

20. Genentech later renounced this admission. Testimony of John McLaughlin, general counsel, Genentech, Hearing before the Subcommittee on Health and the Environment of the Committee on Energy and Commerce, US House of Representatives (February 7, 1990).

21. Holt, R.I.G., Erotokritou-Mulligan, I., Sönksen, P.H., 'The history of doping and growth hormone abuse in sport', *Growth Hormone & IGF Research* (May 24, 2009).

22. Picard, A., 'The Durbin Inquiry: Francis blames slower performances for speedup in athletes' use of drugs', *Globe and Mail* (March 7, 1989).

23. Okie, S., 'New Drug Approved For Anemia; Medicare to Cover Costly Treatment For Kidney Patients', *Washington Post* (June 2, 1989).

24. Testimony of Abbey Meyers before the Subcommittee on Health and the Environment of the Committee on Energy and Commerce, US House of Representatives (February 7, 1990).

25. 'Federal and Private Roles in the Development and Provision of Alglucerase Therapy for Gaucher Disease', United States Congress Office of Technology Assessment (October 1992). Genzyme argued the true figure was closer to $50 million but this included the company's decision to buy back the rights to the drug from investors.

26. Judgment in *Genzyme Limited* v. *The Office of Fair Trading*, Competition Appeal Tribunal, case number 1016/1/1/03 (March 11, 2004).

27. Anand, G., 'Why Genzyme Can Charge So Much for Cerezyme', *Wall Street Journal* (November 16, 2005).

28. Anand, G., 'How Drugs for Rare Diseases Became Lifeline for Companies', *Wall Street Journal* (November 15, 2005).

29. Tanouye, E., 'What Ails Us – What's Fair?', *Wall Street Journal* (May 20, 1994).

30. Interview by the author with Abbey Meyers. Lisa Raines died in the September 11 terrorist attacks.

31. Ibid. Genzyme, now owned by Sanofi, declined to comment on the pricing of Ceredase or Cerezyme.

32. 'Editorial: Sacrificing the cash cow', *Nature Biotechnology* (April 2007).

33. Interview by the author with Mick Kolassa.

34. Reekie, W.D., 'Price and Quality Competition in the United States Drug Industry', *Journal of Industrial Economics* (March 1978).

35. Ibid.

36. Interview with Sir Alfred Shepperd, ex-chairman, Burroughs Wellcome Oral History project, Wellcome Library (November 24, 2001).

37. Interview by the author with Mick Kolassa.

38. These prices persisted even though, over time, major improvements in increasing the yield would significantly reduce the cost of manufacturing biologics.

39. Transcript of BioMarin Pharmaceutical Inc. at SG Cowen Securities 24th Annual Healthcare Conference (March 9, 2004).

40. Interview by the author with Abbey Meyers.

41. Danzon, P.M., Pauly, M.V., 'Health Insurance and the Growth in Pharmaceutical Expenditures', *The Journal of Law and Economics* (October 2002).

42. Smith, G., 'Remembering Dan Nimer', the *Pricing Advisor* newsletter (January 2015).

43. LinkedIn profile of Dan Nimer.

44. Schmookler, A.B., 'Prescription for Reform', *Baltimore Sun* (July 21, 1993).

45. Kronholm, 'Cyclosporine: A Drug With Vast Promise Will Succeed', Associated Press (May 12, 1986).

46. Langreth, R., Tracer, Z., 'The Blues Singer Who Created America's Hated Drug-Pricing Model', Bloomberg News (May 3, 2016).

47. Interview by the author with Fran Leath. Leath first described this incident in an interview with Fran Quigley for CommonDreams.org.

48. Ibid.

49. Frieswick, K., 'Clinical trials: A new kind of pricing pressure puts pharmaceutical FOS in an unfamiliar role: Evangelist', *CFO* (March 1, 2002). The company did not respond to a request for comment on its pricing of Xigris.

50. Burton, T.A., 'Why Cheap Drugs That Appear To Halt Fatal Sepsis Go Unused', *Wall Street Journal* (May 17, 2002).

51. Krauskopf, L., Pierson, R., 'Lilly pulls sepsis drug Xigris, no benefit found', Reuters (October 25, 2011).

52. Interview by the author with anonymous former chief executive of a large drug company.

53. This concern was raised in a recent study which interviewed four anonymous executives on pricing decisions for multiple sclerosis drugs. See Hartung, D.M., Alley, L. et al., 'Qualitative study on the price of drugs for multiple sclerosis', *American Academy of Neurology* (November 25, 2019).

54. Rockoff, J.D., 'Drugmakers Find Competition Doesn't Keep a Lid on Prices', *Wall Street Journal* (November 27, 2016).

55. Kolassa, M., *The Strategic Pricing of Pharmaceuticals* (The PondHouse Press, 2009) p.7.

56. Interview by the author with anonymous former chief executive of a large drug company.

57. As we shall see, some countries use negotiations and, more recently, cost-effectiveness assessments which play a role in setting a ceiling on the price for which a company will be reimbursed.

58. 'Pricing Products for Success in the Pharmaceutical Industry: Interview with Mick Kolassa', ACN Newswire (April 17, 2012).

59. See Loftus, P., 'Backlash Against Drug Prices Hits Manufacturers and Middlemen', *Wall Street Journal* (October 28, 2016) and Werble, C., 'Health Policy Brief: Pharmacy Benefit Managers', *Health Affairs* (September 14, 2017).

60. Baycol, launched in 1997, was cheaper than other statins but struggled to make a significant dent in the market. It was withdrawn from the market in 2001 because it had a potentially lethal side effect.

Chapter Five: Dirty pharma

1. Berenson, A., 'A Long Shot Becomes Pfizer's Latest Chief Executive', *New York Times* (July 29, 2006).

2. 'Alumni Focus: Former CEO of Pfizer Jeff Kindler offers insights from a career in law and business', Harvard Law Today (June 8, 2016).

3. Jimenez, J., 'The CEO of Novartis on Growing After a Patent Cliff', *Harvard Business Review* (December 2012).

4. Rockoff, J.D., 'Merck Names Frazier as CEO', *Wall Street Journal* (December 1, 2010).

5. Interview by the author with William Lazonick, Öner Tulum and Rosie Collington.

6. In August 2019, the organisation shifted to a new definition reflecting a world in which the idea of a corporation having a social purpose and creating long-term value rather than focusing on maximising profits was coming to the fore. It declared that companies should try to serve all stakeholders, including staff, suppliers and customers, and not just shareholders.

7. Drews, J., 'Strategic trends in the drug industry', *Drug Discovery Today* (May 2003).

8. Drews, J., *In Quest Of Tomorrow's Medicines* (Springer-Verlag, 1999) p.234.

9. Interview by the author with Mick Kolassa.

10. Before the United States fell in line with other countries in 1995, US patents lasted for seventeen years but applied from the date they were granted rather than when an application was filed.

11. Berger, J., Dunn, J.D., Johnson, M.M. et al., 'How drug life-cycle management patent strategies may impact formulary management', *American Journal of Managed Care* (January 20, 2017) and Feldman, R., 'May your drug price be evergreen', *Journal of Law and the Biosciences* (December 7, 2018).

12. Aitken, M., Berndt, E.R., Cutler, D.M., 'Prescription Drug Spending Trends In The United States: Looking Beyond The Turning Point', *Health Affairs* (December 16, 2008) and Aitken, M., Kleinrock, M., 'Medicine Use and Spending in the US', IQVIA Institute for Human Data Science (April 2018).

13. Harris, G., 'Fast Relief: As a Patent Expires, Drug Firm Lines Up Pricey Alternative', *Wall Street Journal* (June 6, 2002).

14. Otto, M.A., 'Ads promote Clarinex as a new, improved Claritin, but some doctors aren't so sure', *Seattle Times* (April 16, 2002).

15. Harris, G., 'Fast Relief: As a Patent Expires, Drug Firm Lines Up Pricey Alternative', *Wall Street Journal* (June 6, 2002).

16. Interview by the author with Josh Krieger.

17. Templeton, S-K., 'The money pharm', *Sunday Herald* (August 10, 2003).

18. Jain, D.C., Conley, J.G., 'Patent Expiry and Pharmaceutical Market Opportunities at the Nexus of Pricing and Innovation Policy', INSEAD Faculty & Research Working Paper (2012).

19. Interview by the author with Fran Leath.

20. Armstrong, D., 'FDA Investigating Lilly's Zyprexa Injection After Two Die', *Bloomberg News* (June 18, 2013).

21. Feldman, R., 'May your drug price be evergreen', *Journal of Law and the Biosciences* (December 7, 2018).

22. 'An Unwarranted Patent Stretch', *New York Times* (August 7, 1982).

23. Interview by the author with Tahir Amin.

24. I-MAK has produced a number of reports on this subject including 'Imbruvica's Patent Wall' (revised July 2020) and 'Overpatented, Overpriced Special Edition: Humira' (revised October 2020).

25. Interview by the author with David Maris.

26. Hemphill, C.S., Lemley, M.A., 'Earning Exclusivity: Generic Drug Incentives and the Hatch–Waxman Act', *Antitrust Law Journal* (2011).

27. Other generic companies who might be seeking regulatory approval for their own versions must wait until 180 days after the first generic has hit the market. Rival generic manufacturers can circumvent this if they win a patent lawsuit of their own, but research-led companies can decline to sue when they file for drug approval, meaning they remain stuck in this bottleneck. See Ibid.

28. Carrier, M., 'FTC v. Actavis: Where We Stand After 5 Years', ipwatchdog.com (June 18, 2018) and 'Agreements Filed with the Federal Trade Commission Under the Medicare Prescription Drug, Improvement, and Modernization Act of 2003 – Overview of Agreements Filed in FY 2015', Report by the Bureau of Competition (November 2017).

29. Jones, G.H, Carrier, M.A., Silver, R.T., Kantarjian, H., 'Strategies that delay or prevent the timely availability of affordable generic drugs in the United States', *Blood* (January 27, 2016).

30. Teva and its subsidiary Cephalon were also fined more than €60 million by the European Commission in 2020 for conspiring to fix the price of Provigil. It said it planned to appeal. Rudge, D., 'Teva Plans To Appeal EU Provigil Fine', *Generics Bulletin*, Informa Pharma Intelligence (November 27, 2020).

31. Feldman, R.C., Misra, P., 'The Fatal Attraction of Pay-for-Delay', *Chicago-Kent Journal of Intellectual Property* (February 8, 2019).

32. AbbVie strongly contested the 'pay-for-delay' label applied by critics including two US senators to the settlements it came to over the launch of biosimilar versions of Humira. The company said it had not agreed to pay the companies and would instead receive royalties once their biosimilar products launched at the agreed dates.

33. Graham, S., 'How AbbVie and Humira Avoided "Pay for Delay" Finding', *National Law Journal* (June 8, 2020).

34. Feldman, R., Wang, C., 'A Citizen's Pathway Gone Astray – Delaying Competition from Generic Drugs', *New England Journal of Medicine* (April 20, 2017).

35. Ibid.

36. Citizen Petition from AstraZeneca Pharmaceuticals LP to the Food and Drug Administration (dated May 31, 2016, revised June 21, 2016).

37. Staton, T., 'AstraZeneca's bid to protect Crestor fails as judge refuses to block new generics', FiercePharma.com (July 20, 2016).

38. Silverman, E., 'AstraZeneca loses court battle to prevent generic versions of Crestor', Stat News (July 20, 2016).

39. Davidson, A., 'Why is Allergan partnering with the St. Regis Mohawk Tribe?', *New Yorker* (November 20, 2017).

40. Hurley, L., 'US Supreme Court rejects Allergan bid to use tribe to shield drug patents', Reuters (April 15, 2019).

41. Almashat, S., Lang, R. et al., 'Twenty-Seven Years of Pharmaceutical Industry Criminal and Civil Penalties: 1991 Through 2017', Public Citizen (March 14, 2018).

42. Martina, M., 'GSK used travel agencies for China bribes: police', Reuters (July 15, 2013).

43. Hirschler, B., 'GSK faces new corruption allegations, this time in Romania', Reuters (July 29, 2015).

44. Plaintiff's complaint filed in *US Securities and Exchange Commission* v. *Johnson & Johnson*, United States District Court of Columbia (April 8, 2011).

45. 'Teva Pharmaceutical Industries Ltd. Agrees to Pay More Than $283 Million to Resolve Foreign Corrupt Practices Act Charges', Press release from the US Department of Justice (December 22, 2016).

46. Interview by the author with Donald Macarthur.

47. Wouters, J.O., 'Lobbying Expenditures and Campaign Contributions by the Pharmaceutical and Health Product Industry in the United States, 1999–2018', *JAMA Internal Medicine* (March 3, 2020).

48. Ibid.

49. McCoy, M.S., Carniol, M., Chockley, K. et al., 'Conflicts of Interest for Patient-Advocacy Organizations', *New England Journal of Medicine* (March 2, 2017).

50. O'Donnell, J., 'Patient groups funded by drugmakers are largely mum on high drug prices', *USA Today* (January 22, 2016).

51. Cohen, D., Raftery, J., 'Paying twice: the "charitable" drug with a high price tag', *BMJ* (February 15, 2014).

52. The charities cannot prioritise one drug over another treating the same condition. Donations to charity are tax-deductible up to a limit of 10 per cent of company income in the US.

53. Frerick, A., 'The Cloak of Social Responsibility: Pharmaceutical Corporate Charity', *Tax Notes* (November 28, 2016).

Chapter Six: The trick

1. Interview by the author with Marc Cohodes.

2. Ibid.

3. Interview by the author with Dimitry Khmelnitsky.

4. The equity analyst was interviewed by the author on condition of anonymity.

5. Interview by the author with Dimitry Khmelnitsky.

6. Analysis of UK medicines sales agreed between the Association of the British Pharmaceutical Industry (ABPI) and the Department of Health and Social Care (DHSC) each year. The figures cited represent spend on branded medicines at net prices with a deduction for the annual payment made by the industry to the DHSC under a voluntary scheme.

7. 'AMCo Acquisition Investor Presentation', Concordia Healthcare (September 8, 2015).

8. Concordia Healthcare M&A call (September 8, 2015).

9. Ibid.

10. At the time, the UK system imposed a profit cap across a company's portfolio of branded drugs if they had signed up to a voluntary scheme governing this. If they hadn't, a separate statutory scheme mandated specified price cuts.

11. Patel, S., 'Making £300m before turning 40', *Asian Wealth Magazine* (Autumn 2017).

12. Government lawyers concluded that the UK Department of Health's ability to intervene in the price of generic medicines was hampered in many cases by rules preventing companies who had agreed to participate in a voluntary scheme governing the price of branded medicines from being subject to other price controls. This loophole would be rectified by new legislation in 2017. Existing policy detailed in Barber, S., Harker, R., Rhodes, C., 'Briefing Paper: The Health Service Medical Supplies (Costs) Bill (Bill 72 of 2016–17)', House of Commons Library (October 21, 2016).

13. Auden Mckenzie (Pharma Division) Limited annual accounts, Companies House.

14. Lewis, J., 'NHS doesn't care what drugs cost', *Mail on Sunday* (July 18, 2010).

15. The founder of Auden Mckenzie, Amit Patel, has said that the Department of Health accepted the price changes and did not challenge them, although hydrocortisone tablets were later referred to the Competition and Markets Authority, which opened an investigation into excessive pricing. In June 2014, the more popular 10mg strength was recategorised under NHS pricing rules as a 'category M' drug. Such drugs are priced on the basis of manufacturers' pricing but also include a margin for pharmacists' profits, meaning suppliers cannot fully control the price paid by the NHS. From 2015, Auden Mckenzie was no longer the sole supplier of hydrocortisone tablets in the UK.

16. Oral evidence from Professor Karim Meeran, Deputy Director of Medical Education, Imperial College, to the Commons Public Accounts Committee (July 4, 2018).

17. The claims related to the supply and prices of several antibiotics and the blood thinner warfarin during the 1990s. Goldshield paid £4 million to settle a civil lawsuit brought by the Department of Health without admitting liability. Criminal charges brought by the Serious Fraud Office against five companies and nine executives were thrown out because of a ruling that conspiracy to defraud could not be used in price-fixing cases. Price-fixing had only become a specific criminal offence in 2003, after the start of the case.

18. John Beighton evidence on day five of a Competition Appeal Tribunal hearing in the cases between Flynn Pharma and the Competition and Markets Authority (CMA) and Pfizer and the CMA (November 7, 2017).

19. Slides from presentation by John Beighton and Guy Clark (November 13, 2012). The content of these slides was first reported by the author in Kenber, B., 'Lessons in exploiting a loophole to make millions out of the NHS', *The Times* (June 4, 2016).

20. Beighton did not respond to multiple requests for an interview.

21. Cinven has said that 'debranding' was not a trick but an approach which was an obvious consequence of the UK government's decision to allow market forces to determine prices and ensure an adequate supply of generic drugs. It argues that price rises reflected the value of the products and that health officials were aware of prices and could have raised concerns if they wished.

22. The drugs were carbimazole tablets and dipipanone 10mg / cyclizine 30mg tablets. NHS reimbursement prices are detailed in the monthly Drug Tariff.

23. Kenber, B., '"Extortionate" prices add £260m to NHS drug bill', *The Times* (June 3, 2016).

24. McGee, N., 'How Concordia Healthcare got caught in a stock market storm', *Globe and Mail* (October 2, 2015).

25. McGee, N., 'Concordia Healthcare CEO says pricing controls unlikely', *Globe and Mail* (October 27, 2015).

26. Concordia Healthcare Q3 2015 Earnings Call (November 13, 2015).

27. Concordia Healthcare at CIBC Whistler Institutional Investor Conference (January 20, 2016).

28. Emails obtained under the Freedom of Information Act. Cinven, which owned AMCo at the time, denied that any price rises were linked to the Concordia transaction.

29. Concordia, now known as Advanz Pharma, said that written approval for its price rises were approved by officials at the UK Department for Health. Emails obtained under freedom of information legislation show that National Health Service (NHS) officials did not seek justifications for any price rises before approving them. See Kenber, B., 'NHS failure on medicine prices costs public £125m', *The Times* (August 16, 2016). Advanz Pharma said that health officials had powers to intervene to control prices if there were objections but did not do so. It said it operated a 'portfolio pricing' model which meant that 'whilst the price of some medicines increased (for a number of reasons, including significant investment to ensure continuity of supply and availability of medicines to patients, increase in cost of materials, and regulatory & quality requirements), the majority of medicines decreased in price each year, with around 25 per cent of medicines being sold for no profit or at a loss'. It said the average cost of a month's supply of medicines to UK patients was around £4 and that this represented substantial cost savings for the NHS.

30. Kenber, B., 'Patients pay price as drug soars to £9 a pill', *The Times* (October 31, 2017).

31. Taylor, P.N. et al., 'Liothyronine cost and prescriptions in England', *The Lancet Diabetes & Endocrinology* (January 1, 2019).

32. Interview by the author with Melanie Woodcock.

33. Celarier, M., 'Hacked Printers. Fake Emails. Questionable Friends. Fahmi Quadir Was Up 24% Last Year, But It Came at a Price', *Institutional Investor* (January 9, 2019).

34. Eisinger, J., 'For One Whistle-Blower, No Good Deed Goes Unpunished', ProPublica (June 1, 2011).

35. Interview by the author with David Maris.

36. Khmelnitsky, D., 'Concordia Healthcare Corp.: Changing Strategy, Risky Bet', Veritas Investment Research (March 11, 2016).

37. 'Report: Heightened Risk at Concordia', Pacific Square Research (March 11, 2016).

38. Consolidated financial statements of Concordia Healthcare (December 31, 2015).

39. Shmuel, J., 'Rough ride for Concordia in Valeant's wake', *Financial Post* (March 30, 2016).

40. Interview by the author with Chris Crum.

41. This emerged in August 2016 when a collapse in Concordia's share price resulted in a margin call on the debt, which forced him to sell 505,000 shares.

42. Balgorri, M., Banerjee, D., Porter, K., 'Blackstone reportedly eyeing Concordia Healthcare', Bloomberg News (April 22, 2016).

43. Interview by the author with David Maris.

44. Figures from the Prime Institute, University of Minnesota, presented at a hearing before the Joint Economic Committee, Congress of the United States (July 24, 2008).

45. US Senate Special Committee on Aging, 'Sudden Price Spikes in Off-Patent Prescription Drugs: The Monopoly Business Model that Harms Patients, Taxpayers, and the US Health Care System', US Government Publishing Office (December 2016) pp.44–5.

46. Burnham, T.C., Huang, S., Lo, A.W., 'Pricing for Survival in the Biopharma Industry: A Case Study of Acthar Gel and Questcor Pharmaceuticals', *Journal of Investment Management* (September 22, 2017).

47. Questcor ran a patient assistance programme which gave away supplies of the drug worth $50 million a year at full price to insured and underinsured patients.

48. Prepared statement of Danielle Foltz at a hearing before the Joint Economic Committee, Congress of the United States (July 24, 2008).

49. Ibid.

50. Burnham, T.C., Huang, S., Lo, A.W., 'Pricing for Survival in the Biopharma Industry: A Case Study of Acthar Gel and Questcor Pharmaceuticals', *Journal of Investment Management* (September 22, 2017).

51. Questcor Pharmaceuticals, Inc., Annual Report on Form 10-K (December 31, 2007 and December 31, 2013).

52. Drash, W., 'Whistleblowers: Company at heart of 97,000% drug price hike bribed doctors to boost sales', CNN (April 30, 2019).

53. 'Questcor Pharmaceuticals Acquires Rights to Synacthen', press release from Questcor Pharmaceuticals (June 11, 2013).

54. Deutsch, B., 'Company Profile: Ovation Pharmaceuticals, Inc.', *Pharmacogenomics* (November 2002).

55. Berenson, A., 'A Cancer Drug's Big Price Rise Disturbs Doctors and Patients', *New York Times* (March 12, 2006) and prepared statement of Alan L. Goldbloom, president and CEO of Children's Hospitals and Clinics of Minnesota, at a hearing before the Joint Economic Committee, Congress of the United States (July 24, 2008).

56. Berenson, A., 'A Cancer Drug's Big Price Rise Disturbs Doctors and Patients', *New York Times* (March 12, 2006). Ovation Pharmaceuticals said the price rises were necessary to allow for investment in manufacturing facilities.

57. Walker, J., 'Marathon Pharmaceuticals to Charge $89,000 for Muscular Dystrophy Drug After 70-Fold Increase', *Wall Street Journal* (February 10, 2017). The drug had been taken through FDA approval by Marathon but this required only limited work because the company largely used efficacy data which was

decades old and had been bought for $350,000, the *WSJ* reported. Marathon said it expected to keep an average of $54,000 of the $89,000 list price after allowing for the cost of rebates, free prescriptions and some patients taking fewer pills than recommended.

58. Letter from Representative Elijah E. Cummings and Senator Bernard Sanders to Jeffrey S. Aronin, Chairman and Chief Executive Officer, Marathon Pharmaceuticals, LLC (October 2, 2014).

59. Khot, U.M., Vogan, E.D., Militello, M.A., 'Nitroprusside and Isoproterenol Use After Major Price Increases', *New England Journal of Medicine* (August 9, 2017).

60. El Akkad, O., 'Pharmaceuticals industry puts Valeant's strategy under microscope', *Globe and Mail* (November 5, 2015).

61. US Senate Special Committee on Aging, 'Sudden Price Spikes in Off-Patent Prescription Drugs: The Monopoly Business Model that Harms Patients, Taxpayers, and the US Health Care System', US Government Publishing Office (December 2016).

62. Deutsch, B., 'Company Profile: Ovation Pharmaceuticals, Inc.', *Pharmacogenomics* (November 2002).

63. Crow, D., 'Irish drugmaker Horizon Pharma raises painkiller price to $3,000 in US', *Financial Times* (February 15, 2018) and 'Horizon Pharma Files for IPO', *Venture Capital Journal* (August 4, 2010).

64. Crow, D., 'Valeant – the Harder They Fall', *Financial Times* (March 28, 2016).

65. Forsythe, M., Bogdanich, W., Hickey, B., 'As McKinsey Sells Advice, Its Hedge Fund May Have a Stake in the Outcome', *New York Times* (February 19, 2019).

66. Email sent by Aamir Malik of McKinsey to Mike Pearson and Andrew Davis of Valeant (December 29, 2014). It was obtained by the staff of the United States House Committee on Oversight and Government Reform and released without revealing the name of the consultancy firm or McKinsey. A class action lawsuit filed in 2016 unmasked the names.

67. Bogdanich, W., 'McKinsey Advised Johnson & Johnson on Increasing Opioid Sales', *New York Times* (July 25, 2019). McKinsey told the newspaper that its work for Johnson & Johnson 'was designed to support the legal use of a patch that was then widely understood to be less susceptible to abuse'.

68. Ibid.

69. The plan did not appear to have been adopted, with distributors telling the *New York Times* that they never received rebates for customers who had overdosed. McKinsey stopped advising clients on opioid-specific business in 2019 and has said it is 'cooperating fully with opioid-related investigations'. See Bogdanich, W., Forsythe, M., 'McKinsey Proposed Paying Pharmacy Companies Rebates for OxyContin Overdoses', *New York Times* (November 27, 2020).

70. Open letter from Kevin Sneader, McKinsey's global managing partner, 'Today's settlement on opioids and setting a higher standard' (February 4, 2021).

71. Alpern, J.D., Stauffer, W.M., Kesselheim, A.S., 'High-Cost Generic Drugs – Implications for Patients and Policymakers', *New England Journal of Medicine* (November 13, 2014). Spending by Medicaid on albendazole rose from an

average of $36.10 per prescription in 2008 to $241.30 in 2013. The list price rose by an even greater amount, from $5.92 a day to $119.58.

72. Rockoff, J.D., 'An Old Gout Drug Gets New Life and a New Price, Riling Patients', *Wall Street Journal* (April 12, 2010).

73. Complaint for Injunctive and Other Equitable Relief, *Federal Trade Commission and the State of New York* v. *Vyera Pharmaceuticals, LLC, Phoenixus AG, Martin Shkreli and Kevin Mulleady*, in the United States District Court for the Southern District of New York (January 2, 2020).

74. Lowe, D., 'The Most Unconscionable Drug Price Hike I Have Yet Seen', blog on sciencemag.org (September 11, 2014).

75. US Senate Special Committee on Aging, 'Sudden Price Spikes in Off-Patent Prescription Drugs: The Monopoly Business Model that Harms Patients, Taxpayers, and the US Health Care System', US Government Publishing Office (December 2016).

76. Ibid.

77. Ibid.

78. 'Martin Shkreli: "I Would've Raised Prices Higher"', *Forbes* video (December 3, 2015).

79. Conti, R.M., Nguyen, K.H., Rosenthal, M.B., 'Generic drug price increases: which products will be affected by proposed anti-gouging legislation?', *Journal of Pharmaceutical Policy and Practice* (November 21, 2018).

80. Data from Connecture, cited in O'Brien, E., 'Why drug prices remain insanely high and 6 things you can do to save', MarketWatch (September 21, 2015).

81. Langreth, R., 'Dealmakers Behind Soaring Drug Prices Hit the Jackpot', Bloomberg News (November 2, 2016).

82. 'Valeant Pharmaceuticals International Inc. is becoming the 800-pound gorilla of the TSX – and that should worry index investors', *Financial Post* (May 12, 2015) and Alexander, D., Lam E., 'Valeant passes RBC as Canada's largest company by market value', *Globe and Mail* (July 23, 2015).

83. Khot, U.N., Vogan, E.D., Militello, M.A., 'Nitroprusside and Isoproterenol Use After Major Price Increases', *New England Journal of Medicine* (August 9, 2017).

84. In 2014 alone, drugs which had increased in price by at least 100 per cent accounted for $4.5 billion in Medicare Part D spending. See 'Generic Drugs Under Medicare: Part D Generic Drug Prices Declined Overall, but Some Had Extraordinary Price Increases', United States Government Accountability Office (August 2016).

85. Kenber, B. 'Drug companies' price rises cost NHS extra £370m', *The Times* (April 22, 2017).

86. 'Price increases for cancer drugs up to 1500%: the ICA imposes a 5 million Euro fine on the multinational Aspen', press release by the Italian Competition Authority (October 14, 2016).

87. 'Excessive Prices in Pharmaceutical Markets, Background Note by the Secretariat', Organisation for Economic Co-operation and Development (October 3, 2018).

88. Bannenberg, W., 'Response of the Pharmaceutical Accountability Foundation to the press release of the Dutch Competition Authority (Netherlands

Authority for Consumers and Markets, ACM) on CDCA Leadiant', Pharmaceutical Accountability Foundation (June 29, 2020).

89. The document was obtained as part of an investigation by the Committee on Oversight and Government Reform, US House of Representatives, and disclosed in a memorandum published on February 2, 2016.

90. Quoted in Wasserman, E., 'Valeant comes under fire for timely, dramatic price hike on assisted-suicide drug', FiercePharma (March 24, 2016).

91. Interview by the author with Mick Kolassa.

92. The Association of the British Pharmaceutical Industry press release (June 3, 2016).

93. 'Decision of the Competition and Markets Authority: Unfair pricing in respect of the supply of phenytoin sodium capsules in the UK', CMA (December 7, 2016).

94. 'Particulars of Claim', *Tor Generics Limited* v. *Pfizer Limited*, The High Court of Justice Chancery Division (filed November 6, 2013).

95. 'Decision of the Competition and Markets Authority: Unfair pricing in respect of the supply of phenytoin sodium capsules in the UK', CMA (December 7, 2016).

96. Ibid.

97. Ibid. Steve Poulton told a later Competition Appeal Tribunal hearing in November 2017 that 'we didn't want to just simply raise the price for a couple of years, it wasn't about getting financial benefit; it was about putting this product back on a fair sustainable basis for the longer term'.

98. Email is quoted in 'Decision of the Competition and Markets Authority: Unfair pricing in respect of the supply of phenytoin sodium capsules in the UK', CMA (December 7, 2016). The name of the sender is revealed in 'Re-amended defence', *Tor Generics Limited* v. *Phfizer Limited*, The High Court of Justice Chancery Division (filed May 2015).

99. 'Decision of the Competition and Markets Authority: Unfair pricing in respect of the supply of phenytoin sodium capsules in the UK', CMA (December 7, 2016).

100. Flynn Pharma said it had initially offered to maintain the branded version of the drug in exchange for a 'one-off price increase on the basis that the list price for the branded product was not sustainable' but the Department of Health would not agree to this.

101. Flynn Pharma and Pfizer argue that the price was not unreasonable because the tablet version of phenytoin sodium was more expensive, at £30 for a smaller packet of twenty-eight pills. The companies believed that health officials had approved this price because the UK Department of Health (DoH) had made contact with Teva, the company selling the tablet version, after it increased in price significantly in 2007 and £30 a pack represented a price cut from £60. However, during a meeting with Flynn in November 2012, DoH officials made it clear that the previous discussions over the tablet version did not mean the British health service was 'happy' with the price of the tablets. Clinical guidance meant doctors and pharmacists would not normally move patients between the tablet and capsule versions once stabilised on the drug because of its narrow therapeutic index. See 'Decision of the

Competition and Markets Authority: Unfair pricing in respect of the supply of phenytoin sodium capsules in the UK', CMA (December 7, 2016).

102. Interview by the author with George Jepsen.

103. Ibid.

104. Heritage Pharmaceuticals paid more than $7 million to settle civil and criminal charges in 2019. Two former Heritage executives pleaded guilty to price-fixing charges and agreed to help the investigation.

105. Plaintiff's complaint filed in *The State of Connecticut et al.* v. *Teva Pharmaceuticals USA, Inc et al.* in the United States District Court for the District of Connecticut (May 10, 2019).

106. In March 2020 Sandoz admitted price fixing and paid $195 million in a criminal settlement with the US Department of Justice (DoJ). Teva was charged by the DoJ in August 2020 with conspiring to fix generic drug prices. The company denied the allegations and said it would 'vigorously defend [itself] in court'. Teva has also defended itself against price-fixing claims made in lawsuits brought by forty-four US states which followed Jepsen's investigation, saying in 2019 that it 'has not engaged in any conduct that would lead to civil or criminal liability'. Pfizer, which has been named in the same lawsuits, has said it does not believe it engaged in unlawful conduct.

107. Mylan said it was confident that the claims made against it in civil litigation 'will prove meritless when examined in a court of law'. The company said it had throughly investigated the allegations made against it and had found no evidence of price fixing.

108. Plaintiff's complaint filed in *The State of Connecticut et al.* v. *Teva Pharmaceuticals USA, Inc et al.* in the United States District Court for the District of Connecticut (May 10, 2019).

Chapter Seven: The acquisition game

1. Figures for novel FDA approvals per year are compiled in Mullard, A., '2018 FDA drug approvals', *Nature Reviews Drug Discovery* (January 15, 2019).

2. Singh, D., Desai, R., 'Shaping a Three-Layered Intended Strategy to Realize Benefits for Life Sciences R&D Site Closures', Cognizant 20-20 Insights (December 2012).

3. Schuhmacher, A., Gassmann, O., Hinder, M., 'Changing R&D models in research-based pharmaceutical companies', *Journal of Translational Medicine* (April 27, 2016) and Loftus, P., Falconi, M., Plumridge, H., 'In Drug Mergers, There's One Sure Bet: The Layoffs', *Wall Street Journal* (April 29, 2014).

4. Herper, M., 'A decade in drug industry layoffs', *Forbes* (April 13, 2011).

5. LaMattina, J., 'The impact of mergers on pharmaceutical R&D', *Nature Reviews Drug Discovery* (August 2011).

6. Interview by the author with anonymous former chief executive of a large drug company.

7. Kollewe, J., 'Botox maker Allergan bought by US drug giant for $63bn', *The Guardian* (June 25, 2019).

8. 'World Preview 2020, Outlook to 2026', EvaluatePharma (July 16, 2020).

9. 'PhRMA Annual Membership Survey', published by the Pharmaceutical Research and Manufacturers of America (2010).

10. 'PhRMA Annual Membership Survey', published by the Pharmaceutical Research and Manufacturers of America (2020).

11. Jolls, C., 'Stock Repurchases and Incentive Compensation', The National Bureau of Economic Research Working Paper (March 1998).

12. Tulum, O., Lazonick, W., 'Financialized Corporations in a National Innovation System: The US Pharmaceutical Industry', *International Journal of Political Economy* (2018).

13. Humer C., Pierson, R., 'Obama's inversion curbs kill Pfizer's $160 billion Allergan deal', Reuters (April 5, 2016). Mylan was renamed Viatris in late 2019 after acquiring Pfizer's Upjohn generics division.

14. Hartung, D.M., Alley, L. et al., 'Qualitative study on the price of drugs for multiple sclerosis', *American Academy of Neurology* (November 25, 2019).

15. For companies who don't opt into this voluntary scheme, there is a separate statutory scheme which seeks to limit annual sales growth to 1.1 per cent and does not include an exemption for new medicines.

16. Interview by the author with unnamed former drug industry chief executive.

17. Testimony of Madeline Carpinelli, research fellow, Prime Institute, University of Minnesota, at a hearing before the Joint Economic Committee, Congress of the United States (July 24, 2008).

18. Interview by the author with an anonymous former Big Pharma chief executive.

19. Edwards, J., 'Price of Viagra Has Risen 108% Since Launch; 100 Pills Now Cost $1,400', CBS News (September 10, 2009).

20. Wineinger, N.E., Zhang Y., Topol, E.J., 'Trends in Prices of Popular Brand-Name Prescription Drugs in the United States', *JAMA Network Open* (May 31, 2019).

21. This is based on the list price of the drug, meaning a proportion of that increase is likely to have been paid back to PBMs and insurers in rebates. Data from Truven Analytics cited in Huggett, B., 'America's drug problem', *Nature Biotechnology* (December 2016).

22. The US House of Representatives Committee on Oversight and Reform released a series of staff reports as part of its drug-pricing investigation in October 2020.

23. Marsh, T., 'Live Updates: January 2021 Drug Price Increases', GoodRX.com (January 19, 2021).

24. Merrill, J., 'US Drug Pricing Challenges Poised To Impact Pharma Growth, Leerink Warns', Scrip (October 19, 2018).

25. 'Pharmaceuticals Exit Research and Create Value', Morgan Stanley Research Report (January 20, 2010).

26. Plieth, J., Elmhirst, E., 'If you want blockbuster sales, buy them in', Vantage (April 29, 2019).

27. Schuhmacher, A., Gassmann, O., Hinder, M., 'Changing R&D models in research-based pharmaceutical companies', *Journal of Translational Medicine* (April 27, 2016).

28. Research by Öner Tulum. Pfizer has disclosed sales of seventy-six named drugs in annual reports since 2001, of which four are internally developed and originated. See also Lazonick, W., Hopkins, M. et al., 'US Pharma's Financialized Business Model', Working Paper, Institute for New Economic Thinking (September 8, 2017).

29. Schipper, I., de Haan, E., Cowan, R., 'Overpriced: Drugs Developed with Dutch Public Funding', SOMO in collaboration with Wemos (May 2019).

30. Nayak, R.K., Avorn, J., Kesselheim, A.S., 'Public sector financial support for late stage discovery of new drugs in the United States: cohort study', *BMJ* (October 23, 2019). The study looked at the role of direct public funding and spin-off companies that had their origins in public sector research institutions.

31. Interview by the author with Bernard Munos.

32. Foxman, S., 'Baker Brothers Make $1.4 Billion in Two Weeks on Biotech', Bloomberg (November 1, 2019).

33. Steedman, M., Stockbridge, M, et al., 'Ten years on: Measuring the return from pharmaceutical innovation', Deloitte Centre for Health Solutions (December 20, 2019).

34. Hughes. B., 'An audience with . . . Marc Cluzel', *Nature Reviews Drug Discovery* (January, 2010).

35. Russell, S., 'Antisense Drugs Could Be Medical, Financial Bonanza,' *San Francisco Chronicle* (July 10, 1989).

36. Letter from Dr Michael L. Riordan, founder of Gilead Sciences, to unnamed recipient, Slideshare.net (undated).

37. Russell, S., 'Biotech Firms Open New Era in Bay Area', *San Francisco Chronicle* (September 12, 1988).

38. Loeckx, R., *Cold War Triangle: How Scientists in East and West Tamed HIV* (Leuven University Press, 2017).

39. Gilead Sciences Initial Public Offering Prospectus, Slideshare.net (January 1992).

40. Gellene, D., 'Gilead's Research Goes to Front Lines', *Los Angeles Times* (July 31, 2003).

41. Watts, G., 'Obituary: Antonín Holý', *The Lancet* (September 15, 2012).

42. Liotta, D.C., Painter, G.R., 'Discovery and Development of the Anti-Human Immunodeficiency Virus Drug, Emtricitabine (Emtriva, FTC)', *Accounts of Chemical Research* (October 5, 2016).

43. Ibid.

44. Huggett, B., Scott, C., 'Gilead's deal of a lifetime', *Nature Biotechnology* (May 2009).

45. Berkrot, B., 'Interview – Gilead could have had Pharmasset cheap', Reuters (November 23, 2011).

46. Interview by the author with Victor Roy.

47. Lowe, D., 'The Check Shows Up In The Mail. Really', blogpost on sciencemag. com (July 25, 2005).

48. Cohen, J., 'King of the pills', *Science* (May 8, 2015).

49. US Senate Committee on Finance, 'The Price of Sovaldi and its impact on the US Health Care System', US Government Publishing Office (December 2015).

50. Roy, V., 'The Financialization of a Cure: A Political Economy of Biomedical Innovation, Pricing and Public Health', PhD dissertation, University of Cambridge (June 2017) p.158.

51. US Senate Committee on Finance, 'The Price of Sovaldi and its impact on the US Health Care System', US Government Publishing Office (December 2015).

52. Ibid.

53. Ibid.

54. Responding to the report, Gilead said it had 'responsibly and thoughtfully priced Sovaldi and Harvoni' in line with the previous standards of care. It said they offered significant value by reducing the long-term costs associated with managing chronic hepatitis C.

55. Gilead Sciences FY 2014 financial results.

56. Gilead Sciences FY 2015 financial results.

57. Cohen, J., 'King of the pills', *Science* (May 8, 2015).

58. Gilead repurchased stock totalling $25.8 billion between December 2013 and December 2016.

59. Lazonick, W., Hopkins, M. et al., 'US Pharma's Financialized Business Model', Working Paper, Institute for New Economic Thinking (September 8, 2017).

60. Companies routinely offer discounts on list prices and Gilead struck a commercial agreement with the British health service which lowered the actual price paid.

61. Letter to the *BMJ* by Gregg Alton, Executive Vice President, Gilead Sciences (published July 27, 2016).

62. 'Final report: The Comparative Clinical Effectiveness and Value of Simeprevir and Sofosbuvir in the Treatment of Chronic Hepatitis C Infection', Institute for Clinical and Economic Review (April 15, 2014).

63. Figures on share of generics in pharmaceutical markets compiled by the Organisation for Economic Co-operation and Development (OECD).

64. Lowe, D., 'Big Pharma's Lost Stock Market Decade', blogpost at sciencemag. org (December 13, 2010).

65. US Senate Committee on Finance, 'The Price of Sovaldi and Its Impact on the US Health Care System', US Government Publishing Office (December 2015) p.58.

66. 'Technology appraisal guidance: Sofosbuvir for treating chronic hepatitis C', National Institute of Health and Care Excellence (February 25, 2015).

67. Iyengar, S., Tay-Teo, K. et al., 'Prices, Costs, and Affordability of New Medicines for Hepatitis C in 30 Countries: An Economic Analysis', *PLOS Medicine* (May 31, 2016).

68. Gilead said in 2016 that 'the price of treatment should not be considered as the limiting factor in patient access' in the UK. It said it 'our hepatitis C regimens have been deemed cost effective by NICE at list price and are offered to the NHS with substantial discounts to these already cost-effective prices'.

69. The $1.3 billion does not include any rebates. US Senate Committee on Finance, 'The Price of Sovaldi and Its Impact on the US Health Care System', US Government Publishing Office (December 2015).

70. Barber, J.M., Gotham, D., et al. 'Price of a hepatitis C cure: Cost of production and current prices for direct-acting antivirals in 50 countries', *Journal of Virus Eradication* (September 2020).

71. Freeman, J.D., Hill, A., 'The use of generic medicines for hepatitis C', *Liver International* (June 16, 2016).

72. Chen Q., Ayer T., Bethea E. et al. 'Changes in hepatitis C burden and treatment trends in Europe during the era of direct-acting antivirals: a modelling study', *BMJ Open* (June 11, 2019).

Chapter Eight: A one-sided tug of war

1. 'Speaker: Cost of cancer drugs a "major problem"', Healio (June 2, 2015).
2. Andrews, A., 'Treating with Checkpoint Inhibitors – Figure $1 Million per Patient', *American Health & Drug Benefits* (August 2015).
3. Slides from 'ASCO Plenary Session 2015: Perspectives on Value'. Courtesy of Leonard B. Saltz. Data on cancer drug prices is from Peter Bach and Geoffrey Schnorr at Memorial Sloan Kettering Cancer Center.
4. Interview by the author with Leonard Saltz.
5. Walker, J., 'High Prices for Drugs Attacked at Meeting', *Wall Street Journal* (June 1, 2015).
6. Morgan, S.G., Bathula, H.S., Moon, S., 'Pricing of pharmaceuticals is becoming a major challenge for health systems', *BMJ* (January 13, 2020).
7. Figures are for net spending. See Aitken, M., Berndt, E.R., Cutler, D.M., 'Prescription Drug Spending Trends In The United States: Looking Beyond The Turning Point', *Health Affairs* (December 16, 2008) and Hernandez, I., San-Juan-Rodriguez, A. et al., 'Changes in List Prices, Net Prices, and Discounts for Branded Drugs', *Journal of the American Medical Association* (March 3, 2020).
8. Aitken, M., Kleinrock, M. et al., 'The Global Use of Medicine in 2019 and Outlook to 2023', IQVIA Institute for Human Data Science (January 2019).
9. 'Observations on Trends in Prescription Drug Spending', Office of the Assistant Secretary for Planning and Evaluation, US Department of Health & Human Services (March 8, 2016). An earlier analysis in the US concluded that price increases accounted for around 25 per cent of the increase in prescription drug spending between 1994 and 1999, with the introduction of more expensive products also playing a significant role; see Danzon, P.M., Pauly, M.V., 'Health Insurance and the Growth in Pharmaceutical Expenditures', *The Journal of Law and Economics* (October 2002).
10. Hegele, R.A., 'Correspondence: Insulin affordability', *The Lancet Diabetes & Endocrinology* (May 2017).
11. Figures from Fortune Business Insights (September 30, 2020).
12. A tiny proportion of patients have other types of diabetes, including those related to cystic fibrosis or caused by rare syndromes.
13. Interview by the author with Mindi Patterson.
14. A bipartisan congressional report published in April 2019 by members of the Congressional Diabetes Caucus found that 'the list price of competing insulin formulations has appeared to rise in tandem'.
15. Rajkumar, S.V., 'The High Cost of Insulin in the United States: An Urgent Call to Action', Mayo Clinic Proceedings (January 2020).
16. Interview by the author with Margaret Ewen.
17. Cefalu, W.T., Dawes, D.E. et al., 'Insulin Access and Affordability Working Group: Conclusions and Recommendations', *Diabetes Care* (June 2018).
18. Luo, J. et al., 'Strategies to improve the affordability of insulin in the USA', *The Lancet Diabetes & Endocrinology* (February 8, 2017).
19. Herkert, D., Vijayakumar, P., Luo, J. et al., 'Cost-Related Insulin Underuse Among Patients With Diabetes', *JAMA Internal Medicine* (January 2019).
20. Gotham, D., Barber, M.J., Hill, A., 'Production costs and potential prices for

biosimilars of human insulin and insulin analogues', *BMJ Global Health* (September 25, 2018).

21. Fuglesten Biniek, J., Johnson, W., 'Spending on Individuals with Type 1 Diabetes and the Role of Rapidly Increasing Insulin Prices', Health Care Cost Institute (January 21, 2019).

22. This changed when AbbVie and Merck & Co. (MSD) subsequently launched their own hepatitis C drugs. For interferon-based treatment success rates see Rong, L., Perelson, A.S., 'Treatment of hepatitis C virus infection with interferon and small molecule direct antivirals: viral kinetics and modeling', *Critical Reviews in Immunology* (July 1, 2010).

23. Figure for net spending from Aitken, M., Kleinrock, M. et al., 'Medicine Spending and Affordability in the US', IQVIA Institute for Human Data Science (August 4, 2020) and Aitken, M. and Kleinrock, M., 'Medicine Use and Spending in the US', IQVIA Institute for Human Data Science (May 9, 2019).

24. OECD Pharmaceutical spending indicator (2020).

25. Strongin, R.J, 'The ABCs of PBMs', Issue Brief, National Health Policy Forum (October 27, 1999).

26. Urahn, S.K., Coukell, A., 'The Prescription Drug Landscape, Explored', The Pew Charitable Trusts (March 2019). This figure is for retail prescription drugs, meaning those dispensed in pharmacies. Manufacturers pay rebates to insurers and pharmacies as well as PBMs.

27. 'Second Amended Consolidated Class Action Complaint' in *Anthem* v. *Express Scripts, Inc,* filed in United States District Court Southern District of New York (March 2, 2017).

28. Testimony of Peter Bach, director, Centre for Health Policy and Outcomes, Memorial Sloan Kettering Cancer Center, to the US Senate Committee on Finance (January 29, 2019).

29. 'The Global Use of Medicine in 2019 and Outlook to 2023', IQVIA Institute for Human Data Science (January 2019).

30. Hernandez, I., San-Juan-Rodriguez, A., Good, C.B., Gellad, W.F., 'Changes in List Prices, Net Prices, and Discounts for Branded Drugs in the US, 2007–2018', *JAMA* (March 3, 2020).

31. The American company Merck & Co. (MSD), one of a number of drugmakers which has started publishing details of the average discount it offers on list prices, has disclosed that this amounted to 27.3 per cent in 2010 but rose to 44.3 per cent in 2018. '2018 US Pricing Transparency Report', Merck & Co. (February 2019). In 1992, the weighted average discount across the industry was 16 per cent. See 'Drug Manufacturers Are Giving Discounts of Over 25% From List Price to Majority of the Market, Boston Consulting Group Finds in State-of-the-Industry Study', *The Pink Sheet* (April 5, 1993).

32. Cefalu, W.T, Dawes, D.E. et al., 'Insulin Access and Affordability Working Group: Conclusions and Recommendations', *Diabetes Care* (June 2018).

33. Testimony of Olivier Brandicourt, chief executive officer, Sanofi, to the US Senate Committee on Finance (February 26, 2019). Separately, Novo Nordisk said its net prices were declining as it paid a larger rebates and

discounts in the US, which rose from 68 per cent of sales to 71 per cent between 2018 and 2019. It said these savings weren't being fully passed on to patients.

34. Pear, R., 'He Raised Drug Prices at Eli Lilly. Can He Lower Them for the US?', *New York Times* (November 26, 2017).

35. Howard, D.H., Bach, P.B., Berndt, E.R., Conti, R.M., 'Pricing in the market for anticancer drugs', Working Paper 20867, National Bureau of Economic Research (January 2015).

36. Ibid.

37. It was previously 6 per cent but was reduced in 2019. Lieberman, S.M, Ginsburg, P.B, 'CMS's International Pricing Model For Medicare Part B Drugs: Implementation and Issues', Health Affairs blog (July 9, 2019).

38. Howard, D.H., Bach, P.B., Berndt, E.R., Conti, R.M., 'Pricing in the market for anticancer drugs', Working Paper 20867, National Bureau of Economic Research (January 2015).

39. List and net prices for a bottle of ninety Duexis pills in early 2020 according to data from SSR Health. Because of its high cost, Duexis is no longer covered by many insurance companies.

40. Horizon Pharma annual reports 2012–2016.

41. The company said that 98 per cent of insured patients face out-of-pocket costs of $25 or less for Duexis, which ensured that 'cost is not a barrier for patients'. It said that 'the price of our therapies reflects the value they provide to the people who receive them, and the value we have and will continue to create within the communities we serve'.

42. Sacks, C.A., Lee, C.C. et al., 'Medicare Spending on Brand-name Combination Medications vs Their Generic Constituents', *Journal of the American Medical Association* (August 21, 2018).

43. Sarnak, D.O., Squires, D., Bishop S., 'Paying for Prescription Drugs Around the World: Why Is the US an Outlier?', The Commonwealth Fund, commonwealthfund.org (October 5, 2017).

44. Berchick, E.R, Barnett, J.C., Upton, R.D., 'Health Insurance Coverage in the United States: 2018', United States Census Bureau (November 8, 2019).

45. Schutte, S., Marin Acevedo, P.N., Flahault, A., 'Health systems around the world – a comparison of existing health system rankings', *Journal of Global Heath* (March 15, 2018).

46. Interview by the author with Mark Lindsay.

47. 'FDA approves new breakthrough therapy for cystic fibrosis', press release from FDA (October 21, 2019).

48. Vertex declined to comment.

49. Interview by the author with John Wallenburg.

50. Danzon, P.M., Ketcham, J.D., 'Reference Pricing of Pharmaceuticals: Evidence from Germany, the Netherlands and New Zealand', National Bureau of Economic Research working papers (October 6, 2003).

51. Stargardt, T., Schreyögg, J., 'Impact of cross-reference pricing on pharmaceutical prices: manufacturers' pricing strategies and price regulation', *Applied Health Economics and Health Policy* (2006).

52. Kanavos, P., Fontrier, A-M. et al., 'The Implementation of External Reference

Pricing Within and Across Country Borders', London School of Economics (November 2017).

53. It was called the National Institute for Clinical Excellence until 2013 when the name was changed to reflect a wider remit.

54. Gotham, D., Redd, C. et al., 'Pills and profits: How drug companies make a killing out of public research', report by Global Justice Now and STOPAIDS (October 2017). Genzyme did not respond to a request for comment on its pricing of Lemtrada.

55. Comparisons with existing treatments are not routinely repeated once a previous drug has gone generic and dropped in price, meaning that the British health service will continue to pay for drugs which are no longer more cost-effective than older alternatives for the benefits they offer.

56. Interview by the author with Andrew Stevens.

57. Figures for pharmaceutical spending per capita in 2019 compiled by the OECD.

58. The figures reflect list prices before confidential deals will have reduced the actual price paid by health services. US Senate Committee on Finance, 'The Price of Sovaldi and Its Impact on the US Health Care System', US Government Publishing Office (December 2015).

59. Gornall, J., Hoey, A., Ozieranski, P., 'A pill too hard to swallow: how the NHS is limiting access to high priced drugs', BMJ (July 27, 2016).

60. 'Gilead gets "gold" in England's hepatitis C eradication drive', PMLive (April 30, 2019).

61. Aitken, M., Kleinrock, M. et al., 'The Global Use of Medicine in 2019 and Outlook to 2023', IQVIA Institute for Human Data Science (January 2019).

62. Robinson, J.C., Ex, P., Panteli, D., 'How Drug Prices Are Negotiated in Germany', The Commonwealth Fund, commonwealthfund.org (June 13, 2010).

63. 'Remarks by President Trump on Lowering Drug Prices', whitehouse.gov (May 11, 2018).

64. The author previously revealed details of Aspen's actions in several articles for The Times including Kenber, B., 'Child cancer patients pay the price for "unfair" drug costs' (April 14, 2017). The company said price rises were 'at levels appropriate to promote long-term sustainable supply to patients' and claimed they had been increased from 'a very low and unsustainable base'. Aspen said it had never withheld products but acknowledged supply problems, including from a third-party manufacturer in Italy.

65. Patients were left reliant on imported foreign supplies of the medicines. See Kenber, B., 'Drug giant's secret plan to destroy cancer medicine', The Times (April 14, 2017).

66. Testimony of John Stewart, national director, Specialised Commissioning, NHS England to Commons Health and Social Care Committee (March 7, 2019).

67. Testimony of Sir Andrew Dillon, chief executive, NICE, to Commons Health and Social Care Committee (March 7, 2019).

68. Liu, A., '"Sham" or public interest? ICER suggests 70%-plus discounts on Vertex's cystic fibrosis drugs', FiercePharma (May 4, 2018).

69. Written evidence to Commons Health and Social Care Select Committee,

letter from Simon Lem, vice-president and general manager, Northern Europe Region, Vertex Pharmaceuticals (March 25, 2019). Estimate of deaths is from the campaign group Just Treatment.

70. 'Technical Report: Pricing of cancer medicines and its impact', World Health Organization (December 18, 2018).

71. The New York non-profit Knowledge Ecology International obtained correspondence between Gilead and the Office of the United States Trade Representative under freedom of Information laws. See Love, J., 'Communications between Gilead and USTR regarding Malaysia compulsory license on HCV patents, 2017 to May 2018', keionline.org (November 28, 2018).

72. 'Pharmaceutical Market: Pharmaceutical sales', OECD Health Statistics 2019. Figures for Australia and Germany exclude spending on hospital drugs.

73. Analysis of UK medicines sales agreed between the Association of the British Pharmaceutical Industry (ABPI) and the Department of Health and Social Care (DHSC) each year. The figures cited represent spend on branded medicines at net prices with a deduction for the annual payment made by the industry to the DHSC under a voluntary scheme.

74. Schipper, I., de Haan, E., Cowan, R., 'Overpriced: Drugs Developed with Dutch Public Funding', SOMO in collaboration with Wemos (May 2019).

Chapter Nine: The drugs we get

1. Mullard, A., '2018 FDA drug approvals', *Nature Reviews Drug Discovery* (January 15, 2019).

2. Russell, C., 'Victims of Rare Disorder Get New Relief – "Orphan Drug" wins US Approval', *Washington Post* (August 8, 1984).

3. Alhawwashi, S., Seoane-Vazquez, E., et al., 'Price of Drugs For Chronic Use With Orphan Designation In The United States (1983–2014), *Value In Health* (May 2016).

4. The per patient annual cost of the top 100 orphan drugs in the United States hit $150,854 in 2018, although this did not include off-invoice discounts. See Pomeranz, K., 'Orphan Drug Report 2019', EvaluatePharma (April 25, 2019).

5. See Brennan, Z., 'FDA: 2019 Continues Uptick in Orphan Drug Approvals', *Regulatory Focus* (January 6, 2020) and Orphanet Report Series, 'Lists of medicinal products for rare diseases in Europe', Orpha.net (November 2020).

6. Alhawwashi, S, Seoane-Vazquez, E. et al., 'Prices of Drugs For Chronic Use With Orphan Drug Designation In The United States (1983–2014)', *Value in Health* (May 1, 2016).

7. Ashbury, C.H., 'The Orphan Drug Act: the first 7 years', *Journal of the American Medical Association* (February 20, 1991).

8. Cote, A., Keating, B., 'What Is Wrong with Orphan Drug Policies?', *Value In Health* (December 1, 2012).

9. Jones, N., 'Can't come home: New Zealand a "death sentence"', *New Zealand Herald* (December 6, 2018).

10. Interview by the author with Donald Macarthur.

11. Ibid.

12. Johnson, C.Y., 'This old drug was free. Now it's $109,500 a year', *Washington Post* (December 18, 2017).

13. Ibid.

14. 'Hyper- and Hupokalemic Periodic Paralysis Study (HYP-HOP)', Clinicaltrials. gov Identifier NCT00494507.

15. Johnson, C.Y., 'This old drug was free. Now it's $109,500 a year', *Washington Post* (December 18, 2017).

16. Response to Freedom of Information Request to the Department of Health and Social Care made on WhatDoTheyKnow.com (December 11, 2019). The European Medicines Agency raised concerns about the application and it was withdrawn in October 2019.

17. NHS Drug Tariff June 2020.

18. The prevalence thresholds in the US are approximately 1 in 1,500 people; in Europe they are 1 in 2,000 people and in Japan they are 1 in 2,500 people.

19. Carey, J., Hamilton, J., 'These "Orphans" Don't Need Any Nurturing', *Business Week* (July 2, 1990), quoted in Rin-Laures, L-H., Janofsky, D., 'Recent Developments Concerning The Orphan Drug Act', *Harvard Journal of Law & Technology* (Spring issue, 1991).

20. Gibson, S., Von Tigerstrom, B., 'Orphan drug incentives in the pharmacogenomic context: policy responses in the US and Canada', *Journal of Law and the Biosciences* (April 19, 2015).

21. Interview by the author with Donald Macarthur.

22. Tribble, S.J., Lupkin, S., 'Drugmakers Manipulate Orphan Drug Rules to Create Prized Monopolies', Kaiser Health News (January 17, 2017).

23. Lanthier, M., 'Insights into Rare Disease Drug Approval: Trends and Recent Developments', FDA, Presentation at NORD Rare Diseases & Orphan Products Breakthrough Summit (October 17, 2017).

24. Thomas, S., Caplan, A., 'The Orphan Drug Act Revisited', *Journal of the American Medical Association* (February 15, 2019).

25. Kesselheim, A.S., Treasure, C.L., Joffe, S., 'Biomarker-Defined Subsets of Common Diseases: Policy and Economic Implications of Orphan Drug Act Coverage', *PLOS Medicine* (January 3, 2017).

26. Ahmad, A.S., Ormiston-Smith, N., Sasieni, P.D., 'Trends in the lifetime risk of developing cancer in Great Britain: comparison of risk for those born from 1930 to 1960', *British Journal of Cancer* (February 3, 2015).

27. 'Estimates of Funding for Various Research, Condition and Disease Categories', National Institutes of Health Research Portfolio Online Reporting Tools.

28. Cancer drugs averaged 25 per cent of new drug approvals in the United States between 2014 and 2018. See Mullard, A., '2019 FDA drug approvals', *Nature Reviews Drug Discovery* (January 8, 2020).

29. Mailankody, S., Prasad, V., 'Five Years of Cancer Drug Approvals: Innovation, efficacy, and costs', *JAMA Oncology* (July 2015). The study used average whole-sale prices, which do not reflect discounts offered to wholesalers or purchasers.

30. Howard, D.H., Bach, P.B., Berndt, E.R., Conti, R.M., 'Pricing in the market for anticancer drugs', Working Paper 20867, National Bureau of Economic Research (January 2015).

31. Interview by the author with Leonard Saltz.

32. Saltz, L.B., 'Progress in Cancer Care: The Hope, the Hype, and the Gap Between Reality and Perception', *Journal of Clinical Oncology* (November 1, 2008).

33. Sullivan, R., Peppercorn, J. et al., 'Delivering affordable cancer care in high-income countries', *Lancet Oncology* (September 29, 2011).

34. Vertex finally announced that it was submitting Trikafta for approval in Canada in November 2020.

35. Aggarwal, A., Fojo, T., Chamberlain, C., Davis, C., Sullivan, R., 'Do patient access schemes for high-cost cancer drugs deliver value to society? Lessons from the NHS Cancer Drugs Fund', *Annals of Oncology* (August 2017).

36. The Cancer Drugs Fund has been replaced by a smaller fund which will only cover drugs while they are being appraised by NICE.

37. Kim C., Prasad, V., 'Cancer Drugs Approved on the Basis of a Surrogate End Point and Subsequent Overall Survival: An Analysis of 5 Years of US Food and Drug Administration Approvals', *JAMA Internal Medicine* (December 2015).

38. Davis, C., Naci, H., Gurpinar, E., Poplavska, E., Pinto, A., Aggarwal, A., 'Availability of evidence of benefits on overall survival and quality of life of cancer drugs approved by European Medicines Agency: retrospective cohort study of drug approvals 2009–13', *BMJ* (September 2017).

39. Interview by the author with Peter Bach.

40. Kesselheim, A.S., Myers, J.A., Avorn, J., 'Characteristics of clinical trials to support approval of orphan vs nonorphan drugs for cancer', *JAMA* (June 8, 2011).

41. Jayasundara, K., Hollis, A., Krahn, M. et al., 'Estimating the clinical cost of drug development for orphan versus non-orphan drugs', *Orphanet Journal of Rare Diseases* (January 10, 2019).

42. 'Orphan Drugs in the United States', IQVIA Institute for Human Data Science (December 2018).

43. Interview by the author with Bruce Booth.

44. Roy, A., 'Biologic Medicines: The Biggest Driver of Rising Drug Prices', *Forbes* (March 8, 2019).

45. Urquhart, L., 'Top drugs and companies by sales in 2018', *Nature Reviews Drug Discovery* (March 12, 2019).

46. 'Biosimilars approved in Europe', Generics and Biosimilars Initiative, gabionline.net/Biosimilars/General/Biosimilars-approved-in-Europe

47. 'FDA-Approved Biosimilar Products', US Food and Drug Administration (as of January 2020).

48. Pomeranz, K., Siriwardana, K., Davies, F., 'Orphan Drug Report 2020', EvaluatePharma (March 21, 2020).

49. Kollewe, J., 'GSK to cut drug development projects to focus on "winners"', *The Guardian* (July 26, 2017). GSK subsequently unveiled a strategy to use genetic information to make decisions on which development molecules to pursue in an effort to improve a success rate of less than 10 per cent for drugs that undergo clinical testing becoming medicines. The company said its early-stage research 'is not constrained by therapy areas with teams actively encouraged to follow the science', while its later-stage pipeline is focused on several therapy areas including oncology, infectious diseases and vaccines.

50. Taylor, N.P., 'Sanofi punts 38 R&D projects to narrow pipeline focus',

FierceBiotech (February 7, 2019). Sanofi did not respond to a request for comment.

51. Vaccine Knowledge Project, 'Respiratory Syncytial Virus (RSV)', vk.ovg.ox.ac. uk. GSK said it remained 'committed to R&D for infectious diseases that affect children and young people in developing countries focusing on HIV, malaria and TB' and was one of a handful of companies actively researching new antibiotics.

52. Interview by the author with Josh Krieger

53. Interview by the author with Peter Bach.

54. Wong, C.H., Siah, K.W., Lo, A.W., 'Estimation of clinical trial success rates and related parameters', *Biostatistics* (January 31, 2018) and Steedman, M., Taylor, K. et al. 'Unlocking R&D productivity: Measuring the returns from pharmaceutical innovation 2018', Deloitte Centre for Health Solutions (December 19 2018).

55. 'Are companies developing health products that are urgently needed and offer a clear public health benefit?', Access to Medicine Foundation, accesstomedicinefoundation.org (January 2021).

56. Interview by the author with Aidan Hollis.

57. Clatworthy, A.E., Pierson, E., Hung, D.T., 'Targeting virulence: a new paradigm for antimicrobial therapy', *Nature Chemical Biology* (August 20, 2007).

58. Interagency Coordination Group on Antimicrobial Resistance,'No Time To Wait: Securing the future from drug-resistant infections', Report to the Secretary-General of the United Nations (April 2019).

59. Interview by the author with Jim O'Neill.

60. Ventola, C.L., 'The antibiotic resistance crisis: part 1: causes and threats', *Pharmacy and Therapeutics* (April 2015).

61. Offit, P.A., 'Why Are Pharmaceutical Companies Gradually Abandoning Vaccines?', *Health Affairs* (May 1, 2005).

62. Ibid.

63. Interview by the author with Aidan Hollis.

64. Offit, P.A., 'Why Are Pharmaceutical Companies Gradually Abandoning Vaccines?', *Health Affairs* (May 1, 2005).

65. Merck & Co. (MSD) 2018 annual report and Pfizer Inc 2018 annual report.

66. Wilson, D., 'Vaccine Approved for Child Infections', *New York Times* (February 24, 2010). This is the price on the private market; federally-funded programmes pay a discounted price of $137 per dose. In the United States, Prevnar is administered in four doses, including a booster shot at twelve to fifteen months. Centers for Disease Control and Prevention Vaccine Price List as of September 2019.

67. Sagonowsky, E., 'GSK exits US market with its HPV vaccine Cervarix', FiercePharma (October 21, 2016).

68. Branswell, H., 'Who will answer the call in the next outbreak? Drug makers feel burned by string of vaccine pleas', Stat News (January 11, 2018).

69. 'Lives on the Edge: Time to align medical research and development with people's health needs', Médecins Sans Frontières (May 2016).

70. Grady, D., 'Ebola Vaccine, Ready for Test, Sat on the Shelf', *New York Times* (October 23, 2014).

71. 'Lives on the Edge: Time to align medical research and development with people's health needs', Médecins Sans Frontières (May 2016).

72. Branswell, H., 'Who will answer the call in the next outbreak? Drug makers feel burned by string of vaccine pleas', Stat News (January 11, 2018).

73. 'List of Blueprint Priority Diseases', World Health Organization (February 2018).

74. Interview by the author with Peter Hale.

75. Gallagher, J., 'Oxford vaccine: How did they make it so quickly?', BBC News (November 23, 2020).

76. Baker, S., 'Covid Vaccine Front Runner Is Months Ahead of Her Competition', Bloomberg Businessweek (July 15, 2020). Gilbert and Hill had previously set up a spin-off company, Vaccitech, and raised £30 million in financing in 2016.

77. Open letter from Public Citizen and other groups to Daniel O'Day, chief executive of Gilead (March 25, 2020).

78. Gilead said it had sought the designation to speed up approval of the drug but dropped it when it became confident it would be expedited by regulatory agencies without needing this status.

79. Gilead's chief executive defended the drug's pricing as well below the cost of spending the extra days in hospital and said the company was 'guided by the need to do things differently'. He said the price reflected a balance between ensuring it didn't hinder 'rapid and broad treatment' and supporting ongoing investment in the drug and other research. Gilead said it expected to spend more than $1 billion on the development and manufacture of remdesivir by the end of 2020. As with Sovaldi and Harvoni, Gilead agreed voluntary licensing deals with generic manufacturers which saw the drug sold for less than $66 a vial in lower-income countries. See 'An Open Letter from Daniel O'Day, Chairman & CEO, Gilead Sciences' (June 29, 2020) and Reuters Staff, 'India's Cipla to price remdesivir version for Covid-19 under $66', Reuters (June 23, 2020).

80. Kuchler, H., 'Gilead's Covid drug delivers $2bn boost to revenue in Q4', *Financial Times* (February 4, 2021).

81. Interview by the author with Sir John Bell.

82. A company founded by the Oxford scientists Sarah Gilbert and Adrian Hill, Vaccitech Ltd, explored whether it could manufacture the vaccine without signing over exclusive rights to a large drugmaker, the *Wall Street Journal* reported. It was subsequently persuaded to sign over its rights to the university. See Strasburg, J., Woo, S., 'Oxford Developed Covid Vaccine, Then Scholars Clashed Over Money', *Wall Street Journal* (October 21, 2020).

83. Interview by the author with Sir John Bell.

84. Ralph, A., 'Pascal Soriot put Astrazeneca's star in the ascendant', *The Times* (December 30, 2020).

85. A Moderna representative told the author in January 2021 that the company had 'been negotiating pre-approval potential supply agreements, mostly to governments, with smaller volume agreements executed at $32–37/dose', with 'lower prices for higher volumes'. They said Moderna expected 'to contribute a substantial portion of the value of our vaccine to benefit society, and not to capture all of it in our ultimate pricing model'.

86. The United States paid between $15 and $17 per shot for 200 million doses of Moderna's vaccine in 2020. The amount paid per dose rises to $20.80 if the US government's development funding is also included.

87. The European price of the vaccine was revealed in December 2020 when a Belgian minister briefly tweeted a list showing the prices which the European Union had agreed to pay for different coronavirus vaccines. Moderna sold the US government 200 million doses for around $32 per two-shot course early in the pandemic.

88. Moderna executives were criticised for selling stock shortly after the company announced positive trial data for its Covid vaccine. The company said the stock sales had been previously scheduled and executives didn't benefit from insider information, which would be illegal.

89. Kuchler, H., 'Pfizer expects $15bn in Covid vaccine revenue this year', *Financial Times* (February 2, 2021). Costs and profits for the vaccine are split evenly with the biotech company BioNTech which helped develop the vaccine.

90. Interview by the author with Peter Hale.

91. So, A.D., Woo, J., 'Reserving coronavirus disease 2019 vaccines for global access: cross sectional analysis', *BMJ* (December 15, 2020).

92. 'WHO Director-General's opening remarks at 148th session of the Executive Board', who.int (January 18, 2021).

93. Cheng, M., Hinnant, L., 'Countries urge drug companies to share vaccine know-how', Associated Press (March 1, 2021).

94. Reuters Staff, 'Rich, developing nations wrangle over COVID vaccine patents', Reuters (March 10, 2021).

95. Statement from Ambassador Katherine Tai on the Covid-19 Trips Waiver, https://ustr.gov/about-us/policy-offices/press-office/press-releases/2021/may/statement-ambassador-katherine-tai-covid-19-trips-waiver (May 5, 2021).

96. Interview by the author with Jayasree Iyer.

97. Ibid.

98. 'Access to Medicine Index 2021', Access to Medicine Foundation (January 26, 2021).

Chapter Ten: Hard science

1. Interview by the author with Jack Scannell.

2. Le Fanu, J., *The Rise and Fall of Modern Medicine* (Little, Brown, 1999; Abacus, 2011) p.321.

3. D'Argenio, V., 'The High-Throughput Analyses Era: Are We Ready for the Data Struggle?', *High Throughput* (March 7, 2018).

4. Testimony of Jennifer Taubert, executive vice president and worldwide chairman, Janssen Pharmaceuticals, Johnson & Johnson, to the US Senate Committee on Finance (February 26, 2019).

5. 'Pharma giant Pfizer pulls out of research into Alzheimer's', BBC News (January 10, 2018).

6. Interview by the author with Jack Scannell.

7. Cook, D., Brown, D., Alexander, R. et al., 'Lessons learned from the fate of AstraZeneca's drug pipeline: a five-dimensional framework', *Nature Reviews Drug Discovery* (May 16, 2014).

8. Interview by the author with Bernard Munos.
9. The only Eli Lilly drug approved between August 2004 and April 2014 was the blood thinner Effient, which it had licensed from a Japanese company. It never topped much more than $500 million in worldwide annual sales and was considered a flop.
10. Drews, J., 'Strategic trends in the drug industry', *Drug Discovery Today* (May 2003).
11. Interview by the author with anonymous former chief executive of a large drug company.
12. Morgan, P., Brown, D., Lennard, S. et al., 'Impact of a five-dimensional framework on R&D productivity at AstraZeneca', *Nature Reviews Drug Discovery* (January 19, 2018).
13. Interview by the author with Margaret Kyle.
14. Kyle, M., 'Are Important Innovations Rewarded? Evidence from Pharmaceutical Markets', *Review of Industrial Organization* (June 7, 2018).
15. Interview by the author with Jamie Love.
16. DiMasi, J.A., Grabowski, H.G., Hansen, R.W., 'Innovation in the pharmaceutical industry: New estimates of R&D costs', *Journal of Health Economics* (February 12, 2016).
17. Wouters, O.J., McKee, M., Luyten, J., 'Estimated Research and Development Investment Needed to Bring a New Medicine to Market, 2009–2018' *JAMA* (March 3, 2020).
18. DiMasi excludes these post-approval costs from his estimates. The 2019 PhRMA Annual Membership Survey gave a figure of 11.1 per cent for the proportion of R&D costs accounted for by Phase IV studies.
19. 'PhRMA Annual Membership Survey', published by the Pharmaceutical Research and Manufacturers of America (2010 and 2020 surveys).
20. Steedman, M., Stockbridge, M. et al., 'Ten years on: Measuring the return from pharmaceutical innovation', Deloitte Centre for Health Solutions (December 19, 2018).
21. Steedman, M., Taylor, K., et al., 'Unlocking R&D productivity: Measuring the returns from pharmaceutical innovation 2018', Deloitte Centre for Health Solutions (December 2018).
22. Ringel, M.S., Scannell, J.W. et al., 'Breaking Eroom's Law', *Nature Reviews Drug Discovery* (April 16, 2020).
23. Ibid.
24. It was just within the bounds on an alternative measure of $150,000 per life year gained as assessed by the Institute for Clinical and Economic Review.
25. As we shall see, the manufacturer of Zolgensma has introduced a lottery to give away 100 doses of the drug to patients who are not currently able to access the treatment in their country.
26. Bhangra, K.S., 'Europe's first gene therapy withdrawn', BioNews (April 24, 2017).
27. 'The Global Use of Medicine in 2019 and Outlook to 2023', IQVIA Institute for Human Data Science (January 2019).
28. Kim, T., 'Goldman Sachs asks in biotech research report: Is curing patients a sustainable business model?', CNBC.com (April 11, 2018).

29. Gilead Sciences FY accounts 2014–2018.
30. Silver, E., 'What the "Shocking" Gilead Discounts on its Hepatitis C Drugs Will Mean', *Wall Street Journal* (February 4, 2015).
31. Interview by the author with Victor Roy.
32. Interview by the author with Kelvin Stott.
33. Healthcare spending has roughly doubled as a percentage of GDP over the past four decades in leading economies. It rose from 5 per cent to more than 10 per cent of GDP in the UK between 1980 and 2019, according to figures collected by the OECD. Over the same period, it rose from 8 per cent to nearly 17 per cent in the United States and from 6 to 11 per cent in Japan. Pharmaceuticals account for around 20 per cent of healthcare spending on average, although this can vary significantly between countries. In 2018, the UK and US spent around 12 per cent of healthcare expenditure on retail prescription drugs – those sold in pharmacies – while in 2017 Japan spent 18 per cent, according to the OECD. These figures exclude spending on drugs for patients undergoing hospital treatment, a category that typically includes some of the most expensive drugs. Spending on drugs dispensed in hospitals is responsible for more than half of the drugs bill in England before discounts and rebates, according to NHS Digital, and an estimated one-third of US drug spending. See 'Health at a Glance 2019', OECD (2019) and Conti, R.M., Turner, A., Hughes-Cromwick, P., 'Projections of US Prescription Drug Spending and Key Policy Implications', *JAMA Health Forum* (January 29, 2021).

Chapter Eleven: Fighting back

1. Interview by the author with Deidre Waxman.
2. Jefferys, G., 'Greg's Hepatitis C Diary', courtesy of Greg Jefferys.
3. Interview by the author with Greg Jefferys.
4. Jefferys, G., 'My Hep C Travel Diary: A Journey to India', courtesy of Greg Jeffreys.
5. Interview by the author with 'Demir'.
6. Span, P., 'Medicare's Part D Doughnut Hole Has Closed! Mostly. Sorta.', *New York Times* (January 17, 2020).
7. Reindl, J.C., Shamus, K.J., 'Drugstore trips to Canada aren't happening as much. Here's what changed', *Detroit Free Press* (November 29, 2019).
8. Gambino, L., 'Insulin is our oxygen: Bernie Sanders rides another campaign bus to Canada', *The Guardian* (July 28, 2019).
9. Germano, B., 'Mourning Mothers Protest Cost of Insulin Outside Cambridge Drug Company', CBS Boston (November 16, 2018).
10. YouTube video of protest outside Eli Lilly posted by the Right Care Alliance (November 17, 2019). Earlier that year, in response to a different protest, the company issued a statement saying 'people have a right to be heard, and we agree that real policy changes are needed'. It said it was advocating for changes such as exempting insulin from deductibles owed by patients with health insurance and in the meantime had taken steps to ensure insulin was more affordable, including by introducing a lower-cost version.
11. Interview by the author with Ellen De Meyer.

12. 'Charity and NIH funding related to Zolgensma', Knowledge Ecology International, keionline.org (June 14, 2019). Novartis said it had invested more than $1 billion 'to establish the structure necessary to transform scientific data into a tangible treatment that can be consistently manufactured and delivered to patients.'

13. The price was significantly below the $4 to $5 million which had previously been floated by a Novartis executive. Novartis said Zolgensma 'has the potential to reduce the long-term financial burden for a number of patients, families, and healthcare systems by replacing repeat, lifelong therapies with a single treatment'.

14. Novartis said that it understood the desire of families to help children with SMA to receive treatment as quickly as possible because of the progressive nature of the disease but as Zolgensma was not approved for use in Europe at the time Pia's family were fundraising, 'there were limited options to provide the treatment legally to a Belgian patient'.

15. Interview by the author with Leonard Saltz.

16. Trials showed both improved median overall survival for patients with advanced colon cancer by 1.4 months when compared to standard chemo-therapy treatment alone.

17. Bach, P.B., Saltz, L.B, Wittes, R.E., 'In Cancer Care, Cost Matters', *New York Times* (October 14, 2012).

18. Pollack, A., 'Sanofi Halves Price of Cancer Drug Zaltrap After Sloan-Kettering Rejection', *New York Times* (November 8, 2012).

19. Russell, S., 'New Crusade To Lower AIDS Drug Costs', *San Francisco Chronicle* (May 24, 1999).

20. Cameron, E., *Witness to Aids* (Tafelberg, 2005), p.164.

21. Swarns, R.L., 'Drug Makers Drop South Africa Suit Over AIDS Medicine', *New York Times* (April 20, 2001).

22. Ibid.

23. Speech by Nkosi Johnson at the opening of the 13th International AIDS Conference in Durban, South Africa (July 10, 2000), online at web.sabc.co.za/digital/stage/trufm/Nkosi_speech.pdf

24. McNeil Jr., D.G., 'South Africa's Small Warrior Against AIDS Dies Quietly', *New York Times* (June 2, 2001).

25. The Indian Patent Act of 1970, which came into effect in 1972, did not recognise product patents for pharmaceutical products and process patents – protecting a method of making a particular drug – only lasted for five years. See Sundaram, J., 'India's trade-related aspects of Intellectual Property Rights compliant pharmaceutical patent laws: what lessons for India and other developing countries?', *Information & Communications Technology Law* (March 28, 2014).

26. Interview by the author with Jamie Love.

27. Gellman, B., 'A Turning Point That Left Millions Behind', *Washington Post* (December 28, 2000).

28. Khanna, T., 'Interview with Yusuf Hamied', Creating Emerging Markets Oral History Collection, Baker Library Historical Collections, Harvard Business School (April 29, 2013).

29. Ooms, G., Hanefeld, J., 'Threat of compulsory licences could increase access to essential medicines', *BMJ* (May 28, 2019).

30. Kass, D., 'Israel Defies AbbVie IP To Import Generic Drugs For Covid-19', Law360 (March 19, 2020).
31. Ooms, G., Hanefeld, J., 'Threat of compulsory licences could increase access to essential medicines', *BMJ* (May 28, 2019).

Chapter Twelve: A reckoning

1. Interview by the author with Leonard Saltz.
2. Kleinrock, M., Muñoz, E., 'Global Medicine Spending and Usage Trends', IQVIA Institute for Human Data Science (March 5, 2020).
3. Sarpatwari, A., Kesselheim, A.S., 'Reforming the Orphan Drug Act for the 21st Century', *New England Journal of Medicine* (July 11, 2019).
4. Wouters, O.J., Kanavos, P.G., McKee, M., 'Comparing Generic Drug Markets in Europe and the United States: Prices, Volumes, and Spending', *Milbank Quarterly* (September 12, 2017).
5. Bach, P.B.,Trusheim, M.R., 'The Drugs at the Heart of Our Pricing Crisis', *New York Times* (March 15, 2021).
6. Interview by the author with David Maris.
7. Davis, C.S., 'The Purdue Pharma Opioid Settlement – Accountability, or Just the Cost of Doing Business?', *New England Journal of Medicine* (January 14, 2021).
8. Azar, A.M., 'Remarks on Drug Pricing Blueprint', Speech in Washington, DC, (May 14, 2018).
9. Rind, D.M, Borrelli, E. et al., 'Unsupported Price Increase Report: 2019 Assessment', Institute for Clinical and Economic Review (updated November 6, 2019).
10. Venker, B., Stephenson, K.B., Gellad, W.F., 'Assessment of Spending in Medicare Part D If Medication Prices From the Department of Veterans Affairs Were Used', *JAMA Internal Medicine* (January 14, 2019).
11. A company launching a new drug will not have to include the first three years of those sales when a calculation of its contribution to the rebate is made. However, those sales are included when calculating the health service's overall spending on branded medicines, meaning companies face higher payments when a rival launches a successful new drug.
12. Data from SSR Health published by Drug Channels, drugchannels.net (January 5, 2021).
13. Interview by the author with Jayasree Iyer.
14. Nayak, R.K., Avorn, J., Kesselheim, A.S., 'Public sector financial support for late stage discovery of new drugs in the United States: cohort study', *BMJ* (October 23, 2019). Another study, Stevens, A.J., Jensen, J.J. et al. 'The Role of Public-Sector Research in the Discovery of Drugs and Vaccines', *New England Journal of Medicine* (February 10, 2011), produced an estimate of approximately one in seven drugs for the period 1990–2007. The more recent study covers the years 2008 to 2017.
15. Cleary, E., Beierlein, J.M., 'Contribution of NIH funding to new drug approvals 2010–2016', *PNAS* (March 6, 2018).
16. Gavaghan, H., 'NIH drops reasonable pricing clause', *Nature* (April 20, 1995).
17. OTT Statistics, National Institutes of Health Office of Technology Transfer (2011–2019).

18. 'NIH-Private Sector Partnership in the Development of Taxol', United States General Accounting Office (June 2003).

19. Hampton, P., 'UCLA sells royalty rights connected with cancer drug to Royalty Pharma', UCLA Newsroom (March 4, 2016).

20. 'Abiraterone: a story of scientific innovation and commercial partnership', Institute of Cancer Research, London, icr.ac.uk (May 11, 2014).

21. Gotham, D., Redd, C. et al., 'Pills and profits: How drug companies make a killing out of public research', report by Global Justice Now and STOPAIDS (October 2017).

22. Johnson & Johnson's pharmaceutical division Janssen defended its pricing approach, saying it reflected the value of its medicines in improving patients' lives and sustained the discovery and development of future medicines. It said that 'the story of abiraterone's journey from initial concept at the United Kingdom's Institute for Cancer Research to eventual commercialisation by Janssen exemplifies how the work of public research organisations is translated through private-sector partnerships into medicines for patients'.

23. Schipper, I., de Haan, E., Cowan, R., 'Overpriced: Drugs Developed with Dutch Public Funding', SOMO in collaboration with Wemos (May 2019).

24. Interview by the author with Leonard Saltz.

25. Interview by the author with Steve Pearson.

26. Following the earlier-than-expected launch of rival hepatitis C treatments, Gilead announced shortly after ICER's deliberations that it expected to give an average discount of 46 per cent off its list prices, taking Harvoni within ICER's suggested price. See 'New Lower Prices for Gilead Hepatitis C Drugs Reach CTAF Threshold for High Health System Value', press release from ICER (February 17, 2015).

27. The 'partners and supporters' listed on Patientsrising.org in January 2021 were Pfizer, Amgen, Takeda Oncology, Celgene and Janssen. The organisation's founder, Terry Wilcox, said it 'proudly advocates for a patient-centred health system' and such a system 'must encourage and reward innovation'. She criticised the use of QALYs as 'discriminatory, unethical and arbitrary' and accused the UK and European governments of 'sacrificing long-term health benefits to their citizens for short-term cost controls'.

28. Interview by the author with Karl Claxton.

29. Claxton, K., Martin, S. et al., 'Methods for the estimation of the NICE cost effectiveness threshold', *Health Technology Assessment* (February 19, 2015).

30. Interview by the author with Karl Claxton.

31. Head-to-head trials remain 'very infrequent', Steve Pearson, the ICER founder, says, although in some disease areas (like rheumatoid arthritis) it is no longer considered ethical to compare a new drug to a placebo when patients have a disease which is actively progressing.

32. Interview by the author with Margaret Kyle.

33. Moon, S., Erickson, E., 'Universal Medicine Access through Lump-Sum Remuneration – Australia's Approach to Hepatitis C', *New England Journal of Medicine* (February 14, 2019).

34. Interview by the author with Jamie Love.

35. Frank, R.G., Ginsburg, P.B., 'Pharmaceutical Industry Profits And Research And Development', Health Affairs blog (November 13, 2017).
36. Interview by the author with Peter Bach.
37. Interview by the author with Jack Scannell.
38. Interview by the author with Karl Claxton.
39. Interview by the author with Bernard Pécoul.
40. Cohen, D., Raftery, J., 'Paying twice: the "charitable" drug with a high price tag', *BMJ* (February 15, 2014).
41. Cummings, J.L., Morstorf, T., Zhong, K., 'Alzheimer's Disease Drug-Development Pipeline: Few Candidates, Frequent Failures', *Alzheimer's Research & Therapy* (July 3, 2014).
42. Bell, J., 'Big pharma backed away from brain drugs. Is a return in sight?' BioPharma Dive (January 29, 2020).
43. Novartis said that supply constraints mean there are only 100 doses per year available for its scheme offering free doses to families outside the US who cannot access Zolgensma. It said that it was designed on the principles of 'fairness, clinical need and global accessibility' and 'under conditions where the programme has more requests than doses available, we wanted to ensure that all eligible children had an equal chance to receive therapy'.
44. Interview by the author with Ellen De Meyer.

Epilogue: Concordia's fall

1. The complaint was lodged with the Office of Fair Trading, which, along with the Competition Commission, was replaced by the newly formed Competition and Markets Authority in April 2014.
2. 'Consultation on Changes to the Statutory Scheme to Control the Prices of Branded Health Service Medicines', Department of Health (September 2015).
3. 'Third Affidavit of Mark Thompson', *Concordia Pharmaceuticals Inc. et al.* v. *Lazarus Pharmaceuticals, Inc. et al.*, United States District Court for the District of South Carolina (September 28, 2018, filed October 16, 2020).
4. Second Reading of the Health Service Medical Supplies (Costs) Bill in the House of Commons (October 24, 2016).
5. Interview by the author with Marc Cohodes.
6. Crow, D., 'Novum faces outcry over $10,000 acne cream', *Financial Times* (September 21, 2016) and Sliverman, E., 'The curious case of the $9,500 skin gel', Stat News (September 23, 2016).
7. Schencker, L., 'A Chicago pharma company raised the price of its skin gel to $7,968. Now it's bankrupt', *Chicago Tribune* (February 5, 2019).
8. Details in bankruptcy papers filed by Novum Pharma (February 3, 2019).
9. After the European Commission raised concerns that Aspen had abused a dominant position by imposing unfair prices, the company said it disagreed with this assessment but offered to reduce its prices to settle the case. Under proposed commitments made public in July 2020, the company agreed to continue supplying the medicines for at least five years and to not increase prices for a decade. Aspen said the six drugs had generated sales of €28 million in 2019, meaning the price cuts would save European health systems around €20 million a year.
10. As of early 2021, the case was ongoing. Thompson and his fellow defendants

have denied wrongdoing and argued that the formula for Donnatal and the process for manufacturing such products are not trade secrets.

11. In prepared remarks for an appearance before a Senate committee in 2016, Mr Pearson apologised for the company's pricing strategy, saying that 'the company was too aggressive – and I, as its leader, was too aggressive – in pursuing price increases on certain drugs'. 'Statement of J. Michael Pearson', US Senate Special Committee on Aging (April 27, 2016).

12. US Senate Special Committee on Aging, 'Sudden Price Spikes in Off-Patent Prescription Drugs: The Monopoly Business Model that Harms Patients, Taxpayers, and the US Health Care System', US Government Publishing Office (December 2016).

13. 'FTC and NY Attorney General Charge Vyera Pharmaceuticals, Martin Shkreli, and Other Defendants with Anticompetitive Scheme to Protect a List-Price Increase of More Than 4,000 Percent for Life-Saving Drug Daraprim', press release from the Federal Trade Commission (January 27, 2020).

14. Interview by the author with Sanjeeth Pai.

15. 'Bausch Health agrees to pay $1.21 billion to settle share price lawsuit', Reuters (December 16, 2019).

16. Advanz Pharma 2019 Annual Information Form.

17. Second amended complaint in *City of Rockford and Acument Global Technologies Inc.* v. *Mallinckrodt*, United States District Court for the Northern District of Illinois (filed December 8, 2017). See also Stahl, L., 'The Problem With Prescription Drug Prices', CBS *60 Minutes* (May 6, 2018).

18. Advanz Pharma 2019 Annual Information Form.

19. Cinven denied AMCo's success was due to a debranding strategy and said AMCO's growth was driven by the combination of Amdipharma and Mercury Pharma which gave the new business an international footprint and meant the business was much larger when it was sold than it had been when Cinven first acquired it.

20. Brady, A., 'The Luxury of Wanderlust', *Harpers Bazaar Arabia* (Summer 2017).

21. Patel, S., 'Making £300m before turning 40', *Asian Wealth Magazine* (Autumn 2017).

22. '3 drug firms accused of illegal market sharing', CMA press release (October 3, 2019).

23. 'Pharma company director disqualified for competition law breaches', CMA press release (June 4, 2020).

24. *Auden Mckenzie (Pharma Division) Ltd* v. *Patel* [2019] EWCA Civ 2291 (December 20, 2019). In June 2020, Mr Patel told *The Times* he made an 'error of judgment, which I sincerely regret' and had immediately cooperated with the tax authorities after being contacted by them. See Kenber, B., 'Tories accepted £50,000 gift from tax fraudster who ripped off NHS', *The Times* (June 9, 2020).

25. 'Drug firms accused of illegal market sharing in supply of antibiotic', CMA press release (July 25, 2019).

26. 'Drug firms accused of illegal market sharing over anti-nausea tablets', CMA press release (May 23, 2019).

27. 'Pharma firms accused of illegal agreements over life-saving drug', CMA press release (February 28, 2019).

28. Dyer, O., 'Firm bribed doctors to prescribe overpriced drug, US alleges in suit', *BMJ* (May 2, 2019).

29. Blankenship, K., 'Humana calls Mallinckrodt's Acthar a "billion-dollar golden goose" in $700M fraud lawsuit', FiercePharma (August 12, 2019).

30. 'Three Pharmaceutical Companies Agree to Pay a Total of Over $122 Million to Resolve Allegations That They Paid Kickbacks Through Co-Pay Assistance Foundations', press release from the US Department of Justice Office of Public Affairs (April 4, 2019).

31. The legislation bears the title 'Health Service Medical Supplies (Costs) Bill'.

32. At the time of writing in early 2021, the British government had not used the powers. A spokesman for the Department of Health and Social Care said that the government used competition to drive the price of generic medicines down and said the UK had 'some of the lowest prices in Europe'. They said the department 'has been considering proposals for ways to address high prices of generic medicines, and it will need to consult on any proposals before implementing them'.

33. Author's research based on seventy-one drugs identified by a 2016 investigation for *The Times* into price-hiked generics. Nineteen drugs have seen significant price reductions while three are no longer on the market.

34. NHS Drug Tariff January 2021.

35. Several cases were delayed by issues affecting the landmark phenytoin capsules case. In late 2016, the Competition and Markets Authority (CMA) found that Pfizer and Flynn Pharma had broken competition law by abusing a dominant position by charging excessive prices and handed down a record £90 million fine. This decision was subsequently overturned by the Competition Appeal Tribunal, which concluded that both companies held a dominant position but determined that the CMA had not properly applied the test of excessive pricing set out in the landmark United Brands case. In particular, the tribunal ruled that the CMA had not sufficiently considered the wider economic value of the drug or the price of comparator products, including the tablet version, when determining that the price was unfair. This judgment was largely upheld by the Court of Appeal in March 2020 and the case was sent back to the CMA to reconsider the evidence against the companies and the way it assessed the prices charged as excessive.

36. Thomas, K., 'Patients Eagerly Awaited A Generic Drug. Then They Saw The Price', *New York Times* (February 23, 2018).

37. Crow, D., 'Irish drugmaker Horizon Pharma raises painkiller price to $3,000 in US', *Financial Times* (February 15, 2018).

38. Statement from the Chief Investigators of the Randomised Evaluation of Covid-19 thERapY (RECOVERY) trial on dexamethasone (June 16, 2020). Figures published in March 2021 showed that the drug saved 22,000 lives in the UK and an estimated one million worldwide.

39. Interview by the author with David Maris.

40. Hopkins, J.S., 'BioMarin Explores Pricing Experimental Gene Therapy at $2 Million to $3 Million', *Wall Street Journal* (January 16, 2020).

Index

References to notes are indicated by n.

3TC 202, 204

Abbot Laboratories 34
AbbVie 138, 140, 190, 196, 289
abiraterone 329
Académie Impériale de Médicine 35
Access to Medicine Foundation 257,
    269, 270, 326
ACE inhibitors 48, 278
acetylsalicylic acid 34, 35
Ackman, Bill 21, 174, 349
acquisitions 169–71, 177–9, 195–9,
    209; see also mergers
ACT UP (AIDS Coalition to
    Unleash Power) 50–1, 66–8,
    72–3, 76–9, 81
Actavis 352
Acthar Gel 171–2, 178, 351, 353
Actimmune 178
Addison's disease 154, 352
ADHD 9, 24
Advanz Pharma 350, 351, 380n29
advertising 93–4, 96–7
advocacy groups 81, 144–5
Africa 3; see also South Africa
Ahari, Shahram 86–93, 94, 101, 125
AIDS (acquired immunodeficiency
    syndrome) 52–82, 201, 244
    and compulsory licences 313–14
    and Epogen 112
    and South Africa 309–11
    and trials 251
    and Triomune 311–13

AIDS Action Council 62, 66, 76,
    81
AIDS Drug Assistance Program 66,
    77
albendazole 175
alcohol 33
alemtuzumab 233–4
Alexander, Albert 30
Alexion Pharmaceuticals 190
Allergan 20, 141–2, 190, 191
allergy treatments 133
Alzheimer's disease 275, 344
AMCo (Amdipharm Mercury) 26,
    152–3, 166–7
    and Concordia 156–7, 160–4,
        346–7
    and merger 157–8, 159–60
Amdipharm 157–8, 159–60
Amedra Pharmaceuticals 175, 176
American Civil War 34
American Pharmacological
    Association 35
Amgen 112, 115
Amilco 352
Amin, Tahir 136–8
An Early Frost (film) 67
anaemia treatments 62, 112, 246
animal testing 43–4, 45, 52, 58, 264
animals 48–9
Annan, Kofi 313
anthrax 314
anti-depressants 83, 94, 133, 139,
    278, 354; see also Prozac

anti-inflammatories *see* Acthar Gel;
　Orapred
anti-psychotics　278; *see also* Zyprexa
antibiotics　40–1, 43, 257–9, 331, 340
　and nitrofurantoin　163, 166–7,
　　353
　see also penicillin
antimalarials　3–4, 34, 36
antimicrobials　258
antiretroviral drugs　309–11
antivirals　55, 200–1
Apollo Global Management　168
apothecaries　33–4
Arbor Pharmaceuticals　22
Armstrong, Lance　112
Arno, Peter　65
Aronin, Jeff　172, 173, 178
Aspen Pharmacare　237, 349, 352,
　404n9
aspirin　34, 35, 45, 225, 364n19
assays　56, 58, 241, 273
AstraZeneca　22, 131–3, 135, 136,
　139, 140–1
　and Covid vaccine　266, 268
　and merger　189, 190
　and research　277–8, 279–80
athletic drugs　111, 112
Atorvastatin *see* Lipitor
Auden Mckenzie　154–6, 183, 351–2,
　353
Aureomycin (chlortetracycline)　40–1
Australia 226, 231, 232 239, 281,
　294–6, 298, 339, 393n72
Avastin　308
AveXis　287, 305
Avonex　193
Azar, Alex　221–2, 321–2
AZT (azidothymidine)　52, 56–82,
　116, 144

Bach, Peter　252, 288, 309, 319
　and Patients Rising　335
　and public funding　341

bacterial infections　258
Bailey, Don　171
Baker Bros. Advisors　197–8
Ballou, Dr Rip　262
Banting, Frederick　214, 217
Barbados　9, 13
Barr Laboratories　80
Barré-Sinoussi, Françoise　54–5
Barry, Dr David　54–6, 57, 58, 79,
　116
　and AZT trials　59, 61, 64, 69–70,
　　74–5
　and Triangle Pharmaceuticals
　　201, 202
Bausch Health　350–1
Baycol　126
Bayer　29, 34, 35
Bayh–Dole Act (1980)　45
Beecham　96
Behrens, Lisa　73, 77
Beighton, John　152–3, 157–9
Belgium　303–7
Bell, Sir John　266
benzodiazepines　48, 278
Berndt, Ernst　248
beta blockers　48, 187, 278
Biden, Joe　269
biologics　48, 252–5, 319; *see also*
　Humira
BioMarin　117, 356–7
BioNTech　265, 267
biotechs　48, 191, 197–8, 289–90
　and orphan drugs　109–15,
　　116–17
　see also Gilead Sciences; Triangle
　　Pharmaceuticals
Biovail　9, 10–11, 12, 165
Bischofberger, Norbert　207
Blackstone Group　167–8
Blair, Dr Henry　113
blockbuster drugs　83–6, 94, 95–9,
　101, 120, 168–9
　and biotechs　112

and orphan status 246–7
and profits 317
blood-pressure treatments 23, 83, 93, 278
blood thinners *see* Plavix
Bolar Pharmaceuticals 109
Bolognesi, Dr Dani 58, 61
Booth, Bruce 253
Borkowski, Ed 24
Botox 190
Boyer, Dr Herbert 109–10, 327
Brady, Dr Roscoe 113
brain drain 190–1
brand name drugs 44, 46, 153–6, 322, 325–6; *see also* debranding
Brandicourt, Olivier 221
Brazil 314
bribes 142–3, 353
Bristol-Myers Squibb 81, 190, 202, 327–8
Britain *see* National Health Service
British Technology Group (BTG) 329
Broder, Dr Sam 53–4, 56, 58, 80
and AZT trials 59, 60–1, 65
Brydon, Bruce 12
Burroughs Wellcome 35, 41, 198
and AIDS 54, 55, 56–7, 58, 60, 61, 64–5, 68–72, 73–7, 81, 82
Bush, George H. W. 112
Bush, George W. 220
buybacks 191–2, 283
buyers' clubs 73, 298, 308, 309

Campath 233–4
Campostar 223
Canada 10–13, 21, 25, 27, 84, 105, 167, 178, 218, 227–231, 232, 250, 261, 293, 300–1, 324
cancer drugs fund 250–1
cancer treatments 52–3, 247–51, 255, 257
and Aspen 349

and cervical 260
and co-payments 323
and Epogen 112
and genes 273
and Imbruvica 138
and immune system 287–8
and insurance 223
and lenalidomide 314
and lung 196, 240, 247, 254
and prices 178
and prostrate 328–9
and skin 211–13
and surrogate endpoints 252
and Taxol 327–8
and Zantrap 308–9
Caribbean *see* Barbados
Carlyle Group 168
Celexa 133
Celgene 190
Cephalon 139
CEPI (Coalition for Epidemic Preparedness Innovations) 263, 264, 268
Cerberus Capital Management 22, 23
Ceredase 113–14, 117, 118
Cerezyme 114–15, 117, 118, 243
Chain, Ernst 30, 38
charities 342
Chemie Grünenthal 43
chemists 34
children 9, 36, 104, 110, 303–7
chloroform 34
Chloromycetin (chloramphenicol) 41
Choi, Woo-Baeg 203, 204
cholesterol treatments 83, 93, 96–7, 141; *see also* Lipitor
Christopher Moraka Defiance Campaign 310
Cialis 193
Cinven 26, 27, 157, 159–60, 351, 352, 379n21

Cipla 311–13
ciprofloxacin 314
Civica RX 318
Clarinex 133
Claritin 133
Clark, Guy 157, 158
Claxton, Karl 335, 336, 342
clinical value 331–2, 338
clinical testing 44, 95
  and Alzheimer's disease 344
  and AZT 69–70
  and costs 190
  and drug discovery 276–7
  and efficacy 251–2
  and old drugs 342
  and orphan drugs 109
  see also animal testing; assays;
    human testing
Clinton, Bill 118, 310
Clinton, Hillary 160, 348
Clinton Foundation 313
closed distribution systems 176
Clozaril 119
CMA (Competition and Markets
  Authority) 352, 353, 354, 406n35
co-payment schemes 170–1, 323,
  348
cocaine 33
Coe, Fred 71
cognitive behavioural therapy 342
Cohen, Stanley 326–7
Cohodes, Marc 148–50, 167
Colcrys 176
Cole, Mike 184
combination drugs 224–5, 311–13
Combs, Kevin 16–18
competition 252–3, 316–17, 318,
  323, 346; see also CMA
compulsory licences 42, 313–14
Concordia Healthcare x, 8, 10,
  13–15, 20–7
  and AMCo 156–7
  and Donnatal 17–18, 175–6

and equity research 151–2
and fall 346–9, 351
and Morningside 353
and prices 193–4, 380n29
and rebranding 350
and share price 160–4, 174
and short selling 150, 164–6
and takeover 167–8
and Zonegran 19–20
consultancy firms 174–5
Cooper, Ellen 62
Copaxone 143
CorePharma 176
coronavirus see Covid-19 pandemic
corticosteroids 48
Cougar Biotechnology 329
COVAX 268, 269
Covid-19 pandemic 260, 264–70,
  314, 319, 326
  and public funding 331
  and steroids 355
  and vaccine 1–2, 3, 330,
    397–8n85–8
Covis 22–3, 24
Crestor 140–1
Creutzfeldt-Jakob disease 110
CRISPR-Cas9 286
Crum, Chris 166–7
Cuatrecasas, Pedro 54, 55, 57
cures 289
Cystic Fibrosis Foundation 145,
  343–4
cystic fibrosis treatments 227–30,
  237–8, 250
cytochrome P17 328

Dainippon Pharmaceutical 19
Daranide 244–5
Daraprim 176–7, 255–6, 350
ddC 81–2
ddI (didanosine) 81
De Meyer, Ellen 293–4, 303–4,
  303–7, 345

debranding 154, 159–60, 180–4,
    346–7
deductibles x, 323
dementia *see* Alzheimer's disease
dengue fever 260
Department of Veterans Affairs
    323, 334
dexamethasone 355
dextran sulphate 73
diabetic treatments 14, 48, 96, 257;
    see also insulin
Dibenzyline 23
dichlorphenamide 244–5
dietyhlene glycol 36
DiMasi, Joseph 283
Diovan 83
discounts x, 125, 337
Disease X 262, 263–4
dividends 283
DNA 48, 52, 55, 199, 200
    and embryos 286
    and recombinant 326–7
DNDi (Drugs for Neglected
    Diseases initiative) 343
doctors 88–93, 225–6, 290–1, 346,
    371n14
    and bribes 142–3, 353
Dole, Bob 98
Domagk, Gerhard 29–30
donations 49
Donnatal 15–19, 27, 162, 175–6,
    347
dosage 73–4, 79
Drews, Jürgen 84, 99, 129–30, 279
drug discovery 58, 272–3, 274–86,
    290–2, 338–9, 341
    and clinical value 332
    and collaboration 344
    and competition 317
    and costs 320
    and public funding 326–7
drug reps 86–93
drug-resistant diseases 258

Duchaine, Dan: *The Underground
    Steroid Handbook* 111
Duexis 224–5
Duke University 58, 60, 65, 80
Dutoprol 23
dwarfism 110
dyes 34

Ebola virus 261, 262, 263, 265
efficacy 42, 44, 47, 175–6, 276–7
    and AZT 79
    and trials 251–2
Egypt 209
Ehrlich, Paul 30, 34
Eisai 19, 20
Elan Pharmaceuticals 19
Elovich, Richard 77
embryos 286
Emory University 201–2, 203, 204,
    328
Epanutin 180–4
epilepsy treatments 19–20, 180–4,
    346
Epogen 112, 115, 117, 118, 243,
    246
equity research analysts 151–2, 165
ER (TV series) 97
E.R. Squibb 32, 34
erectile dysfunction treatments 93;
    see also Viagra
Eroom's Law 272–3, 282, 285–6
Essential Pharma 354
ethical drugs 33–4
evergreening 316–17
Ewen, Margaret 217–18
exclusivity period 317
experimental drugs 109
Express Scripts 351
eye treatments 141–2, 160, 167

F. Bayer & Co. *see* Bayer
famotidine 224–5
Fauci, Dr Tony 76, 79

FDA (Food and Drug
    Administration) 16–17, 42, 54,
    114–15, 175
    and advertising 93, 97
    and AZT 58, 59, 62–3, 68, 73, 79
    and petition schemes 140
    and thalidomide 44
Feldman, Robin 139, 140
fentanyl patches 175
fexinidazole 343
Finance Act (1944) 37
financialisation 128, 147, 356
fines 142, 172, 317, 321, 406n35
First World War 35, 36, 42
FixHepC 298
Fleming, Alexander 29, 30, 32, 37
Florey, Howard 30–1
flu vaccines 260, 261
fludrocortisone acetate 352
Flynn Pharma 182–4, 346, 384n102
Foltz, Danielle 171–2
Food, Drug and Cosmetic Act
    (1938) 37
Forest Laboratories 133
Foundation for Vaccine Research
    262–3
Frazier, Ken 127–8
Freeman, James 298
FTC (emtricitabine) 201–3, 204, 328
FTC (Federal Trade Commission)
    24–5, 139
Fucithalmic 160
Fusidic acid 167

Gallo, Robert 56, 68
Garrett, Benj 9
Gates, Bill 260
Gavi Vaccine Alliance 260
GDP (gross domestic product) 291,
    322, 400n33
gene therapies 286–90, 199–201,
    356–7
Genentech 48, 109–11, 112, 115

generic medicines 7, 14, 46–7,
    130–1, 252–4, 317
    and AZT 80
    and Covis 22
    and hepatitis C 295–9
    and insulin 299–303
    and Kapvay 24–5
    and margins 146–7
    and names 44
    and non-profit 318
    and patents 136
    and 'pay-for-delay' 138–9, 140
    and prices 153–6, 184–7
    and Prozac 121
    and taxation 178
    and useage 319, 342
    and Zonegran 19–20
genetics 48
genomics 273–4
Genzyme 113, 114–15, 117, 233
Germany 29–30, 33–4, 35, 37, 43–4,
    131, 231, 232, 234–6, 239, 364n22
Gilbert, Sarah 264
Gilead Sciences 199–201, 202–8,
    209–10, 234–5, 397n79
    and Ebola 265
    and hepatitis C 321, 323, 333,
        339
    and HIV 289
    see also Sovaldi
GlaxoSmithKline (GSK) 22, 82,
    139, 142–3, 202, 395n49
    and merger 189
    and vaccines 260
Glybera 288
Gold, Griffin 67
Gold Standard Drug Database x
Goldman Sachs 24, 26, 149, 160,
    289
Goldshield 157
GoodRx 194
Gordon, Charles 122
gout treatments 176

governments ix, 2, 15, 143–4
  and AZT 67–8, 77, 79–80
  and Covid-19 330
  and generic medicines 318
  and legislation 316–17
  and orphan drugs 107–8
  and prices 155, 222–3
  and spending 326
  and vaccines 259, 260
Great Britain see National Health
  Service
Greenberg, Herb 165
Greenstone 186
GSK see GlaxoSmithKline

Haddad, Bill 311
haemophilia treatments 357
Haigler, Ted 64, 68, 69, 72
Hale, Peter 262–3, 267
Hamied, Yusuf 311–13
Harrington, Mark 66, 73, 74–5, 79
Harvoni 106–7, 205, 210, 235, 333,
  334
Hatch, Orrin 108
Hatch–Waxman Act (1984) 47
head-lice treatments see Ulesfia
head-to-head trials 337
Health Action International
  217–18
health insurers ix, 15, 18, 226–7,
  323
  and coverage 222–3
  and managed care networks
  125
  see also Medicaid; Medicare
health systems 318–19, 331–2,
  336–7, 338, 339; see also National
  Health Service
health technology assessments
  (HTAs) 233, 335–6
Heatley, Norman 30–1
Heckler, Margaret M. 109, 242
hedge funds 5, 20, 21, 151–2, 174

hepatitis B treatments 200
hepatitis C treatments 203–8,
  209–10, 234–5, 295–9, 343
herbs 33
Herceptin 234
Heritage Pharmaceuticals 185
heroin addicts 154, 295
herpes 33, 63, 82, 200
Hg Capital 157
HGH (human growth hormone)
  110–11, 112, 116, 117, 118
Hilferty, Robert 50–1, 77
Hill, Adrian 264
HIV (human immunodeficiency
  virus) 55, 58, 60, 65, 66, 68–9
  and FTC 201–3, 204, 328
  and Gilead 200, 289
  and positivity 76
  and South Africa 309–11
Hodgins, James 20
Hoffmann, Felix 34
HoFH (homozygous familial hyper-
  cholesterolemia) 141
Hollis, Aidan 257, 259, 261
Horizon Pharma 174, 224–5, 355
hormone replacement treatments
  154, 369n41
Horwitz, Jerome 51–2, 65
Humalog 216, 253
Human Genome Project 273
human testing 45, 58–62
Humira 138, 140, 190, 194
Humulin 48
Hunt, Jeremy 347–8
hydrocortisone 154–6, 183, 353
Hydrocortone 154–6
hydroxycarbamide 245
hypertension see blood-pressure
  treatments

I-MAK (Initiative for Medicines,
  Access and Knowledge) 137–8
ibuprofen 224–5

ICER (Institute for Clinical and Economic Review) 332–5, 338

ICI (Imperial Chemical Industries) 41

ICR (Institute of Cancer Research) 328–9

illegality 142–3

Imbruvica 138

immune systems 3–4

impotence *see* erectile dysfunction treatments

incentives 316, 319–20, 342

Incivek 204–5

India 209–10, 293, 295–7, 298, 311–13

insulin 48, 100, 214–19, 221, 299–303, 323

insurance *see* health insurers

intellectual property *see* patents

interferon 204, 205, 299

iodine 34

Irinotecan 223

irritable bowel syndrome (IBS) treatments 15–19, 27, 162, 349

Isaly, Samuel 69

Israel 314

Isuprel 173, 179

ivermectin 48–9

Iyer, Jayasree 269, 326

Janssen Pharmaceuticals 266, 274, 328, 403n22

Jarman, Mike 328

Jeffreys, Greg 293, 294–8, 299, 307, 308

Jenner Institute 265–6

Jensen, Michael 128–9

Jepsen, George 184–6, 187

Jimenez, Joe 127–8

Johnson, Ben 111

Johnson, Nkosi 311

Johnson, Robert Wood 39

Johnson & Johnson (J&J) 39, 134, 143, 175, 329

Jones Pharma 169

J.P. Morgan Healthcare Conference 17, 22, 25

Kalydeco 228, 237–8

Kaposi's sarcoma 52–3

Kapvay 9, 10, 13–14, 24

Kaspar, Brian 305

Kefauver, Estes 42, 43, 44, 46, 116

Keiper, Roland 150

Kelsey, Frances 44

Kennedy, John F. 44

Kennedy, Tom 61–2, 64, 73

Kessell, Lori 16, 18–19, 27

ketoconazole 328

Keveyis 245

Keytruda 329

Khmelnitsky, Dimitry 150–3, 164–5

kickbacks 142–3

kidney treatments 112

Kindler, Jeff 127

King Pharmaceuticals 169

Kite Pharma 207, 288

Klugman, Jack 106, 107, 108

Klugman, Maurice 106, 108

Kolassa, Mick 115–16, 117, 118, 119, 130, 179–80
　The Strategic Pricing of Pharaceuticals 124–5, 126

Kramer, Larry 66, 68

Kreppner, Wayne 13, 17

Krieger, Josh 132, 256, 281–2

Kruif, Paul de: *Microbe Hunters* 51

Kyle, Margaret 281, 338–9

L-5-HTP 105–6, 108–9

LaMattina, John 189

Lanoxin 24

Lantus 217, 218, 221

Lassa fever 270

lawsuits 351, 353

layoffs 189, 208
Lazarus Pharmaceuticals 349
Lazonick, William 128, 129
LDL (bad cholesterol) 97
Le Fanu, James 273
Leath, Fran 120–1, 122, 123, 133–4
Lederle 32
Legacy Pharma 11–12
legislation 36–7, 353–4
Lemtrada 234
lenalidomide 314
leukaemia treatments 233–4
Levitra 193
Lexapro 133
licences 42, 44, 46, 80, 282; see also
    compulsory licences
lifestyle drugs 98–9
Lilly, Eli 34, 36, 99–101, 120–3
    and HGH 110, 112
    and insulin 214, 217
    and reps 86–92
    and research 278–9
    and Zyprexa 133–5
Lindsay, Chantelle 227–30, 250
liothyronine 156, 159, 163–4, 354
Liotta, Dennis 203, 204
Lipitor 83, 85, 96–7, 188, 253
lithium 278, 354
lobbying 143–4, 226, 327
Lonsurf 249
Losec 132
lotteries 345
Love, Jamie 282, 311–13, 339–40, 344
Lundbeck 178
Luxturna 287
Lydia E. Pinkman's Vegetable
    Compound 33

Macarthur, Donald 144, 243, 244,
    246
McCleery, John 13
McGuire, Jean 62, 66, 76
McHutchison, John 203

McKesson & Robbins 46
McKinsey 174–5, 284
Macleod, John 214
McNeil Laboratories 104, 108
malaria 257
Mallinckrodt Pharmaceuticals 172,
    350, 351, 353
managed care networks 125
Manning, Paul 15, 16
manufacturing costs 116, 124, 135
Marathon Pharmaceuticals 173, 179,
    350
Maris, David 138, 165, 169–70, 321,
    355
market research 124
marketing 36–7, 44, 85–6, 95; see
    also advertising; drug reps
Martin, John 200, 201, 205, 207
Max Planck Institute 58
May, Theresa 238
May & Baker 41
Mbeki, Thabo 310, 311
'me-too' drugs 94–5, 101, 193,
    281–2
Médecins Sans Frontières 312, 343
Medicaid 65–6, 113
Medical Marketing Economics
    (MME) 179–80
Medical Research Council 35, 38
Medicare 113, 146, 210, 220
    and cancer treatments 288
    and insulin 300
    and Part B 223
    and Part D 222, 323
Medicines Act (1968) 44
Meeran, Karim 156
Mellanby, Edward 38
Melnyk, Eugene 10–11, 12, 21
Merck, George 32, 36, 39, 356
Merck, Heinrich Emanuel 33–4
Merck & Co. 39, 99, 101–2, 127–8
    and research 198, 356
    and vaccines 260

Mercury Pharma 157–8, 159–60
mergers 157, 159–60, 189–90, 208
MERS (Middle East respiratory
    syndrome) 262
methadone 154
Meyers, Abbey 103, 106–7, 112,
    117, 145, 242
    and NORD 108, 109, 113–15
MHRA (Medicines and Healthcare
    products Regulatory Agency) 59,
    183
microbiology 37, 39
Milligan, John 207
Mitsuya, Hiroaki 'Mitch' 56, 58, 65
Moderna 265, 266–7, 330
monopolies 47, 71, 316–17, 318
Morgan Stanley 195–6
Morningside 353
morphine 33, 34
Moyer, Andrew 31
MSD (Merck Sharp & Dohme)
    39–40, 48–9, 85, 154–5, 263
multiple sclerosis treatments 143,
    171–2, 193, 273
Munos, Bernard 99–101, 197, 278–9
Mylan 24, 141, 187, 191, 297
myoclonus 105–6, 108–9

nadolol v
National AIDS Network 81
National Association of People with
    AIDS 81
National Authority for Health
    (France) 281
National Health Service (NHS) 37,
    43, 133, 155, 318
    and Concordia 347
    and cystic fibrosis 237–8, 308
    and liothyronine 354
    and NICE 235
    and spending 152, 153–4, 324–5
National Institutes of Health (NIH)
    45, 53, 113, 331, 327–8

    and AZT 59–60, 66, 74, 80
    and cancer treatments 247
National Pharmaceutical Council 46
National Research Development
    Corporation (NRDC) 38
NCI (National Cancer Institute) 53,
    58, 61, 65, 80
Netherlands 232, 234, 240, 318, 329
'Netflix model' 339, 340
neurodegenerative diseases 275
New Drug Application (NDA) 62
new drugs see drug discovery
NewLink Genetics 261
Nexium 83, 132–3, 136, 139
NHS see National Health Service
NICE (National Institute for Health
    and Care Excellence) 232–3,
    234–5, 238, 240, 243
    and cancer treatments 250–1, 288
    and cost effectiveness trials 329,
        336
Nielsen, Joe 184
NIH see National Institutes of
    Health
Nimer, Dan 118–19
nitrofurantoin 163, 166–7, 353
Nitropress 173
non-governmental organisations
    (NGOs) 314
NORD (National Organization for
    Rare Disorders) 108, 109, 113–15
Northern Regional Research
    Laboratory (NRRL) 31
Novartis 127–8, 305, 307, 345,
    404n43
Novo Nordisk 217
Novum Pharma 348–9

Obama, Barack 192, 226
off-patent drugs 11–12, 26, 169–73
Offit, Dr Paul 260
old drugs 3–4, 7–10, 11–12, 13–19,
    342

omeprazole 132, 225
onchocerciasis (river blindness) 48–9, 198
oncology *see* cancer treatments
O'Neill, Jim 258
Operation Warp Speed 266, 267
opioids 154, 175, 321, 356
opium 33
Orapred 9, 10
Orkambi 228, 238
Orphan Drug Act (1983) 65, 107–8, 110, 112, 145, 242
orphan drugs 57, 103–15, 141, 242–7, 317
  and prices 116–18, 119–20, 255
Ostertag, Wolfram 58
Ovation Pharmaceuticals 172–3, 174, 178
Oxford University 264, 265–6
OxyContin 175

Pacific Square Research (PSR) 24
Pai, Sanjeeth 350
pain relief treatments 154
Palin, Sarah 226
Palmeiro, Rafael 98
pandemics *see* Covid-19 pandemic
Par Pharmaceuticals 14, 24
parasitic diseases 176
Parke-Davis 34, 36
Parkinson's disease 275
Pasteur Institute 54
Patel, Amit 154–6, 351–2, 379n15
Patel, Hasmukh 154
Patent Act (1949) 42
Patented Medicine Prices Review Board 231
patents 3, 8, 13–14, 33, 35, 37–8, 45, 130
  and Allergan 141–2
  and antibiotics 41
  and AZT 58, 82
  and Britain 36, 42–3

and Covid vaccine 269
and Germany 364n22
and incentives 342
and India 296, 311
and law 282
and lengths 339–40, 376n10
and nature 39–40
and protection 131–42, 146–7, 344
and Prozac 101, 120
and Zonegran 19–20
and Zyprexa 121
  see also off-patent drugs
patient assistance schemes 81, 145–6, 170–1
Patients Rising 335
Patterson, Meaghan 215–16, 222
Patterson, Mindi 215–17
'pay-for-delay' settlements 138–9
payment terms 339
PBM Pharmaceuticals 15, 16–17
PBMs *see* pharmacy benefit managers
Pearson, Mike 21, 167, 173, 174–5, 349
Pearson, Steve 332–5
Pécoul, Bernard 343
Peisert, Dan 17–18, 22
penicillin 29, 30–3, 37–8, 40, 41, 363n5
pentamidine 112, 244
Perfitt, Jason 180, 181
periodic paralysis 244–5
Pershing Square 21, 174, 349
petition schemes 140
Pfizer 20, 32, 43, 85, 101
  and buyback 192
  and Covid vaccine 265, 267
  and Epanutin 180–4
  and Kindler 127
  and Lipitor 96–7
  and merger 189
  and neurodegeneratives 275

Pfizer (*cont'd*)
　　and new drugs 196
　　and origins 34
　　and phenytoin 180–184, 346,
　　　　384n102
　　and reps 87
　　and tetracycline 41
　　and vaccines 260
　　and Viagra 98–9, 193
Pharmaceutical Research and
　　Manufacturers of America 350
Pharmacia 189
pharmacists ix, 18, 318
pharmacoeconomics 118–20
pharmacy benefit managers (PBMs)
　　ix, 125–6, 219–22
Pharmasset 203–4, 206, 207
phenindione 163
phenytoin sodium 181, 346,
　　384n102
philanthropy 342
Philidor 161
Phillips, Dr Berkeley 182
Pimozide 103–5, 107, 108
placebo trials 61
Plavix 83, 188
polio 40
Poulton, Steve 182
poverty x, 81, 261, 268
Powell, Enoch 43
pregnant women 3–4, 44
prescription drugs 14, 18–19, 23–4,
　　27, 66, 116
　　and brands 46
　　and prices 213–14
　　and reps 89, 90
Prevnar 260
Priadel 354
prices 3–5, 41–2
　　and acquisitions 169–71, 178–9
　　and AMCo 166–7
　　and AZT 63–6, 68–72, 74–7,
　　　　78–9, 80–2

and Britain 43
and ceilings 339–40
and company practice 321–2
and Concordia 346–9
and Covid vaccine 266–7
and doctors 225–6
and Donnatal 17–18
and drug discovery 290–2
and gene therapies 287–8
and generic medicines 153–4,
　　184–7
and ICER 333
and increases 4, 10, 17, 20, 23–4,
　　28, 82, 155–6, 158, 162–4,
　　171–3, 175–6, 178–80, 187,
　　192–6, 213, 217–8, 221, 245, 348,
　　352–5, 306n1, 363n51, 383n85,
　　384n102, 392n64, 406n33
and insulin 214–19, 300
and Kolassa 115–16, 124–5
and legislation 353–4
and Lilly 120–3
and monopolies 318
and net rates 325–6
and new drugs 280
and NICE 232–3
and old drugs 12, 14
and orphan drugs 109, 110, 112,
　　113–14, 116–18
and PBMs 219–22
and penicillin 40
and prescriptions 23–4, 213–14
and R&D 123–4
and reference 231–2, 235–40
and Saltz 211–13
and secrecy 337–8
and shares 160–4
and strategy 116–120, 124–6, 130,
　　179–80, 192–6, 205–8
and Thompson 10
and USA ix–x, 322–5, 354–5
and value-based 118–20
and Zonegran 20

price hikes *see prices . . . and increases*
Prilosec 132–3, 136
prize funds 340
profits 2, 3, 41–3, 84, 317, 328
  and Covid vaccine 266
Project Silver 352
Prontosil 29–30
protease inhibitor drugs 82
Protropin 110–11, 369n41
Provigil 139
Prozac 83, 98–9, 101, 121, 122
  and patent 120, 133–4
  and reps 86, 91
PSI-7977 203–7
psychiatric treatments 278; *see also*
  anti-psychotics
Public Citizen 142
public funding 47, 326–31, 341
Purdue Pharma 175
Pure Food and Drugs Act (1906) 33
pyrimethamine 3–4

QALY (Quality-Adjusted Life Year)
  232, 234, 238, 325, 335–6
quack doctors 33
Quadir, Fahmi 150
Questor Pharmaceuticals 171–2,
  173, 178, 351, 353
Quincy, M.E. (TV series) 106, 108
quinine 34, 36
Quinnan, Dr Gerald 58

Rafuse, Joseph 60–1
Rajagopalan, Supraj 27, 159
Ranbaxy 139
rare diseases 104–15, 172, 242–7,
  255
  and co-payments 323
  and QALY 336
  and surrogate endpoints 252
RBC Capital Markets 23
R&D (research and development) 5,
  8, 41, 196–9, 356

and AZT 79–80
and costs 195–6, 320
and discontinued 343
and drug discovery 272–3
and gene therapies 289–90
and lifestyle drugs 98–9
and prices 123–4
and public funding 326–7
and tax credits 317
see also drug discovery
Reagan, Ronald 67, 129, 242
'reasonable pricing' clauses 80, 81,
  327
reference pricing 231–2, 235–40
regulation 317
Reines, Lisa 114
Relprevv 134, 135
remdesivir 265
reps *see* drug reps
research *see* R&D
research-led businesses 7, 46–7
Restasis 141–2
Retrophin 176
retroviruses *see* HIV
Revive Pharmaceuticals 17
rheumatoid arthritis treatments
  224–5
ribavirin 204, 205
Richards, Alfred 31
Rideout, Janet 56
Rift Valley fever (RVF) 270
Right Care Alliance 301
Riordan, Michael 199, 200
Risperdal 134
river blindness 48–9, 198
Robbe, Scott 50–1
Roberts Pharmaceuticals 169
Roche 84, 99, 129, 234, 279, 356
Roth, Bruce D. 96
Roy, Victor 203, 207, 289
royalties 327, 328, 330
Rumsfeld, Donald 200, 201
Russia 314

Rwanda 314
Ryan White CARE Act (1990) 65

safety 36–7, 44, 47
St Clair, Marty 56, 57, 59
St Regis Mohawk Tribe 141–2
sales reps *see drug reps*
salicylic acid 34
Salk, Jonas 40
Saltz, Dr Leonard 211–13, 225,
    248–9, 308–9, 315, 332
Salvarsan 30, 34, 35
Sanders, Bernie 301
Sandimmune 119
Sandoz 119, 186, 187, 385n107
Sanford Bernstein 271, 272
Sanofi-Aventis 22, 198–9, 255, 260,
    309
    and insulin 217, 221, 301
SARS (severe acute respiratory
    syndrome) 262, 270
Scannell, Jack 271–3, 274–7, 285–6,
    290, 337, 342
Schatz, Albert 365n37
Schering-Plough 133
Schinazi, Raymond 203, 204
schizophrenia treatments 104, 119,
    275
Scilipoti, Anthony 151
S.E. Massengill 36
Searle 189
Second World War 30, 31, 32, 35–6
seizure treatments 171–2
Seligman, Adam and Muriel 105
septicaemia treatments 121–3
Seroquel 135
Seroxat 139
Servier 249
Shapiro, Dr Arthur 103–4
shareholders 128–30, 271
Shark Fin project 131, 132
Shaw, Jenny 180, 181
Shepperd, Sir Alfred 71–2, 116

Shionogi 9, 13, 19
Shirkey, Harry C. 104
Shkreli, Martin 4, 176–7, 291,
    349–50
Shore, Michael 142
short selling 148–50, 164–6
side effects 109
    and advertising 93
    and AZT 62
    and reps 88
    and ulcer treatments 85
    and Viagra 98
sleep treatments 139
sleeping sickness 343
SMA (spinal muscular atrophy)
    303–7
small molecule drugs 252–3, 327
SmithKline Beckman 83, 95–6
social contract 3, 5, 47–8, 65, 146,
    218, 253–4, 316, 319
societal responsibility 39–40, 326
sofosbuvir 204–5
Soliris 243
Soon-Shiong, Dr Patrick 197–8
Soriot, Pascal 266
South Africa 309–11, 313
Sovaldi 205–6, 207, 209–10, 235,
    295–9
specialty pharmaceutical companies
    169–71, 173–4, 175
Spinraza 304, 307
Squibb, Edward Robins 34
SSR Health x
Staley, Peter 66–7, 72–3, 74–5, 76,
    79
    and New York Stock Exchange
        demonstration 50–1, 68, 77–8
Staphylococcus aureus 29
state-owned pharmaceuticals
    318–19
statins 94, 96–7, 126, 140–1
Stavros, Stephanie 229
Stemcentrx 196

steroids 41, 48, 111, 355
Stevens, Andrew 234
Stevenson, Alison 180–1, 183
Stivarga 249
stomach ulcer treatments 83, 85–6, 95–6, 132–3
Stott, Kelvin 290
streptococcus 29
streptomycin 39–40, 41
Strimvelis 288
Strongbridge Biopharma 245
subscription models 339, 340
Sullivan, Bill 55, 63, 71
sulpha drugs 29–30, 36
Sun Pharmaceutical Industries 245
surrogate endpoints 251–2
'sustained-release' drugs 11
Sustiva 202
swamp fever 55
Switzerland 34
Symbyax 134
Symkevi 238
Synastone 154
syphilis 30, 34
Syprine 355

T-cells 60–1, 288
Tagamet 83, 85–6, 95–6, 125
Tai, Katherine 269
Taiho Pharmaceutical 249
Taubert, Jennifer 274
taxation 9, 13, 20, 65, 178
Taxol 327–8
Terramycin (oxytetracycline) 41
testing see animal testing; clinical testing; human testing
testosterone treatments 13
tetracycline 41, 43
Teva 139, 141, 143, 157, 352
    and beta blockers 187
    and phenytoin 181
    and Syprine 355
thalidomide 43–4

Thiola 176
Thompson, Mark 7–13, 15, 19, 152, 168
    and AMCo 156–7, 161–3
    and Donnatal 17
    and expansion 22, 23, 24, 25, 27
    and Lazarus 349
    and resignation 348
    and short selling 150, 166
    and Zonegran 20, 21
thyroid treatments 156, 163–4, 354
Tiofarma 352
Tor Generics 180–1, 182, 183
Torbay Pharmaceuticals 318
Torreya Partners 8, 14, 19, 20, 22
Tourette's syndrome 103–5, 106–7
toxicity 44, 58, 62, 79, 82
transparency 323, 337–8
treatments for heart conditions 24, 63, 173, 256, 278
    and Valeant 178, 179–80, 354–5
trials see animal testing; clinical testing; human testing; placebo trials
Triangle Pharmaceuticals 201–3
Tribute Pharmaceuticals 12
Trikafta 228–30, 231, 250
Trimel Pharmaceuticals 12–13, 14
Triomune 311–12
TRIPS agreement 313
tropical diseases 198
Trump, Donald 236
Truvada 202
Turing Pharmaceuticals 176–7, 350
TV adverts 93–4, 96–7
type 1 Gaucher's disease 113–14
typhoid 35
typhus 36

Ubben, Jeffrey 21, 174
ulcers see stomach ulcer treatments
Ulesfia 9, 10, 13
UniQure 288

universities 328
Upjohn 34, 119
URL Pharma 176
US Department of Agriculture 31, 38

Vaccine Research Center 330
vaccines 36, 48–9, 259–70
  and Covid-19 1–2, 3, 330
  and polio 40
  and yellow fever 54, 55
Vagelos, Roy 48, 49, 101
Valeant 21–3, 349–51
  and off-patent drugs 173
  and prices 161, 193–4, 354–5
  and research 272–3
  and share price 174
  and short selling 150
  and treatments for heart
    conditions 178, 179–80
Valium 136
value-based approach 118–19, 120,
  122, 124, 207–8, 291
ValueAct Capital 21, 174
Van Woert, Melvin 105–6, 108–9
Varmus, Harold 327
Veritas Investment Research 151
Vernook, Dr Alan 212–13
Vertex Pharmaceuticals 145,
  228–30, 231, 238–9, 308, 344
Vestager, Margaret 349
Viagra 98–9, 193
Vimovo 355
Vioxx 101–2
viruses see Covid-19 pandemic;
  Ebola virus; HIV; SARS; Zika
  virus
Visium Asset Management 174
Vistide 201
Vyera Pharmaceuticals 350

Waksman, Selman 37, 40, 365n37
Wallenburg, John 230
Walmsley, Emma 255
Warner Chilcott 140
Warner–Lambert 85, 96–7, 189
Waxman, Deirdre 293, 299–303, 307
Waxman, Henry 64–5, 69, 105, 254
wealth 256–7, 268
Wellcome Plc 63–4, 82
Wells, Percy 31
whistleblowers 353
Wilson, Paul 182
Windum, Dr Robert 61
Wirtz, Hermann 43
Wolfe, Dr Sid 76
World Health Organization (WHO)
  239, 262, 263–4, 338
  and Covid vaccine 268, 269, 270
Worsham, Antoinette 301
Wyden, Ron 65, 69

Xigris 121–3
Xtandi 328

Yarchoan, Robert 53, 60–1, 68
yellow fever 54, 55
Yescarta 207, 288
Yosprala 225
Young, Frank 68

Zantac 85–6, 95–6, 125
Zantrap 308–9
Zidovudine see AZT
Zika virus 261–2, 263, 270
Zolgensma 287, 304–7, 345, 356
Zonegran 19–20
Zovirax 82
Zyprexa 120, 86, 91, 121, 133–5,
  188
Zytiga 328–9